The Pathology of
Violent Injury

KU-245-076

The Pathology of Violent Injury

Edited by

J. K. Mason, CBE, MD, FRCPath, DMJ

Regius Professor of Forensic Medicine
Department of Forensic Medicine, University of Edinburgh.

THE BRITISH SCHOOL OF OSTEOPATHY
14 SUFFOLK STREET, LONDON SW1Y 4HG
TEL: 01-930 9254-8

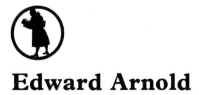

Edward Arnold

J EKF

© Edward Arnold 1978

First published 1978
by Edward Arnold (Publishers) Ltd
25 Hill Street, London W1X 8LL

All Rights Reserved. No part of this publication may be
reproduced, stored in a retrieval system, or transmitted
in any form or by any means, electronic, mechanical,
photocopying, recording or otherwise, without the prior
permission of Edward Arnold (Publishers) Ltd.

British Library Cataloguing in Publication Data
The pathology of violent injury.
  1. Medical jurisprudence
  I. Mason, John Kenyon
  614'.19   RA1051
ISBN 0–7131–4307–X

Printed in Great Britain by
Fletcher & Son Ltd, Norwich

Contributors

Ashton, S. J., MSc, Research Associate, Department of Transportation and Environmental Planning, University of Birmingham.

Brown, R. F., Group Captain, MA, BM, BCh, FRCS, Cade Professor of Surgery and Consultant in Plastic Surgery, Royal Air Force; Princess Mary's RAF Hospital, Halton, Aylesbury, Bucks.

Childs, C. M., MD, Senior Registrar and Clinical Lecturer, Accident and Emergency Department, Aberdeen Royal Infirmary and University of Aberdeen.

Cullen, S. A., Wing Commander, MB, MRCPath, Consultant in Pathology and formerly Officer i/c Department of Aviation and Forensic Pathology, Royal Air Force; RAF Institute of Pathology and Tropical Medicine, Halton, Aylesbury, Bucks.

Flynn, C. T., MBE, MB, MRCP, Director, Renal Dialysis Unit, Iowa Lutheran Hospital, Des Moines, Iowa, and lately Consultant in Medicine and Director of Renal Dialysis Unit, Royal Air Force.

Gordon, A., MD, Consultant Neuropathologist, Lothian Health Board; part-time Senior Lecturer, Department of Pathology, University of Edinburgh.

Green, M. A., MB, DCH, DObstRCOG, DMJ, Senior Lecturer in Forensic Medicine, Department of Forensic Medicine, University of Leeds.

Gresham, G. A., TD, MA, MD, DSc, FRCPath, Professor of Morbid Anatomy, University of Cambridge; The John Bonnett Clinical Laboratories, Addenbrooke's Hospital, Cambridge.

Gunn, J. C., MD, MRCPsych, DPM, Director, Special Hospitals Research Unit; Department of Forensic Psychiatry, London.

Hendry, W. T., MB, ChB, MRCGP, Senior Lecturer in Forensic Pathology, Department of Forensic Medicine, University of Aberdeen.

Johnson, H. R. M., MA, MB, BChir, FRCPath, DMJ, Reader in Forensic Medicine and Honorary Consultant in Forensic Medicine to the St. Thomas' Group of Hospitals; St. Thomas' Hospital Medical School, London.

Knight, B. H., MD, BCh, FRCPath, DMJ, Barrister-at-law, Reader in Forensic Pathology, The Welsh National School of Medicine,

University of Wales; Department of Pathology, The Royal Infirmary, Newport Road, Cardiff.

Macaulay, R. A. A., MB, ChB, MRCPath, Lecturer in Forensic Medicine and Honorary Senior Registrar, Lothian Health Board; Department of Forensic Medicine, University of Edinburgh.

Mackay, G. M., BSc, SM, PhD, MIMechE, Reader in Traffic Safety, University of Birmingham.

McLay, W. D. S., MB, ChB, LLB, FRCS(Glas), Chief Medical Officer, Strathclyde Police; Police Headquarters, Glasgow.

Maloney, A. F. J., MB, ChB, FRCP(Edin), FRCPath, Senior Lecturer in Neuropathology and Honorary Consultant in Pathology, Lothian Health Board; Department of Pathology, University of Edinburgh.

Mant, A. K., MD, MRCP, FRCPath, Professor of Forensic Medicine, University of London at Guy's Hospital; President, International Association for Accident and Traffic Medicine, 1972–78; Guy's Hospital Medical School, London.

Marshall, T. K., MD, FRCPath, Professor of Forensic Medicine, The Queen's University of Belfast; State Pathologist, Northern Ireland; Consultant in Pathology to the Northern Ireland Health and Social Service Boards; Institute of Pathology, Grosvenor Road, Belfast.

Mason, J. K., CBE, MD, FRCPath, DMJ, Regius Professor of Forensic Medicine and formerly Consultant in Aviation Pathology, Royal Air Force; Department of Forensic Medicine, University of Edinburgh.

Petty, C. S., MD, Professor of Forensic Sciences and Pathology, University of Texas, Southwestern Medical School at Dallas and Director, Southwestern Institute of Forensic Sciences, Dallas, Texas.

Proctor, D. M., MB, ChB, FRCS(Edin), Clinical Senior Lecturer in Traumatic Surgery, Department of Surgery, University of Aberdeen.

Rich, N. M., MD, FACS, Colonel, MC, USA, Chief, Peripheral Vascular Surgery Service; Walter Reed Army Medical Center, and Professor of Surgery Uniformed Services University of the Health Sciences, Washington, D.C. 20012.

Smith, R. A., BSc, Chief Field Agent (Death Investigator), Office of the Dallas County Medical Examiner; Southwestern Institute of Forensic Sciences, Dallas, Texas.

Stalker, A. L., TD, DL, MD, FRCPath, Regius Professor of Pathology, University of Aberdeen.

Watson, A. A., MA, MB, BS, MRCPath, DMJ, DTM&H, Senior Lecturer in Forensic Medicine, Department of Forensic Medicine, University of Glasgow.

Preface

Injury and death due to trauma are inseparable from the modern way of life and, although crimes against the person are increasing, the greater proportion of the violence to which we are exposed is of industrial or accidental type. The emphasis of forensic pathology is, for this reason, turning increasingly from the study of criminality to the more widely based happenings of community medicine.

The Royal College of Pathologists has recently stressed the importance of trauma to our society. Its working party stated in 1972 that 'the amount of attention being paid to the pathology of injury is not commensurate with its size as a medical problem. It would seem that disproportionate amounts of money and time are being devoted to topics of far less urgency.'* Accidents, poisoning and violence, in fact, constitute the fifth largest grouping of causes of death in the United Kingdom.

Much of the work involved in the interpretation of violent death has fallen on the shoulders of full-time forensic pathologists whose number is too few to cope with the flow of cases. To overcome this, the Brodrick Committee recommended, as did the College, that hospital pathologists should become increasingly involved in work for the coroners—and, by implication, for procurators fiscal—and, whether the Brodrick recommendations are implemented as a whole or not, such a solution is already being imposed by circumstances.

The time therefore seemed ripe for a fresh look at forensic pathology, and that is what this book sets out to provide. It is intended not so much for the established expert in legal medicine as for those handling the treatment and pathology of trauma whose practice will inevitably contain an increasing proportion of medico-legal problems. Rather than follow the conventional format, the publishers have attempted to achieve their object by a series of reviews of contemporary themes which illustrate the many aspects of violence. The inclusion of a number of chapters which deal with more academic matters is intended to widen the interest of general pathologists and, perhaps, to encourage research in this field. The greater part of the book is, however, essentially practical and it is hoped that it will thus be of value to lawyers, coroners, fiscals and police officers concerned with injury and unnatural deaths.

* Hunt, A. C. (Ed.) (1972). 'Pathology of Injury', London: Harvey Miller & Medcalf Ltd.

The editor is grateful to the publishers for giving him this unusual opportunity to express his own views on the role of forensic pathology today. I must thank especially my personal secretarial assistant, Mrs. Gladys Hamilton, for facing a daunting project with unstinting co-operation and, as always, my wife who made no complaint over the many extra hours of work involved—we were, in fact, involved together in the final stages of preparation during her terminal illness. But the book is, of course, the collective work of the individual contributors and it is to them that major credit is due. I thank them all most sincerely for their forbearance and I hope that they will regard the completed whole as worthy of their efforts. Any opinions expressed in the text are, of course, personal to the author concerned.

Edinburgh 1977

JKM

Acknowledgements

The Editor and Publishers have thought it invidious to make acknowledgements to individuals. Suffice it to say that the contributors all wish to thank most sincerely those who have helped in the preparation of their chapters.

Contents

I

Injuries and death in motor vehicle accidents

Road traffic accidents are the most common cause of death in adults up to 50 years of age. The greatest number of deaths is in the age group 15–24 (Table 1.1) and the highest death rate occurs between 20 and 25 years.

Table 1.1   Fatal road traffic accidents, England and Wales 1973

Ages	0–4	5–14	15–24	25–44	45–64	65–74	Over 75	Total
Motor-cyclists	—	6	478	110	71	19	1	685
Other motor vehicles	52	73	1042	1000	775	258	148	3348

Figures abstracted from the Registrar-General's Statistical Review

The economic and social implications have stimulated research at both governmental and university level in many countries into the incidence and causes of road traffic accidents, the injuries sustained and how these may be alleviated or treated; in the United Kingdom, the work of Sevitt has been outstanding in this field.[17] Although the results may vary considerably, not only from country to country but also within different regions of one country, such research has produced many developments in road and vehicle safety; perhaps one of the greatest advances has been in the field of restraint systems such as the seat belt, the use of which is described in detail in Chapter 2.

The present purpose is to describe the fatal injuries sustained by unrestrained vehicle occupants and motor-cyclists in road traffic accidents and to discuss some of the causes. Those surviving will have injuries which are of similar distribution but of less severity, an aspect of applied pathology which is of major importance in designing treatment; death resulting from the late sequelae of injury is, however, outside the scope of this chapter.

The distribution and severity of the injuries sustained in an accident will depend upon:

1. where the casualty was seated;
2. the direction of the impact;

3. the design of the cabin;
4. the speed or force of impact;
5. the behaviour of the vehicle after impact—e.g. overturning;
6. ejection of the casualty;
7. the intervention of some other hazard—e.g. fire.

The use of motor vehicle space varies from country to country and between age groups within a country. In some areas, and particularly where young persons are involved, the vehicle often contains more persons that it was designed to carry. In the United Kingdom, by contrast, there is frequently either only a driver in the motor vehicle or a driver and a front-seat passenger; the driver was alone in 33 per cent of a series of fatal accidents studied personally.

Seating position

After pedestrians, the driver of the vehicle is the most frequent fatal casualty in road traffic accidents. This does not imply that he is exposed to more trauma; it merely reflects how often the driver is the only occupant of the vehicle.

Next in frequency is the front-seat passenger, followed far less frequently by rear-seat passengers. In the series here reported involving 100 fatal driver accidents, 74 passengers were also killed and, of these, 55 occupied the front seat.

Impact injuries

The impact is frontal in 80 per cent of fatal motor vehicle accidents and this applies whether there is a collision between two vehicles or whether it is a one-vehicle accident, i.e. the vehicle has struck a relatively solid or unyielding obstruction.

Although autopsy may show that the lethal injury is similar, the distribution of injuries will differ as between the driver and front-seat passenger owing to the different layout of the front of the cabin. Certain areas of the cabin may inflict specific injuries.[6]

It must not be forgotten that about 20 per cent of impacts are not frontal, and side or rear impacts produce their own special patterns of injury. The driver and front-seat passenger will be dealt with separately and according to the direction of force.

Unrestrained occupants of a vehicle which is suddenly halted will be thrown upwards and forwards until their progress is arrested by some part or parts of the vehicle or, if they are thrown out, by contact with the ground or some other object.

The mechanism of injury production is illustrated in Chapter 2. As the driver is thrown forward, his chest will come into contact with the steering-wheel and column. Unless the column is of the collapsing type, it will suddenly arrest the forward momentum of the body and may inflict fatal injury to the internal thoracic structures. The head may be thrown into contact with the windscreen or with the upper windscreen surround and the roof. The legs, and especially the knees, may strike the fascia or dashboard.

Although the violence in many fatal impacts is such that any other factor has little relevance, the external injuries are influenced to some extent by the clothing, age and physical state of the deceased.

With regard to skeletal injuries, the only significant differences are those to the head and neck (Fig. 1.1). Forty-two per cent of car drivers

SKELETAL INJURIES

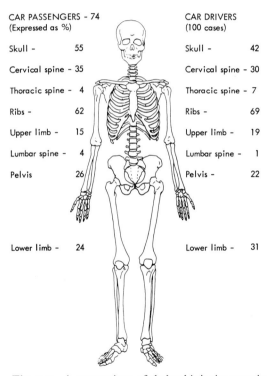

CAR PASSENGERS - 74
(Expressed as %)

Skull -	55
Cervical spine -	35
Thoracic spine -	4
Ribs -	62
Upper limb -	15
Lumbar spine -	4
Pelvis	26
Lower limb -	24

CAR DRIVERS
(100 cases)

Skull -	42
Cervical spine -	30
Thoracic spine -	7
Ribs -	69
Upper limb -	19
Lumbar spine -	1
Pelvis -	22
Lower limb -	31

Fig. 1.1 A comparison of skeletal injuries sustained by drivers and passengers resulting from accidents involving 100 consecutive fatal driver casualties.

suffered fractured skulls as compared with 55 per cent of the passengers. Cervical spine injuries occurred in 30 per cent and 35 per cent respectively. Fractured ribs were 7 per cent more common among the drivers; otherwise, there were only minor variations.

The occurrence of major visceral injuries is shown in Fig. 1.2. As would be anticipated from the distribution of the skeletal injuries, the passengers showed a higher incidence of brain damage—64 per cent compared with 53 per cent in drivers. Injuries to the lungs, aorta and

PRINCIPAL VISCERAL INJURIES

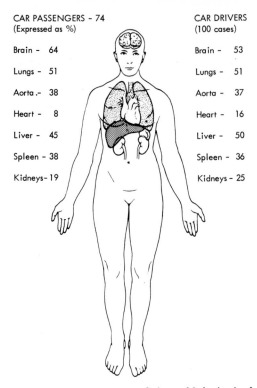

CAR PASSENGERS - 74 (Expressed as %)		CAR DRIVERS (100 cases)	
Brain -	64	Brain -	53
Lungs -	51	Lungs -	51
Aorta .-	38	Aorta -	37
Heart -	8	Heart -	16
Liver -	45	Liver -	50
Spleen -	38	Spleen -	36
Kidneys-	19	Kidneys -	25

Fig. 1.2   A comparison of visceral injuries in drivers and passengers.

spleen were virtually identical but drivers sustained proportionately more injuries to the heart, liver and kidneys.

Some description and discussion of the distribution of the regional injuries is necessary for the proper understanding of these fatal injuries. Only the usual patterns of injury will be discussed, but it must be appreciated that, sometimes, these may be most bizarre.

Injuries to the head and neck
Serious injury to the head and neck is present in over 50 per cent of all fatal road accidents involving motor vehicle drivers or their passengers.

Glass injuries due to shattered windscreens are usually more widespread on the head and neck of the front-seat passenger (Fig. 1.3); they are rarely responsible for more than superficial damage but often cause injury to the eyes.

Skull fractures are conditioned by the form of impact. Drivers' movement may be restricted by the steering-wheel, which will prevent their ejection from the car upon impact and may materially lessen the force of any impact with the interior of the cabin or the windscreen.

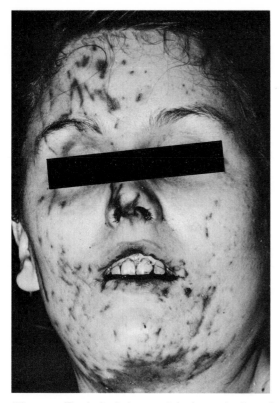

Fig. 1.3   Typical windscreen injuries to the face of a front-seat passenger.

Passengers are not rarely ejected from the car, either through the wind-screen or the door, sustaining severe fractures to the skull from impact with the roadway or some other object such as tree or wall. Fractures of the skull are sometimes depressed, especially following ejection from the vehicle, but most frequently they are basal, involving the middle fossae of the skull. Should the vehicle overturn, ring fractures of the base are not uncommon. Brain injuries are not remarkable, following the expected pattern and distribution of the skull fracture.

Cervical spinal injuries are common. The most important, and frequently the fatal, injury is a dislocation of the atlanto-occipital joint. This injury is found in about one-third of all fatal motor vehicle accidents and may easily be overlooked unless it is specifically sought. There may be no haemorrhage around the joint and, although extreme laxity with wide separation is occasionally seen, this dislocation is often only apparent on rotating or moving the skull in a horizontal plane. Rigor mortis may mask the injury and sometimes the ligaments are only torn or stretched on one side. Macroscopic injury to the medulla may be absent and the injured area may be incised during removal of the

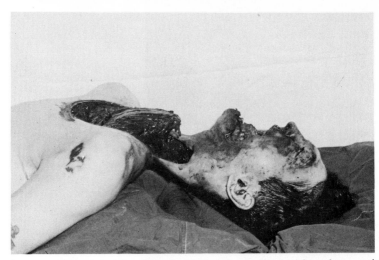

Fig. 1.4   Massive facial and cervical injuries associated with under-running a heavy goods vehicle.

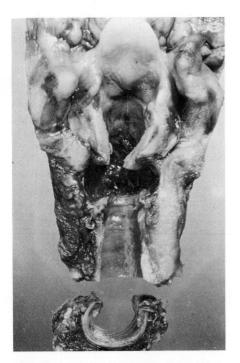

Fig. 1.5   Injuries in a motor-cyclist due to under-running the lowered tailboard of a stationary goods vehicle.

brain at autopsy. Dislocation of the cervical spine between vertebrae is less common and may, also, easily be overlooked. Frequently there is no macroscopic injury to the underlying cervical cord although the function of the cord has been virtually destroyed at the level of the dislocation.

One cervical spine injury, which is now becoming less common, is caused when a motor vehicle driver runs under the tail of a heavy goods vehicle and is virtually beheaded (Fig. 1.4). This injury is prevented by a transverse bar now being fitted below the tailboard. Severe and instantly fatal injuries to the soft tissues of the neck may occur when motor-cyclists or pedal-cyclists travelling at speed undershoot the tail-board of a lorry (Fig. 1.5).

Injury to the vertebral artery, leading to rapidly fatal subarachnoid haemorrhage, is rare—it has been found in only 1 of over 200 fatal cases. Traumatic subarachnoid haemorrhage is becoming more frequently recognized following blows to the side of the upper neck[10]— a part of the body unlikely to be exposed to danger, except possibly from a side impact or when the vehicle rolls over.

Injuries to the chest
Chest injuries resulting from impact with the steering column or fascia occur frequently and are a very common cause of immediate death. The visible external injury to the chest from fatal steering-wheel impact may be minimal, or even absent, or it may be gross. In Fig. 1.6a, the imprint of the lower rim of the steering-wheel can be seen on the left chest and extending on to the arm whereas, in Fig. 1.6b, part of the column is actually in the chest. The appearances are greatly influenced by the clothing and by the age of the deceased. In young adults, the aorta or even heart may be extensively ruptured and yet the ribs and sternum are intact. Fractured ribs are slightly more frequent among car drivers than among their passengers.

It is of interest that severe injuries are often paired when a driver and his front-seat passenger are killed. The fatal and major injuries were similar in all but 1 of 11 such cases. This suggests that the design of the interior of the cabin has little influence on the injuries when the impact has been of great violence; by contrast, the interior design may be of great significance when the impact is slight.

In this series, the number of deaths from rupture of the aorta was virtually the same in the drivers and in the passengers. In the majority of cases, the lesion occurs where the transverse becomes the descending part but the aorta may occasionally rupture in the transverse or ascending section. The laceration may be complete—the severance is sometimes so clean that the ruptured ends appear to have been cut. In these cases death, or at least loss of consciousness, is immediate. All degrees of rupture may occur and sometimes the initial rupture may extend only to the adventitia or be very small. In both cases, the rising blood pressure after recovery from the initial shock may cause fatal haemorrhage which can be delayed for several days. More rarely,

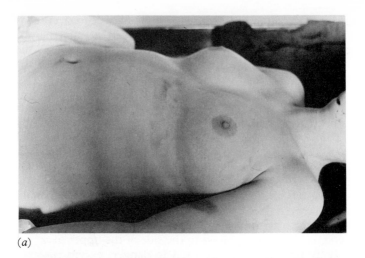

(a)

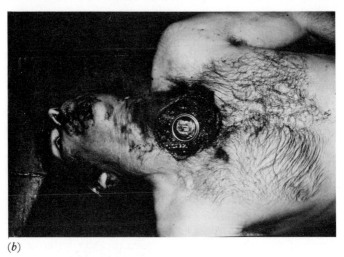

(b)

Fig. 1.6 Two steering-wheel injuries. (a) Minor bruising of the skin of the chest. (b) A major injury in which the centre of the steering column has penetrated the upper chest.

mediastinal haematomas are due to injuries involving the intercostal arteries at their origins.

Injuries to the heart occur in some 16 per cent of car drivers involved in fatal accidents. The traumatic heart rupture is rarely the only fatal lesion; more usually it is merely one of many injuries incompatible with life. The right atrium is the part most frequently ruptured, followed by the right ventricle. Occasionally, the violence is such that all chambers are damaged and bizarre injuries may occur if a rib impales the heart. Figure 1.7 shows extensive injuries to the heart and the aorta.

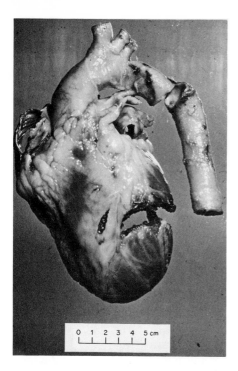

Fig. 1.7 Multiple injuries to the cardiovascular system. Both atria are ruptured and the aorta is torn. The left ventricle has been penetrated by a broken rib.

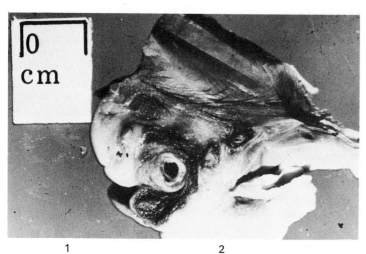

Fig. 1.8 Coronary thrombosis associated with perivascular trauma due to frontal chest impact.
(1) Coronary artery completely occluded and surrounded by bruising.
(2) Fresh area of bruising of the myocardium.

Bruising of the heart wall may result in a traumatic coronary thrombosis. These thromboses, causing death within a short time of injury, are rare but the distribution of bruising in and around the wall of the vessel leaves no doubt as to the aetiology (Fig. 1.8); however, the association of chest injury with subsequent coronary artery disease remains highly speculative.

Injuries to the lungs occurred in just over 50 per cent of both the fatally injured passengers and drivers in this series. Such injuries are due to:

1. sudden changes in intrathoracic pressure;
2. fractured ribs.

A sudden severe impact to the chest wall may rupture a main bronchus even in the absence of any fractures of the thoracic cage. This type of injury is rare except in young persons with highly mobile chest walls.

Traumatic bullae are among the more common pulmonary injuries; their formation is due to the sudden increase in negative intrathoracic pressure following an impact. The bullae are thin-walled and are confined to the immediate subpleural area; they usually occur beneath the site of the impact and along the lung edges. Unlike the emphysematous bullae, their rupture rarely produces any significant pneumothorax.

Contusion of the lung is common and may be severe. The lung may be partly torn from its attachments to the bronchi and extensive haemorrhage may take place within the contused organ. Laceration of the central areas of a lobe or lobes is not uncommon in fatal cases.

Pulmonary laceration may occur with or without penetration of the substance by fractured ribs. Laceration in the absence of a penetrating injury is more frequent when the lung is adherent. In rare cases, a road accident casualty may sustain a fatal haemorrhage arising from torn branches of the pulmonary artery. Fatal intrathoracic haemorrhage which is not associated with injury to the heart or aorta usually arises from torn intercostal vessels. It is unusual for death to be due to a pressure haemopneumothorax as this usually takes some time to develop and is almost invariably relieved upon admission to hospital.

Abdominal injuries
Abdominal visceral injuries are found in the order of frequency: liver, spleen and kidney. There is injury to the pancreas or mesentery in a relatively small number of cases.

The injury to the liver will depend upon the direction of the impact; as this is usually from the front, the central area is most commonly damaged by having been crushed against the spine. There may be severe hepatic injury without immediate rupture of the capsule, a rupture occurring hours later due to an enlarging haematoma. The diaphragm will often have been ruptured when liver injuries are severe, and abdominal viscera will be herniated into the pleural cavity.

The spleen is injured in over one-third of cases but the injury is rarely major, small lacerations being commonly present around the hilum. Severe injury to a normal spleen is seldom seen except following direct impact.

In spite of their protected position the kidneys are injured in 20–25 per cent of cases, the injury usually consisting of transverse lacerations.

Bony injuries

Pelvic injuries are not uncommon and may be due to direct impact or to forces transmitted through the femora when the forward movement of the knees is arrested by the fascia board. The classical injury is a posterior fracture dislocation of the hip joint. Sometimes there will be a dislocation of both sacroiliac joints when the hip joints remain intact following such an impact. This injury may be overlooked if the pelvic ring is otherwise intact; its presence may be suspected when an apparently isolated retroperitoneal haematoma is found over the upper part of the joint.

Very severe comminution of one-half of the pelvis occurs following a lateral impact. The lesion usually includes a central fracture dislocation of the hip joint together with laceration of the pelvic vessels on that side. Fatal haemorrhage, other than from the thoracic aorta, is rare but is occasionally seen after laceration of the iliac or femoral arteries.

The lower limbs are fractured in 25–30 per cent of accidents and the upper limbs in 15–19 per cent. Injuries to the spine, other than the cervical spine, are relatively infrequent.

Principal fatal sequelae to injury

It is not proposed to deal with these in depth but their frequency demands some description.

Haemorrhage

Delayed haemorrhage from incomplete rupture of the aorta or liver has been described above. The possibility of secondary haemorrhage should never be overlooked even with adequate antibiotic coverage. Fatal haemorrhage may rarely occur when the femoral artery is torn in association with a closed fracture of the femur.

Fat embolism

Massive fat embolism may occur quite unexpectedly, especially in the elderly following rib fractures and in young persons following soft tissue crushing as, for instance, sustained when being run over. The forensic significance of fat embolism is described in Chapter 20.

Pneumonia

Fatal pulmonary infection is a common termination of any injury in the aged. It may occur at any age but is most frequent following thoracic or abdominal injuries which interfere with respiratory movement and after serious head injuries.

Pulmonary embolism

This is more common among the elderly but may still occur in the young patient in spite of preventive measures.

Cardiovascular sequelae

Coarse endocardial haemorrhages are seen in cases where there is a period of profound hypoxia following head injury. Endocardial fibrosis and hypertrophy, followed by arrythmias and sudden death, are recognized as occurring in cases which eventually recover but there are few cases reported in the literature. Plueckhahn and Cameron[14] reported 3 cases of 'traumatic myocarditis', 2 of which were fatal, and, more recently, there have been small series reported of cases of sudden death from myocardial lesions in young persons occurring up to 10 years after 'head' injury.[15,16]

Death from burning in road traffic accidents

Many members of the public express reluctance to wear seat belts lest they should die from burning having survived the impact of a crash. It is, therefore, worth assessing how uncommon is this mode of death. A recent survey from Canada[2] showed that only 24 out of 1297 persons fatally injured in motor-car accidents died through incineration; only 3 of these were riding in passenger cars. The authors concluded that the fear of being burned in a crash is greatly over-emphasized.

Fatal injuries to motor-cyclists

If a motor-cyclist should be involved in a traffic accident, he is more likely to suffer injuries to the upper part of his body because of his unprotected position. Some injuries result from impact while the rider is still seated but many occur after he has been thrown off when he strikes the roadway. Other deaths may occur when the cyclist is thrown into the path of a vehicle, the wheel of which goes over his head, crushing the protective headgear which has been compulsory in the United Kingdom since 1973.

In these crushing cases, there may be exceptional bony injuries unaccompanied by any break in continuity of the scalp. The most common fatal head injury in the protected motor-cyclist is, however, a ring fracture of the base of the skull. This occurs when he is thrown off the machine and hits the ground, or some other unyielding object, with the top of his head. Brain injury was present in nearly 80 per cent of fatal motor-cycle accidents compared with 53 per cent in car drivers. Injuries to other areas outside the head and neck were less than those found in car drivers or passengers, except for lower limb injuries.

A recent survey of the distribution of injuries to motor-cyclists has been given by Lahti.[9] The distribution of injuries in 47 fatal cases examined by the author is illustrated in Fig. 1.9.

The effect of safety equipment in motor-cycle accidents is discussed further in Chapter 2. It must, however, be appreciated that a number of accidents occur when the motor-cyclist gets into difficulty while travelling at a very fast speed and, in such conditions, the wearing of even the most efficient protective headgear may have little influence upon the outcome of the accident.

Some causes of fatal road traffic accidents

The two main indisputable causes of fatal road accidents are alcohol and speed, acting either alone or in combination. The majority of countries have introduced legislation during the last 30 years setting an arbitrary blood alcohol level above which it is an offence to drive. The advantages of this legislation over the earlier laws which required clinical proof of insobriety are manifest to all who have seen both systems

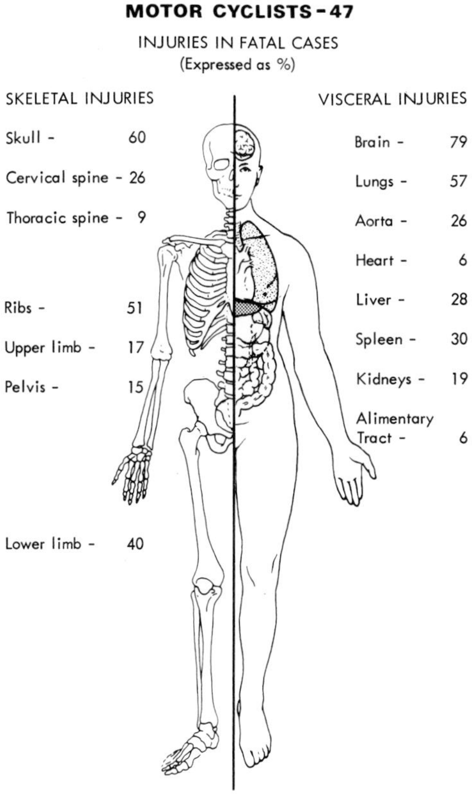

MOTOR CYCLISTS - 47

INJURIES IN FATAL CASES
(Expressed as %)

SKELETAL INJURIES

VISCERAL INJURIES

Skull – 60	Brain – 79
Cervical spine – 26	Lungs – 57
Thoracic spine – 9	Aorta – 26
	Heart – 6
Ribs – 51	Liver – 28
Upper limb – 17	Spleen – 30
Pelvis – 15	Kidneys – 19
	Alimentary Tract – 6
Lower limb – 40	

Fig. 1.9   Skeletal and visceral injuries in 47 consecutive motor-cyclist fatalities.

in operation.[8] The levels of alcohol in the blood permitted in various countries or states varies greatly, the limits lying between 50 mg/100 ml and 150 mg/100 ml. Penalties for driving with a blood alcohol concentration above the statutory limit also vary from little more than a nominal fine to loss of permit to drive and even detention. Regrettably, these laws in the long term have not had the deterrent effect which was anticipated when the legislation was first introduced. Figures taken from personal files of fatal road traffic accidents reveal that, since the introduction of the Road Safety Act 1967, not only has there been an increase in the number of dead drivers with blood alcohol levels above the statutory limit but also higher levels were present.

These personal observations have been supported by the Annual Reports of the Transport and Road Research Laboratory,[19,20] who have shown that the drop in the numbers of drivers killed with blood alcohol levels over 80 mg/100 ml which followed the 1967 Act has not been maintained over the nation. Indeed, during the main drinking hours, the number of dead drivers with blood alcohol concentrations over the statutory limit is higher in the 20–30-year age group than it was before the legislation was introduced.

Pathologists in Great Britain now routinely estimate the blood alcohol level in all persons over the age of 14 years killed in road traffic accidents and who die within 12 hours of the injuries having been received. Ideally such estimations should always be made on urine also when this is available as it is recognized that a driver's behaviour is more erratic when the blood alcohol is rising.

Personal experience in Great Britain has shown that drugs do not

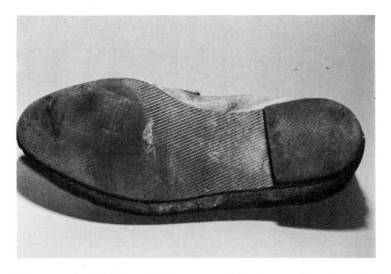

Fig. 1.10   A suicidal crash. The pattern of the depressed accelerator is clearly seen on the sole of the right shoe.

present the problems which are reported elsewhere.[5] Routine drug screening of drivers aged 18–40, killed in road traffic accidents over a 12-month period, revealed no surprises. One driver who was known to have taken some amphetamine had a low therapeutic blood level.

The influence of speed upon the outcome of a highway accident is self-explanatory. The force of impact of a moving vehicle varies with the square of the speed. All those who have worked in the field of traffic medicine know of the dramatic drop in accident rates which may follow the imposition of a speed limit on a particular stretch of road.

Fatigue is important, especially among commercial vehicle drivers driving across continents rather than countries and where no limits as to the time the driver is on the road are laid down or enforced. Sicard[18] estimated that human factors were involved in 90 per cent of accidents and that 40 per cent of these were due to fatigue. The number of accidents in the United Kingdom due to fatigue would appear to be very small compared with those occurring on the continent of Europe. Suicide by driving a motor vehicle into some unyielding object is also very rare in Great Britain. It undoubtedly occurs, and Edland[4] has reported several cases; it is possible that a retrospective study would reveal that it is not as uncommon as it seems. An indication of suicide may sometimes become apparent from an examination of the driver's shoe (Fig. 1.10).

Shoes may themselves be the apparent cause of road traffic accidents. Figures 1.11 and 1.12 illustrate shoes or boots worn by dead drivers and thought to have been contributory to, if not the cause of, the

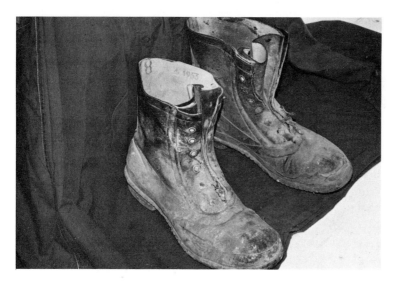

Fig. 1.11   An exceptionally heavy pair of boots. The possibility of fouling the accelerator while braking is obvious. In addition, in this particular case, the boots were worn without laces.

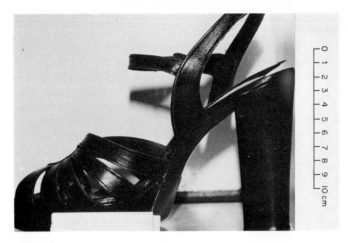

Fig. 1.12 The wearer of these shoes with 11·4 cm (4·5 in) heels was driving home from work on her usual route when she failed to stop at a busy junction and was struck and killed by a lorry.

accident. High heels, built-up soles and boots all affect the driver's sense of touch. Sandals may catch the adjacent pedal when one is being depressed. The significance of the examples shown is clear from the legends to the illustrations.

Natural disease, causing sudden fatal collapse of the driver of the vehicle, is potentially dangerous but is probably exaggerated in the lay mind because of the publicity which surrounds such an occurrence when someone other than the driver is killed. The problem has been investigated by a number of pathologists and others interested in traffic medicine in the USA, the UK and Scandinavia.[1,3,7,11,12,13,21,22,23] In all the collected series it is clear that sudden natural death at the wheel is not uncommon (about 1 per cent of all sudden deaths investigated by HM Coroners in England and Wales) but that injury to any other person as a result of the fatal collapse is rare. Herner et al.[7] also investigated accidents caused by non-fatal collapse; epilepsy and diabetes were found to be the most important underlying conditions.

References

1. Baker, S. P. and Spitz, W. U. (1970). An evaluation of the hazard created by natural death at the wheel. *New Engl. J. Med.* **283**, 405.
2. Bako, G., Mackenzie, W. C. and Smith, E. S. O. (1976). What is the risk of being burned in a motor vehicle crash? A survey of crash fatalities in Alberta, USA,* 1970–1972. *J. Traffic Med.* **4**, 20.

* This must surely be a printers' error in the original—*Editor.*

3. Di Maio, D. J. (1971). A survey of sudden unexpected deaths in automobile drivers. In: *Proc. 3rd Congress Int. Ass. Acc. Traffic Med.*, p. 75. Ann Arbor: University of Michigan.

4. Edland, J. F. (1971). The suicide crash. In: *Proc. 3rd Congress Int. Ass. Acc. Traffic Med.*, p. 81. Ann Arbor: University of Michigan.

5. Gorriott, J. C. (1976). Driving under the influence of drugs; toxicologic and case findings in an 18 month study (abstract). *J. Traffic Med.* **4**, 29.

6. Grattan, E., Wall, J. G. and Hobb, J. A. (1973). The investigation of injuries in road traffic accidents. In: *Modern Trends in Forensic Medicine—3*, Chap. 7. Ed. A. K. Mant. London and Boston, Mass: Butterworths.

7. Herner, B., Smedby, B. and Ysander, L. (1966). Sudden illness as a cause of motor vehicle accidents. *Brit. J. industr. Med.* **23**, 37.

8. Israelstam, S. and Lambert, S. (Eds.) (1975). *Proc. 6th Int. Conf. Alcohol, Drugs and Traffic Safety.* Toronto: House of Lind.

9. Lahti, R. A. (1976). Fatal motor cycle accidents (abstract). *Forensic Sci.* **8**, 187.

10. Mant, A. K. (1972). Traumatic subarachnoid haemorrhage following blows to the neck. *J. Forens. Sci. Soc.* **12**, 567.

11. Mant, A. K. (1977). Natural death whilst in charge of transportation. In: *Legal Medicine Annual—1977*. Ed. C. H. Wecht. New York and London: Appleton-Century-Crofts.

12. Mant, A. K. and Paul, D. M. (1972). Sudden death whilst in charge of transportation. Paper read at *4th Congress Int. Ass. Acc. Traffic Med.*, Abstracts, p. 79.

13. Petersen, B. J. and Petty, C. S. (1962). Sudden natural death among automobile drivers. *J. Forensic Sci.* **7**, 274.

14. Plueckhahn, V. D. and Cameron, J. M. (1968). Traumatic myocarditis or myocarditis in trauma. *Med. Sci. Law* **8**, 177.

15. Rajs, J. (1976). Relation between craniocerebral injury and subsequent myocardial fibrosis and heart failure. Report of three cases. *Brit. Heart J.* **38**, 396.

16. Rajs, J. and Jakobsson, S. (1976). Severe trauma and subsequent cardiac lesions causing heart failure and death. *Forensic Sci.* **8**, 13.

17. Sevitt, S. (1973). Fatal road accidents in Birmingham: times to death and their causes. *Injury* **4**, 281.

18. Sicard, A. (1976). La fatigue au volant. *J. Traffic Med.* **4**, 26.

19. Transport and Road Research 1973 (1974) Annual Report of the Transport and Road Research Laboratory. 0 11 550273 4, London, HMSO.

20. Transport and Road Research 1974 (1975) Annual Report of the Transport and Road Research Laboratory, 0 11 550274 2, London, HMSO.

21. Voigt, J. (1971). Traffic deaths from natural causes. *Proc. 3rd Congress Int. Ass. Acc. Traffic Med.*, p. 71. Ann Arbor: University of Michigan.

22. West, I., Nielsen, G. L., Gilmore, A. E. and Ryan, J. R. (1968). Natural death at the wheel. *J. Amer. med. Ass.* **205**, 266.
23. Ysander, L. (1966). The safety of drivers with chronic disease. *Brit. J. industr. Med.* **23**, 28.

2

The Prevention of Injury in Vehicular Accidents

It has been estimated that the total cost of road traffic accidents in Great Britain during 1973 was £615 million. Accidents involving serious injury or fatality contributed some £360 million to this total. The toll in loss of life and serious injury is vast; throughout 1973 some 7400 persons were killed in such accidents and a further 89 467 were seriously injured. Table 2.1 shows the distribution of these casualties between different classes of vehicle.[5, 10]

Table 2.1 Casualties in vehicular accidents, 1973

	Killed	Seriously injured
Pedestrians	2806	22 865
Pedal-cyclists	336	4 421
Moped riders	76	2 051
Motor-scooters	69	1 604
Motor-cycles	605	10 136
Cars and taxis	3048	40 975
Public service vehicles	57	1 596
Other road vehicles	409	5 819
Aircraft crew	28	10
Aircraft passengers	116	41
Total	7550	89 518

Since motorized transport and frequent accidents are apparently inseparable, an important way to improve safety is to protect the travellers physically against injury and death. A knowledge of the incidence and distribution of these injuries is an essential prerequisite for adequate protection.

The previous chapter has detailed this information with respect to motor vehicle accidents; aviation accidents have been analysed elsewhere.[8] Table 2.2 shows a simplified analysis of the cause of death in fatal motor vehicle, motor-cycle and aircraft accidents.[2, 8, 15] The importance of head and chest injury is emphasized. Sixty-five per cent of the deaths in motor vehicle accidents result from head and/or chest injury alone.[15] Facial injury is accompanied by trauma to the eyes in a

Table 2.2   Causes of death in transport accidents

	Motor-cars (%)	Motor-cycles (%)	Aircraft (%)
Head and neck injury	28	80	22
Chest injury	27	8	15
Multiple injuries	22	12	25
Asphyxia	7		10
Head and chest injury	12		
Other	4	0	28

significant number of cases.[32] The proportion of asphyxial deaths without potentially fatal injury is alarming. Motor-cyclists have two areas at main risk: the head and the legs.

The injuries sustained by the victims of vehicular accidents have two basic causes—either impact of the body against solid structures which are part of the vehicle or ejection from the vehicle at the time of impact. The latter is the cause of death in 27 per cent of automobile accidents.[16] The direction of the impact forces may be in the horizontal, lateral or vertical planes. The impact is in the horizontal direction in most motor vehicle accidents (Table 2.3) and the horizontal vector is an important component of the impact of survivable aircraft crashes.

The mechanism of injury production

Unrestrained front-seat occupants of automobile and aircraft subjected to head-on impact have been studied cinematographically.[28, 33] It has been shown that, on impact, the lower half of the body is thrust forward, possibly injuring the knees on the lower edge of the instrument panel (Fig. 2.1a). The whole body then lifts and the head strikes the windscreen while the abdomen may impact against the lower edge of the steering-wheel or the control column. After recoil of the head, the chest comes into contact with the steering-wheel and the head again strikes the windscreen (Fig. 2.1b). Front-seat passengers who have no steering-wheel or control column in front of them are commonly thrown through the windscreen.

Unrestrained passengers in the rear of motor vehicles or aircraft may suffer one of three fates.[19] They may be thrown forward striking the

Table 2.3   Frequency of types of impact in motor-car accidents

	(%)
Head-on or front corners	60·3
Side	16·0
Rear end	6·2
Roll-over	17·5

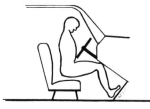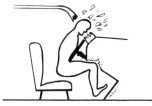

Fig. 2.1 Movement of unrestrained front-seat occupants in head-on crashes: (*a*) initial contact areas, and (*b*) the final resting position.

head, face and chest on the rear of the front seat or the back of front-seat passengers. Alternatively, they may continue forward and come to rest in the front of the vehicle, sustaining injury from fixed objects in this area; this result is particularly common with children. Lastly, they may be thrown completely clear of the vehicle.

'Whiplash' injuries to the cervical spine are caused by a combination of hyperextension and hyperflexion—the former being the most important. They are particularly common in multiple crashes when a vehicle is rammed from the rear, causing hyperextension of the occupant's neck over the seat back; immediately afterwards, when the vehicle cannons into the car in front, there is abrupt deceleration with hyperflexion of the victim's neck. The reverse situation arises in the common head-on crash when hyperflexion is the primary neck displacement; hyperextension occurs as the victim's head strikes the windscreen or instrument panel. Repeated flexion and extension may occur in roll-over accidents.

Motor-cycle riders who are subjected to sudden deceleration are thrown off their machine and fly on, frequently head first. Their injuries are determined by the objects they strike, the angle of impact and the area of the body that sustains the impact. If the rider falls sideways from his machine the major influence on injury is whether he has one leg pinned between the motor-cycle and the ground. Injuries may also be caused by the rider's legs striking the handlebars as he leaves his machine and by his hands being trapped in the handlebars at impact. Protective extension of the arms causes wrist and forearm fractures.

Rationale of protection from impact injury

Injuries sustained in vehicular accidents may be modified in the following ways:

1. by reducing the impact forces;
2. by distributing these forces over a large body area, preferably to areas best able to withstand the impact;
3. by reducing the rate of application of the impact forces and damping down irregularities that may occur during their application.

The magnitude of the force applied to the victim depends upon his weight and the rate of the deceleration. The decelerative force can be calculated in terms of gravitational force (G):

$$G = K v^2 / d$$

where v is the speed of the body just before impact and d is the stopping distance; K is a constant which is 0·0039 if v is measured in kilometres per hour and d in metres; when v is measured in miles per hour and d in feet, K is 0·034.

If a vehicle collides with a fixed object at 50 km h^{-1} (31 m.p.h.) which brings it to a halt with a stopping distance of 1 m (3·28 ft) the deceleration is:

$$G = 0.0039 \times 50^2 / 1$$
$$= 9·75 \quad G$$

The critical factor in this relatively low force is the considerable stopping distance of the cabin associated with deformation of the front of the vehicle. The unrestrained occupant will continue at the same speed as the vehicle until he suffers secondary impact on fixed structures within the car or aircraft. The deformation (stopping) distance of the victim will only be 5 cm (0·16 ft) and his deceleration will be 1·9 km s^{-2} (195 G) which is equivalent to a force of 136 kN (30 800 lbf) for a man weighing 70 kg (154 lb). This is beyond the impact tolerance of the human torso. If the occupant is securely strapped to a seat which remains secure, he will suffer the same deceleration as the vehicle: 97·5 m s^{-2} (9·75 G) in the above example. It is impossible to achieve this ideal situation in practice but the provision of a safety harness will increase the stopping distance to 0·5 m (1·64 ft) by virtue of the stretching of the harness. In the example quoted the man would suffer a deceleration of 195 m s^{-2} (19·5 G), which is equivalent to a force of 13·6 kN (3800 lbf).

The restraint harness distributes the impact forces over a wide surface area. The unrestrained occupant may have an initial contact area of 25 cm^2 (3·9 in^2) and, in the example, this would result in the application of a force of 54 MPa (7900 p.s.i.) to the impact area of the victim. The area of support offered by restraint harnesses varies according to their type. The lap strap and diagonal harness with 7·5 cm (2·9 in) straps offers 900 cm^2 (139 in^2) which, if used in our example, would reduce the force applied to the occupant to 152 kPa (22 p.s.i.). Thus the effect of the restraint harness is to reduce the force on the occupant by a factor of 360.

The optimal redistribution of the impact forces requires a knowledge of the impact tolerance of both the whole body and its various parts. Studies [30] have shown that the body can withstand a deceleration of 300 m s^{-2} (30 G) without injury. The tolerance of specific body areas varies considerably; the fracture tolerance of the frontal bone is 800 m s^{-2} (80 G) while those of the nose, mandible and zygoma are 300, 400 and 500 m s^{-2} (30, 40 and 50 G) respectively; the thoracic cage can withstand 400 m s^{-2} (40 G) without injury. Harness restraint systems serve to redistribute the force of impact from the face to the chest; although the impact tolerance of the chest is not much more than that of the face and head, the concomitant reduction of the decelerative force makes it acceptable.

Moreover, the elasticity of the restraint harness webbing reduces the rate of application of the impact forces and irons out the irregularities in their application.

Types of restraint harness

Since restraint harnesses were first patented in 1885[26] many different forms have been investigated. Chest belts and shoulder belts received only transient interest and attention is now concentrated on:

1. the lap strap;
2. the single diagonal belt;
3. the lap strap and diagonal (the three-point belt);
4. the lap strap with double shoulder harness;
5. the lap strap with air bag restraint.

There have been many studies of the type and severity of injury when these systems are used.[31]

The lap strap was the original equipment designed to protect the occupants of aircraft and motor vehicles against contact injury but it soon became apparent that injuries to the head and upper torso occurred even with such restraint.[25] Cinematographic studies of the behaviour of the human body in simulated crashes demonstrated that the main reason for these injuries was the torso flailing over the strap and impact against fixtures within the vehicle[33] (Fig. 2.2). Specific facial injuries can frequently be related to the presence of projecting controls on the instrument panel (Fig. 2.3). The asphyxial deaths shown in Table 2.2 are due in part to facial injury, concussion and subsequent inhalation of blood.

The evidence that the lap strap acted as a fulcrum for flailing is supported by the high incidence of leg injuries in all relevant accident statistics. Despite this the lap belt can effectively prevent ejection of the body, which has been implicated as a major cause of injury in automobile accidents.[16]

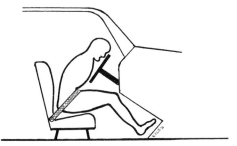

Fig. 2.2 The effect of the lap strap, showing the flexion that occurs in head-on impact.

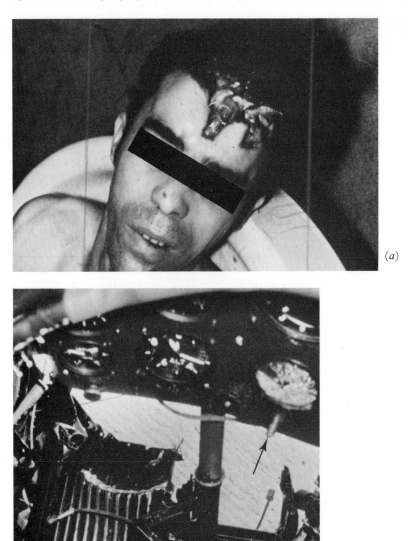

Fig. 2.3   (*a*) A penetrating wound on the forehead of a pilot who died as a result of head injury only. The injury was clearly related to the knob on the control panel shown arrowed in (*b*); note the isolated damage to the instrument above the knob which has been bent downwards.

Single diagonal belts provide no pelvic restraint; on impact, the victim's lower torso swings forward and rotates out of the belt. In lateral impact a whipping action occurs in which the body rotates about and then out of the belt.

The three-point restraint system is used extensively in the United Kingdom. Its principal advantage is that it offers protection against upper torso flexion while, at the same time, providing pelvic restraint. The main problem associated with the system is that correct adjustment is essential for effective restraint. Full upper torso restraint with a lap strap and double shoulder harness has been shown to be very effective[36] but its use seems to be confined to aircraft and racing cars.

The system consisting of a lap belt and an air bag which is folded into a panel in front of the subject has been evaluated by Snyder and his colleagues.[31] The bag is inflated at impact before the subject moves forward and is slowly vented as it is contacted by the subject who is thus gradually decelerated. Animal experiments have shown that decelerations above 570 m s^{-2} (57 G) can be tolerated. Indeed, the lap belt and air bag gave the occupants maximum protection against deceleration, particularly against tertiary collision which has been defined as the trauma resulting from the interaction of the occupant with his restraint system and is particularly common with badly adjusted harnesses.

The examination of fatalities from survivable light aircraft accidents who were provided with shoulder harness showed that failure of the harness or of its attachments accounted for nearly one-quarter of the deaths.[8] The investigation of these cases of harness failure suggested that the provision of adequate harness with shoulder restraint should have prevented the fatalities. Harness failure is relatively unusual in

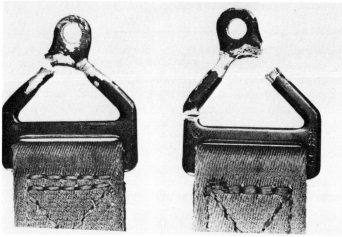

Fig. 2.4 An example of defective harness mounts, showing the dangers of do-it-yourself repairs. This failed at impact and caused the death of the occupant. (Reproduced by courtesy of Chief Inspector of Accidents, Department of Trade.)

motor vehicle accidents and occurs in less than 0·01 per cent of impacts, usually associated with high speeds.[11] Figure 2.4 shows an example of inadequate harness attachment.

The effect of harness restraint

The value of seat belts can only be proved by a reduction in the number of deaths and injuries in vehicular accidents which is directly attributable to their usage. In the United States, despite much publicity and the fact that seat belts have been fitted as standard equipment in cars manufactured since 1964, seat-belt usage has only risen from 3 per cent in 1958 to 40 per cent in 1971.[26]

In the United Kingdom, the statistics for seat-belt usage are not accurately known but casualties in front seats of cars and vans have been so analysed.[10] Table 2.4 shows the details of this study and it is significant that only 14·2 per cent of the casualties were wearing seat belts. Some would say that this figure is itself sufficient endorsement for the use of seat belts but the antagonists suggest that it merely mirrors the rate of seat-belt use.*

Table 2.4   Casualties and seat-belt usage in the United Kingdom, 1973

Use of belt	Killed	Seriously injured	All casualties
	(%)	(%)	(%)
Fitted and worn	9·5	11·3	14·2
Fitted but not worn	63·7	60·7	60·1
Not fitted to vehicle	12·8	13·7	13·6
Not known	14·0	14·3	12·1

Australia is the only country to have accurate statistics of injury rates which have been collected both before and after the introduction of legislation making the wearing of seat belts compulsory. Compulsory use of seat belts was introduced in the State of Victoria, Australia, in 1970 and subsequently in the State of New South Wales. It was observed that 90 per cent of drivers and 80 per cent of front-seat passengers wore seat belts after this legislation. The immediate effect was a 15–20 per cent reduction in the predicted number of deaths in Victoria and a reduction of 25 per cent in New South Wales.[14, 34] In frontal collisions a significant decrease in head and facial injuries was observed; they accounted for 79 per cent of hospital admissions after such collisions previously but only 23 per cent of similar admissions after legislation. A similar but less dramatic reduction in chest and spinal cord injuries was observed.[3]

* An important review of British experience, which confirms the value of restraint, has appeared since this chapter was completed (Christian, M. S. (1976) Non-fatal injury sustained by seat belt wearers; a comparative study. *Brit. med. J.* **2**, 1310).

Not surprisingly, the experience in Australia showed that the effects of seat belts were less obvious in side impacts. However, a reduction in the number of injuries due to ejection was observed and there was also a significant decrease in the number of admissions for head injury (49 per cent before legislation, 17 per cent after). The reason for this reduction in head injuries is not apparent. Severe chest, abdominal and pelvic injuries are common in side impact crashes and it is important that these accidents are studied to discover what limits the effectiveness of seat-belt restraint.

The provision of seat belts for other passengers

Despite legislation, only 3 per cent of rear-seat passengers in Australia wear seat belts and fewer do so in the United Kingdom, where rear seat belts are seldom fitted. A recent study[4] of injuries sustained by rear-seat passengers in motor vehicle accidents demonstrated that 14 per cent of these sustained severe injuries and another 35 per cent moderately severe injuries, the great majority being to the head, face and thorax. No adult in this study was wearing any form of restraint harness and only 2 children were so equipped. The arguments that apply to the front-seat passengers and drivers in cars and aircraft apply equally to rear-seat passengers and there is no doubt that a dramatic reduction in the injuries sustained by them would be achieved if belts were worn. The author has three-point harnesses fitted to the front and rear seats of his car and insists that his passengers use them!

Children and pregnant women pose particular problems in seat-belt restraint. Children are as likely to suffer injury as are any other passengers but standard seat belts do not fit those under the age of 5 years. Although most parents wish to protect their children, there is considerable uncertainty about the best method of restraint. A recent survey[23] showed that only 17 per cent of children under 6 months and 37 per cent of those between 6 months and 4 years were properly equipped. An infant carrier strapped down with a normal seat belt is regarded as the safest form of restraint for infants under the age of 6 months, while those between 6 months and 5 years are best protected in a special child's car seat or harness which is belted to the structure of the car. Children's car seats that clip to the back of the normal seat are unsafe. Over the age of 5 years a standard seat belt can be used.

Doubts have been expressed as to whether a pregnant passenger should wear a lap strap for fear that uterine compression caused by flexion over the lap strap might increase rather than reduce both maternal and fetal injury;[6] traumatic rupture of the pregnant uterus due to seat-belt injury has indeed been reported.[27] However, the forces in those accidents in which fetal death or uterine injury were attributable to seat belts were so severe that both the mother and child would have received fatal injuries had they not been worn.

A Committee of the American Medical Association has concluded that, despite the possibility of injury to the pregnant woman or her fetus being caused by seat belts in severe accidents, the woman's overall chances of surviving without serious injury are much better with a restraint system.[1] The three-point system was considered superior to the lap strap alone because of the likelihood of flexion over the latter. Another study[7] of 208 pregnant victims of motor-vehicle accidents showed 50 per cent fewer maternal deaths in the group who were wearing seat belts. There was no reduction of the fetal death rate. However, this group were only provided with lap straps and the problem of flexion was still present. The use of a full upper torso restraint should lead also to a decreased incidence of fetal injury and death.

Injuries caused by seat belts

All safety equipment must be evaluated to ensure that it does not actually contribute to injury when used in practice. Since the general adoption of restraint harness in cars and aircraft, it has become clear that seat belts themselves may on occasion cause major injury.[29] These injuries vary with the type of harness in use. Intra-abdominal injury and trauma to the pelvis and lower spine are described with lap straps alone; diagonal belts can cause thoracic, intra-abdominal and upper spinal injuries, while combined lap strap and diagonal belts can be associated with fractures of the thorax and upper spine and with intra-abdominal injuries.

Abdominal injuries are of three main types—abdominal wall damage, gut trauma and injury to the mesentery. Bruising, contusion and muscular injury along the line of the seat belt are commonly found in those casualties who were wearing only a lap strap (Fig. 2.5a). These injuries are caused by a direct blow from the lap strap and, although themselves unimportant, they may be the external markers of more severe internal injuries (Fig. 2.5b). These are frequently found after flexion over the lap belt and include rupture of the small or, less commonly, large intestine. Mesenteric rupture and vascular injuries are also reported in these circumstances. They may occur with any type of harness but are most common with a simple lap strap.[22]

Lumbar spinal injury has been described in 1 per cent of those patients with seat-belt injuries.[11] The main mechanism that has been postulated is, again, acute flexion over a lap strap. This may result in horizontal splitting and separation of the posterior vertebral arch, involving the pedicles, lamina, transverse processes or spinal processes.[9] The main site of these injuries is the mid-lumbar region and they are sometimes associated with pelvic fractures.

Upper torso restraint will prevent these flexion injuries. However, simple diagonal belts have been associated with hyperextension–hyperflexion whiplash strains of the cervical spine, which may be severe enough to fracture or dislocate the cervical or upper thoracic spine. Upper spinal whiplash injuries have also been recorded with three-point belts.

Thoracic injuries are mainly confined to fractures of the ribs, ster-

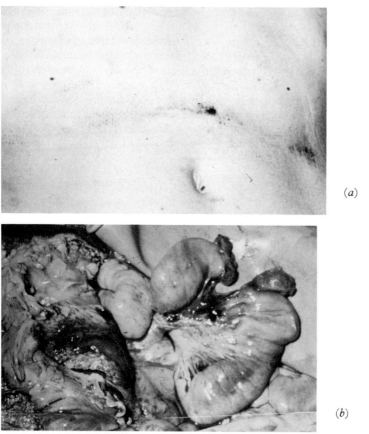

(a)

(b)

Fig. 2.5 (a) Superficial bruising along the line of the lap belt. These injuries may be external markers of trauma to the gut or mesentery shown in (b).[8]

num or clavicle, usually caused by tertiary impact with a diagonal belt or the diagonal component of a combined lap strap and diagonal. The clavicle is fractured on the side of the diagonal belt and the sternum where the belt crosses it.

It has been suggested that the shoulder harness carries a specific hazard in the form of 'submarining' which can cause death comparable with judicial hanging.[8] This risk probably arises only in aircraft accidents when the vertical and horizontal impact forces combine to cause the victim to slide through his harness. It is easily prevented by incorporating a crutch strap in the harness.

The difficulty with most of the reports of 'seat-belt injury' in the literature is that the authors, who are usually surgeons, provide a detailed description of the injuries allegedly caused by restraint harness but they provide insufficient data to evaluate the mechanism of injury. The medical and anthropometric data of the patient, the type of vehicle and harness and the details of the accident are vital if a complete picture of the accident is to emerge. It is only then that the safety equipment can be properly evaluated. The minimum environmental, vehicular and medical data required for such an evaluation are detailed elsewhere.[17] Despite the variety and severity of injuries that have been ascribed to seat belts, rarely, if ever, is the belt responsible for a more severe injury than would have been sustained if the belt had not been worn. It is clear that the occupants of motor vehicles and aircraft should wear a safety harness, preferably with upper torso restraint, no matter at what speed they are travelling nor how short the journey.

Head and neck injuries

The importance of head and neck injury has already been emphasized. It has been shown that the major head injury in light-aircraft accident victims was above the eyes in only one-third of cases.[8] These represent deaths or injuries that could have been prevented by a protective helmet. The other 66 per cent of head injuries are mainly facial and are amenable to protection by a shoulder harness. The large number of asphyxial deaths shown in Table 2.2 are partly due to concussion which prevented the victim from escaping a lethal environment—such as a light aircraft crashing into the sea or a burning car. Again, the majority of these injuries could be minimized by a helmet. The use of helmets in cars other than racing cars is not seriously advocated but light-aircraft pilots and passengers would have increased protection against concussion and against head injury caused by being thrown out of the aircraft at impact.

Whiplash injuries to the cervical spine result from a combination of hyperextension and hyperflexion. The provision of upper torso restraint prevents the impact with fixed structures and the hyperextension which accompanies recoil of the head. In these circumstances the head is subjected to hyperflexion but this infrequently results in serious injury.

A safety harness does not prevent either phase of the whiplash injury in the multiple crash where the car is rammed from behind and cannons into the car in front. The hyperextension occurs in the first phase of the accident when the vehicle is accelerated faster than the occupants. This causes hyperextension of the neck, the fulcrum being the top of the victim's seat. Prevention consists of raising the seat back to the level of the occiput and thus supporting the neck. The design of these 'anti-whiplash seats' requires care if the visibility is not to be impaired. It is essential that these devices are integral parts of the seat; a number were produced that slipped over the back of the standard seat and raised this to an appropriate anti-whiplash height. However, many of these did not stand up to the strain produced by the impact from the rear and were ineffective in preventing hyperextension. The combination of high-back seats and upper torso restraint should be effective in preventing the whiplash injury to the cervical spine of forward-facing vehicle occupants.

The design of seats

The question of seat orientation has bothered aircraft designers for many years and merits consideration here as the problem applies not only to aircraft but also to motor coaches and other high-speed passenger-carrying vehicles.

Since the Second World War, observations suggested that the mortality and morbidity of forward-facing passengers in aircraft was double that of rearward-facing passengers. The advocates of high-back rearward-facing seats claim that in abrupt deceleration the force applied to the occupant is resisted over the whole area of contact between the seat and the back of the body from shoulders to buttocks together with the back of the head. This increases the contact area fourfold with a similar reduction in the forces applied to the body.

Rearward-facing seats were made mandatory for Royal Air Force passenger-carrying aircraft in 1946. The United States Air Force followed this example in 1951 for their transport aircraft. An improvement in survival after accidents was reported and a reduction of passenger fatalities from 18·9 to 5·3 per cent was ascribed to the installation of rearward-facing seats.[13]

The opponents of rearward-facing seats claim that they will fail at lower forces than forward-facing seats because the centre of gravity of the former when occupied is higher. While this is obviously true for forward-facing seats which have been mounted in the opposite direction, it is not true for a seat which has been specifically designed to face rearwards. There may be some small weight penalty but it is felt that, ideally, commercial considerations should play no part in passenger safety.

It has been suggested that all the advantages of rearward-facing seats can be obtained by better design of forward-facing units. While this contention is partially true, such measures cannot prevent the problem of 'jack-knifing' over the lap strap nor the hyperflexion–hyperextension which leads to whiplash injury of the neck.

The efficiency of any seat and its restraint harness depends upon the integrity of the floor fastenings. Most aircraft seat anchorages are stressed to a tolerance of about 120 m s^{-2} (12 G). Once this force has been exceeded and the seat breaks away from the floor of the vehicle, the seat orientation and harness restraint are immaterial. Modern passenger-carrying aircraft are so constructed that crashes with impact forces of less than 120 m s^{-2} (12 G) are rare and so the orientation of seats is becoming less important. High vertical forces are another hazard of crashes involving newer aircraft against which rearward-facing seats offer no protection. Such points do not apply to high-speed passenger-carrying motor coaches, whose accident rate is causing concern in the United Kingdom. There can be no scientific objection to rearward-facing high-back seats for increased passenger safety in these vehicles. It is also imperative to provide them with safety belts; simple lap straps would be adequate if rearward-facing seats were fitted.

The increased tolerance to crash forces is sufficient reason for the introduction of rearward-facing seats into motor coaches but there are many other equally valid reasons. The initial forces in many accidents are in the fore-and-aft direction but the vehicle slews round after impact. In this situation the rearward-facing passenger is partially protected by virtue of being forced back into his seat by the initial deceleration. In a similar situation, the forward-facing passenger is free to swing laterally about the fulcrum of the lap belt anchorages—this results in injury to the head and upper torso.

In motor coaches special safety harnesses are not provided for children and they are poorly protected by standard seat belts. Rearward-facing seats overcome this disadvantage. Similarly, babes-in-arms are more likely to be held fast and protected if their mothers are in rearward-facing seats.

The case is often put that passengers do not like to travel in rearward-facing seats. While this may be true, it should not be beyond the expertise of the advertising industry to convince motor coach passengers that the advantages of rearward-facing seats outweigh their disadvantages.

Other safety features

The three main factors causing injury in transport accidents are ejection, displacement of the occupants within the vehicle with impact against internal structures and distortion of the passenger compartment resulting in direct impact injuries.

Seat belts offer protection against ejection; they also inhibit movement within the passenger compartment provided that the seat stays anchored to the floor. Failure of the floor anchorage has been demonstrated in both aircraft[20] and motor vehicle[12] accidents and must be prevented by good design.

Design is also important to minimize the effects of impact against fixed structures within the vehicle and of deformation of the passenger compartment. The majority of impacts on fixed objects within the vehicle are against the steering column, instrument panel or the windscreen. Safety features such as collapsible steering columns and improved instrument panels with padding and countersunk instruments and switches are beyond the scope of this chapter but it is the duty of pathologists and accident investigators to demonstrate the causes of specific impact injuries so that hazards may be identified.

The increase in the number of facial injuries[18] and, in particular, eye injuries has helped to demonstrate their cause.[32] The mechanism is shown in Fig. 2.1b. The best way to prevent these injuries is to provide effective restraint systems. However, 90 per cent of eye injuries are caused by the victim's head striking and perforating a tempered glass windscreen. The gravity of these injuries can be reduced by laminated glass windscreens which are resistant to penetration.

It is essential that vehicles are strong enough to remain intact after impact but they should incorporate energy-absorbing devices which decrease the decelerative forces applied to the cabin and its occupants. The difficulty lies in the design compromise between providing collapsible components outside the passenger compartment while still protecting against distortion within the compartment.

The high incidence of ejection coupled with the relative failure of seat belts in the prevention of lateral impact injuries suggest that vehicles would be more crashworthy with increased lateral strengthening. However, stronger doors with thick door pillars may well reduce visibility and thus make these vehicles more liable to accidents.[35] The provision of anti-burst locks does not pose such a dilemma.

It is very difficult to provide open sports cars with protection against impacts from without. The fitting of 'roll bars' to these motor vehicles has improved their safety particularly in the roll-over crash.

Methods of increasing the use of safety devices

The value of restraint harnesses for persons travelling in motor vehicles and aircraft is evident but not all ways of increasing their use are equally successful. Publicity has had some effect but seat belts are still used by the minority of road users. Although 85 per cent of the casualties in car accidents in Great Britain during 1973 had safety belts provided, 92 075 of these casualties (80 per cent) had chosen not to use them.[10] Methods other than publicity campaigns are clearly needed.

In the United States, automatic devices which warn that the seat belts are unfastened are commonly fitted in cars; in the future, seat belts may be wired into the ignition circuit so that the engine will not start unless the belt is fastened.

In Great Britain, parliamentary discussions of the Road Safety (Seat Belts) Bill which will enable the Government to make the wearing of seat belts compulsory have been deferred. Despite the experience in Australia, there is a considerable section of the community opposed to such a law. In the absence of legal sanction, the most effective method of increasing the use of seat belts would be to reduce the insurance status of persons who failed to wear them when they have been fitted. Cases have arisen in the United Kingdom where a Court found that failure to wear a seat belt amounted to contributory negligence;[24] it seems probable that it will become standard judicial procedure to reduce damages by some 25 per cent in such cases. It should also be easy for insurance companies to introduce limiting clauses into their policy but it is to be hoped that sensible legislation will be passed.

A very important point in the Bill is that, with the exception of front seat belts, not one safety feature has to be included in a new motor vehicle design. Additional safety features, such as high-back seats, rear seat belts, etc., are readily available but have to be provided by the motorist at additional voluntary cost to himself. This leads to the equipment being omitted or sometimes being fitted by the vehicle owner in an unapproved and amateur way for the sole purpose of saving money. The danger of this practice in private aircraft has been demonstrated.[8] The solution is Government legislation to ensure that all vehicles are made to comply with a minimum safety standard and this standard is kept under constant review. Such action has already been taken in the United States of America.

The problem of motor-cycles

Motor-cycles and other two-wheeled motor vehicles pose particular problems in the prevention of injury. Firstly, they have a high rate of accidents. The death rate for motor-cycle accidents during 1973 was 36 per 100 million miles while the similar rate for cars was 1·4; the serious injury rate was 642 for motor-cycles and only 18 for cars.[10] The second problem is that motor-cycles have less stability than four-wheeled vehicles and are much more likely to skid. The third difficulty relates to the behaviour of the vehicle and rider in accidents. The vehicle does not remain upright; the motor-cyclists receives little or no protection from it and he is frequently thrown off, to sustain further injury on striking the ground.

The parts of the body chiefly at risk in motor-cycle accidents are the head and legs. Head injury accounted for 50 per cent of all casualties and 80 per cent of fatalities in motor-cycle accidents, while trauma to the legs comprised 27 per cent of all injury.[2] The importance of head injury has led to improvements in the design of safety helmets and the standardization of their manufacture. So overwhelming has been the evidence that safety helmets prevent injury in motor-cycle accidents that many countries, including the United Kingdom, have introduced legislation to make their use compulsory for motor-cyclists and their passengers.

The vulnerability of the legs can be reduced with front and rear crash bars fitted just before and behind the rider's legs. More elaborate protection can be provided with fairings similar to those used by police and racing motor-cyclists. These bars and fairings should be sufficiently strong to withstand direct impact and not to trap the rider's legs.

Conclusions

It is essential that minimum standards for the safety of vehicle occupants are defined if the Government is to introduce legislation to ensure that all vehicles offer the maximum protection against injury in accidents.

All vehicles must be designed with the travellers' safety in mind. Cars should be of a crashworthy design with an appropriate steering-wheel and instrument panel: the windscreen should have laminated, penetration-resistant glass; seats should be of the high-back 'anti-whiplash' type; and safety harness with upper torso restraint must be available for all occupants including those in the rear.

The safety of passengers in motor coaches can be improved by providing safety belts. The speed of impact is such that rearward-facing seats must be an advantage and such seat orientation would obviate the need for upper torso restraint.

Motor-cycles should be provided with some form of leg guard and the riders must wear crash helmets.

The problems of light aircraft are similar to those of motor vehicles and the solutions are the same, with the rider that safety helmets provide further protection particularly against concussion caused by buffeting.

The most difficult case is that of the passenger-carrying aircraft. The high speed of travel, and therefore of impact, means that safety measures must aim at maintaining the integrity of the passenger compartment in general and the seat-floor connections in particular.

Accidental death and injury increase each year. The efforts to reduce accidents have achieved some success but considerable energy must also be expended to prevent injury when accidents are inevitable. It is apparent that there are many safety devices available but their use is limited to the minority of travellers. Publicity has only a limited effect in encouraging the use of these devices. The results of regulations making safety helmets compulsory for motor-cyclists have not yet been analysed statistically but evidence from Australia demonstrates that the most effective way to increase the use of safety equipment is by legislation.

Safety equipment must evolve to cope with the changing means of modern travel. The only way it can develop properly is to ensure that the designers of this equipment are provided with information on the causes of death and injury in vehicular accidents. It is the duty of pathologists, casualty surgeons and accident investigators—and also coroners and procurators fiscal—to acquire this information and to ensure that it is made widely available.

References

1. AMA Committee on Medical Aspects of Automotive Safety (1972). Automobile safety belts during pregnancy. *J. Amer. med. Ass.* **221**, 20.
2. Bothwell, P. W. (1962). The problem of motor-cycle accidents. *Practitioner* **188**, 475.
3. Burke, D. C. (1973). Spinal cord injuries and seat belts. *Med. J. Aust.* **2**, 801.
4. Christian, M. S. (1975). Non-fatal injuries sustained by back seat passengers. *Brit. med. J.* **1**, 320.
5. Civil Aviation Authority (1974). *Accidents to Aircraft on the British Register 1973*, p. 59. London: Civil Aviation Authority.
6. Crosby, W. M. (1968). Pathology of obstetric injuries in pregnant automobile accident victims. In: *Accident Pathology*. Ed. K. M. Brinkhous. Washington, DC: US Government Printing Office.

7. Crosby, W. M. and Costiloe, J. P. (1971). Safety of lap-belt restraint for pregnant victims of automobile accidents. *New Engl. J. Med.* **284**, 632.
8. Cullen, S. A. (1973). Death in general aviation accidents and its prevention. In: *Aerospace Pathology.* Eds. J. K. Mason and W. J. Reals. Chicago: College of American Pathologists Foundation.
9. Dehner, J. R. (1971). Seat belt injuries. *Amer. J. Roentgenol.* **111**, 833.
10. Department of the Environment (1974). *Road Accidents in Great Britain, 1973.* London: HMSO.
11. Garrett, J. W. and Braunstein, P. W. (1962). The seat belt syndrome. *J. Trauma* **2**, 220.
12. Gissane, W. and Bull, J. (1964). Motorway fatalities. *Brit. med. J.* **1**, 75.
13. Gronow, D. C. G. (1954). *Backward Facing Seats in Aircraft for Increased Passenger Safety.* Air Ministry Flying Personnel Research Committee, Report No. FPRC 807a.
14. Henderson, M. and Wood, R. (1973). Compulsory wearing of seat belts in New South Wales, Australia. An evaluation of its effect on vehicle occupant deaths in the first year. *Med. J. Aust.* **2**, 797.
15. Hossack, D. W. (1972). The pattern of injuries received by 500 drivers and passengers killed in road accidents. *Med. J. Aust.* **2**, 193.
16. Huelke, D. F. and Gikas, P. W. (1968). Causes of death in automobile accidents. *J. Amer. med. Ass.* **203**, 1100.
17. Huelke, D. F. and Snyder, R. G. (1975). Seat belt injuries: the need for accuracy in reporting of cases. *J. Trauma* **15**, 20.
18. Huelke, D. F., Grabb, W. C. and Dingmann, R. O. (1966). Facial injuries due to windshield impacts in automobile accidents. *Plast. reconstruc. Surg.* **37**, 324.
19. Mackay, G. M. (1969). Some features of traffic accidents. *Brit. med. J.* **4**, 799.
20. Mason, J. K. (1970). Passenger tie-down failure: injuries and accident reconstruction. *Aerospace med.* **41**, 781.
21. *Medical Journal of Australia* (1975). Editorial. Impact—seat belt performance in traffic crashes. *Med. J. Aust.* **1**, 26.
22. Michelinkas, E. (1971). Safety belt syndrome. *Practitioner* **207**, 77.
23. Neumann, C. G., Neumann, A. K., Cockrell, M. E. and Banani, S. (1974). Factors associated with the child use of automobile restraining devices. *Amer. J. Dis. Child.* **128**, 469.
24. Pasternack v Poulton (1973). 1 W.L.R. 476.
25. Pearson, R. G. (1962). Relationship between tie-down effectiveness and injuries sustained in lightplane accidents. *Aerospace Med.* **33**, 5.
26. Pyle, H. (1973). Safety belts—the real preventive medicine in automotive safety. *Prev. Med.* **2**, 3.
27. Rubovits, F. E. (1964). Traumatic rupture of the pregnant uterus from 'seat-belt' injury. *Amer. J. Obstet. Gynec.* **90**, 828.

28. Severy, D. M. and Mathewson, J. H. (1956). Automobile-barrier impacts. *Clin. Orthop.* **8**, 275.
29. Shennan, J. (1973). The seat-belt syndrome. *Brit. J. Hosp. Med.* **10**, 199.
30. Snyder, R. G. (1971). Occupant impact injury tolerances for aircraft crashworthiness design. SAE Paper 710406. National Business Aircraft Meeting, Wichita.
31. Snyder, R. G., Snow, C. C., Young, J. W., Crosby, W. M. and Price, T. G. (1968). Pathology of trauma attributed to restraint systems in crash impacts. *Aerospace Med.* **39**, 812.
32. Soni, K. G. (1973). Eye injuries in road traffic accidents. *Injury* **5**, 41.
33. Swearingen, J. S., Hasbrook, A. H., Snyder, R. G. and McFadden, E. B. (1962). Kinematic behaviour of the human body during deceleration. *Aerospace Med.* **33**, 188.
34. Trinca, G. W. and Dooley, B. J. (1975). The effects of mandatory seat belt wearing on the mortality and pattern of injury of car occupants in motor vehicle crashes in Victoria. *Med. J. Aust.* **1**, 675.
35. Wilks, P. M. (1967). Safety in car design. *Proc. roy. Soc. Med.* **60**, 955.
36. Young, J. W. (1966). *Recommendations for Restraint Installation in General Aviation Aircraft*. Report AM 66.33, Oklahoma: Federal Aviation Agency.

3

Pedestrian injuries and death

Introduction

In global terms, pedestrians are numerically the largest single group of road users killed in accidents. Although no satisfactory statistics are collected in Asian, African or South American countries, there are enough sources of data to suggest that traffic fatalities worldwide total some 300 000 annually and at least half of these are pedestrians. In Western countries the proportion of pedestrian to other road user deaths ranges from 39 per cent for Britain, through 28 per cent for the EEC countries as a whole, to 19 per cent for the United States.[16]

For every pedestrian fatality there are approximately 8 pedestrian casualties who receive significant injuries, but international comparisons are difficult to make because of differences of definition of injury severity.

In the United Kingdom data are collected routinely by the police on every injury-producing road accident. From a medical viewpoint the data collected are of limited use as the injuries are described using three broad overall injury classes:

1. Slight injury: an injury of a minor character such as a sprain, bruise, cut or laceration not judged to be severe.

2. Serious injury: an injury for which a person is detained in hospital as an in-patient, or any of the following injuries whether or not detained in hospital: fractures, concussion, internal injuries, crushings, severe cuts and lacerations, severe general shock requiring medical treatment.

3. Killed: died within 30 days of an accident.

Specific sample studies have to be carried out when more detailed information is needed. For example, Sevitt[22] has described injuries sustained in fatal road accidents, and Gissane et al.[7] have reported on the injuries of one year's admissions to an accident hospital. Hospital-based studies, while describing the injuries, give little information on their causes or the nature of the accident. The combination of police data and medical data can provide valuable information, for instance, on the differences in injuries sustained from impacts by different vehicle types. Because of the limited information collected by the police on the damage to the vehicle, however, it is not possible to determine the specific cause of injury from this type of study.

A detailed examination of the scene of the accident and the vehicle involved in the accident has to be made as soon as possible after the accident if the causes of the injuries are to be determined with precision. The information available from at-the-scene investigations consists of a series of marks on the vehicle from contacts by the pedestrian, the injuries sustained by the pedestrian and usually, but not always, the position of the pedestrian when struck, the final position of the vehicle and the final position and attitude of the pedestrian. It is still a complex task to reconstruct the dynamics of the accident and determine the specific causes of injury.

In order to provide information on the movement of pedestrians when struck by vehicles, experimental tests have been carried out using anthropometric dummies or cadavers. Mathematical models have also been developed to simulate pedestrian accidents and thus give an insight into how changes in vehicle design can influence the movement of the pedestrian when struck.

The aim of this work, be it real accident studies, experimental reconstruction or mathematical modelling, is to enable vehicles to be so designed that they are less likely to cause serious or fatal injuries.

People at risk

In Great Britain in 1973, pedestrians accounted for 23 per cent of all road accident casualties and 40 per cent of all road accident fatalities.[4]

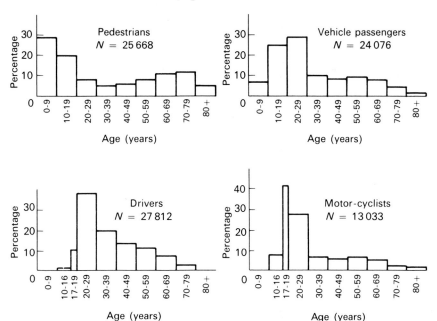

Fig. 3.1 Age distribution of seriously and fatally injured road accident casualties, 1973.

During the decade 1963–73 the relative involvement, and also the total number of pedestrian casualties, remained fairly constant with approximately 20 per cent of casualties and 40 per cent of fatalities being pedestrians.

However, the introduction of measures to protect vehicle occupants will result in a reduction in the number of such persons killed or injured and, consequently, in a relative increase in the importance of pedestrian casualties. Thus it can be expected that, in the future, pedestrians will become the road users most frequently killed as a result of a road accident.

The people most at risk as pedestrians are the young child and the elderly adult. This contrasts with other road users where the young adult is the person most exposed to injury. Figure 3.1 shows the age distribution for different road users sustaining serious or fatal injury. It can be seen that, for pedestrians, the age distribution is U-shaped, with peaks in the 0–10-year age group and 71–80-year age group, whereas, for other types of road user, there are single peaks in the 21–30-year age group for vehicle occupants and in the 17–20-year age group for motorcyclists.

It is perhaps more appropriate when considering people at risk not to use absolute numbers but rather the casualty rate per 100 000 population of the same age groups (Table 3.1). In 1973 there were 118 casualties per 100 000 population in the 5–9-year age group, 82 in the 70–79-year age group and 98 in the 80 + age group. For the 25–49-year age group there were approximately 20 casualties per 100 000 population.

The comments above refer only to serious and fatal injuries. How-

Table 3.1   Pedestrian casualties sustaining serious or fatal injury, 1973

Age group	Number	Casualty rate per 100 000 population	Percentage of all casualties
0–4	2069	50	73·1
5–9	5316	118	78·5
10–14	3137	73	55·7
15–19	1887	49	10·5
20–24	1133	29	7·7
25–29	827	21	9·3
30–39	1200	19	11·9
40–49	1376	21	17·1
50–59	1924	30	23·7
60–69	2727	47	36·7
70–79	2816	82	61·3
80+	1251	98	72·9

From Department of the Environment.[4]

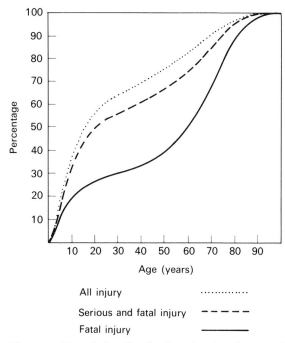

All injury   ··············

Serious and fatal injury   – – – – –

Fatal injury   ————

Fig. 3.2 Cumulative distribution of pedestrian casualties by age and injury severity.

ever, to put the people at risk in pedestrian accidents in the correct perspective, it is necessary to consider all severities of injury.

The cumulative age distribution for different levels of injury severity is shown in Fig. 3.2. It can be seen that, for all severities of injury, children account for a large proportion of the casualties; approximately 50 per cent of all pedestrian casualties are under 16 years of age and approximately 15 per cent are adults aged over 60 years. This is in contrast to the age distribution for fatal pedestrian accidents; only 25 per cent of pedestrian fatalities are children and 50 per cent are adults aged over 60 years.

The influence of age on injury severity can be highlighted by considering the frequency of injuries of different severity by age of pedestrian. In the 11–20-year age group approximately 8 per cent of those sustaining a serious or fatal injury die, while for the 61–70-year age group the figure is 15 per cent, rising to over 25 per cent for those aged over 80 years (Fig. 3.3). The proportional increase in serious and fatal injuries with age is partly explained by the lowering of injury tolerance to impact with age and by the greater susceptibility of the old person to die when once injured.

In contrast to vehicle-occupant casualties, males are involved in pedestrian accidents only slightly more frequently than females. In 1973, 57 per cent of all serious and fatally injured pedestrians were

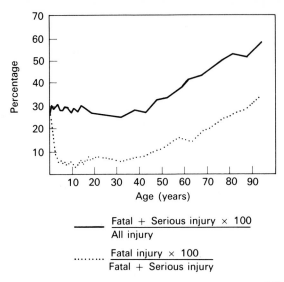

Fig. 3.3   Susceptibility of injured pedestrians to different levels of injury severity according to age.

male. Age influences the proportion of males and females involved: in the 5–9-year age group 68 per cent of serious and fatally injured pedestrians were male, while for the over-60-year age group only 43 per cent were male.

Pedestrian accidents are essentially an urban problem; 95 per cent of all pedestrian accidents in 1973 occurred in built-up areas. Accidents in rural areas tend to be more severe than those in urban areas; 42 per cent of rural accidents involved serious injury and 12 per cent fatal injury, while in urban accidents only 28 per cent resulted in serious injury and 3 per cent in fatal injury. Adults are involved relatively more frequently than children in rural compared with urban accidents; 70 per cent of the former and 54 per cent of the latter concerned adults.

Vehicles involved

In 1973, only 9 per cent of the pedestrian casualties stemmed from accidents which included either more than one vehicle or more than one pedestrian. The majority of pedestrians (92 per cent) were injured in single vehicle to single pedestrian impacts (Table 3.2). Of pedestrians involved in this type of accident, 74 per cent were struck by cars or taxis. The involvement rate of different vehicle types varies; for example, it has been shown that public service vehicles are six times more likely, and good vehicles are twice as likely, to be involved in a pedestrian accident than is a private car.[24]

A better measure in terms of vehicle design is the relative risk of striking a pedestrian throughout the total operating life of the vehicle.

Table 3.2 Vehicles involved in single vehicle pedestrian accidents, 1973

Type of vehicle	Number	Percentage of total	Percentage fatal
Pedal-cycles	554	0·8	1·1
Mopeds	661	0·9	0·8
Motor-scooters	776	1·1	1·0
Motor-cycles	3 143	4·3	3·2
Cars and taxis	54 590	74·0	3·2
Public service vehicles	2 799	3·8	5·5
Goods vehicles:			
< 1524 kg (1·5 tons) u.w.	7 029	9·5	3·6
1524–3048 kg (1·5–3 tons) u.w.	870	1·2	6·7
3048–4572 kg (3–4·5 tons) u.w.	525	0·7	9·0
> 4572 kg (4·5 tons) u.w.	1 091	1·5	12·7
Other	1 714	2·3	2·9

From Department of the Environment.[4]

Then, a bus is some twelve times more likely to injure a pedestrian than is a car. Other similar high risk situations can be detected—for example, the average Manhattan taxi has a 1 in 8 chance of injuring a pedestrian in 2 years; taxis in other large cities, such as London and Paris, may well have equivalent involvement rates. The chance of being killed also varies with the type of vehicle; in Britain only 3 per cent of pedestrians struck by cars or taxis were killed in 1973 while, for goods vehicles, the percentage killed rises from 4 per cent for vehicles of less than 1524 kg (1·5 tons) to 13 per cent for those over 4572 kg (4·5 tons) unladen weight.

Location of contacts

Data from national statistics have been used in the preceding sections to describe pedestrian accident epidemiology. To appreciate such accidents in more detail it is necessary to use the results from the 'in-depth' studies which have been carried out.

Ashton et al.,[3] reporting on an at-the-scene study of pedestrian accidents in Birmingham, noted that pedestrians were most frequently struck by the front of the vehicle; this was found in 84 per cent of the accidents investigated where the location of the first contact was known (Fig. 3.4). The front nearside wing was contacted more frequently than was the front offside wing. Pedestrians are more frequently struck on the side than on the front or back. Appel et al.[1] reported that the left

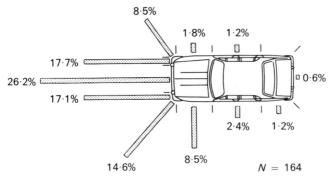

Fig. 3.4   Location of first contact of pedestrian on vehicle.[3]

side of the body was struck in 47 per cent and the right side in 46 per cent of the cases.

Pedestrian dynamics during impact

The most frequent type of pedestrian accident, as discussed above, is that in which the pedestrian is struck by the front of a car. The initial contacts are from the bumper, which strikes the lower leg, and from the leading edge of the bonnet which strikes the upper leg or pelvis. The exact location of these contacts depends on the relative heights of the pedestrian and of the parts of the vehicle. The pedestrian then rotates about the leading edge until the head, shoulders and chest strike the vehicle bonnet, windscreen or windscreen frame. At high impact speeds, the pedestrian rotates about the second contact of the head or shoulders, and the legs may strike the roof. By this time, the casualty is travelling at approximately the same speed as the car.[21]

Should there have been little or no braking during the accident it is likely that, at high speeds, the pedestrian will pass over the top of the car. If, however, the vehicle is being braked—and this is the most frequent accident condition—the car slows down faster than does the pedestrian who thus continues to move forward and lands on the road in front of the vehicle. The person struck will finally come to rest after sliding along the road surface.

The extent of the contacts on the vehicle depends on its speed and on the relative heights of the pedestrian and front structure of the vehicle. The initial contact results in the pedestrian being pushed forward and at the same time rotated about his centre of gravity. These two types of motion are commonly called translation and rotation; their relationship determines the actual movement of the pedestrian.

The influence of the location of the first contact can be shown by the use of a simple model (Fig. 3.5) in which the pedestrian is considered as a rigid body and friction between him and the ground is neglected. Then, if the location of the contact is below the pedestrian's centre of gravity, he will receive both translational and rotational motion, the head moving towards the vehicle. If the contact is at the centre of

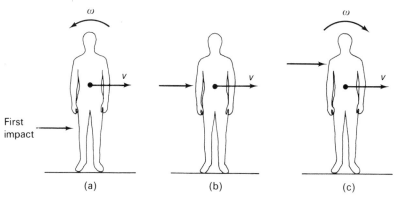

Fig. 3.5 Influence of location of contact on pedestrian motion: (*a*) contact below centre of gravity; (*b*) contact at centre of gravity; (*c*) contact above centre of gravity. *v*, translation velocity; *w*, rotational (angular) velocity.

gravity, he will receive only translational motion; if it is above the centre of gravity, both translational and rotational motion will be transmitted with the pedestrian's head moving away from the vehicle. The motion of a pedestrian in a real accident is, however, much more complex than is indicated by this simplified model.

The motion of an adult struck by a conventional car is usually of the first type—i.e. translation and rotation with the pedestrian's head moving towards the car and, given sufficient angular velocity (i.e. rotation), the head and upper torso will strike the vehicle. At less than 19 km h^{-1}

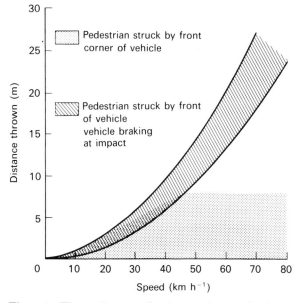

Fig. 3.6 Throw distance of pedestrian by speed at impact.

(12 m.p.h.), there is frequently only contact with the bumper, leading edge and ground. At higher speeds, the pedestrian will strike the bonnet or windscreen frame before sliding off the front of the vehicle.[15]

The pedestrian will finally come to rest some way from the point of impact; this distance, commonly called the throw distance, depends on the speed of the vehicle at impact and the level of braking. There is good correlation between the speed of the vehicle at impact and the throw distance when the vehicle is under heavy braking at or immediately after impact (Fig. 3.6). However, the throw distance is not related to impact speed when there is only light or no braking.

It will thus be appreciated that pedestrians are not as a rule 'run over' but are 'run under'. The former is a fairly rare occurrence unless the pedestrian is lying in the road before the accident.[18]

Impact speeds

In general, the higher the speed of the vehicle at impact, the more severe are the injuries sustained by the pedestrian. Ashton[2] found that the incidence of fatalities in adults rose from 10 per cent in the impact speed range 30–39 km h^{-1} (19–24 m.p.h.), through 47 per cent in the range 40–48 km h^{-1} (25–30 m.p.h.) to 73 per cent in the range 49–58 km h^{-1} (31–36 m.p.h.).

There is, however, great variation in impact speed for a given level of injury; in the same study Ashton noted that adult fatalities had occurred at impact speeds of less than 9·7 km h^{-1} (6 m.p.h.) and that only

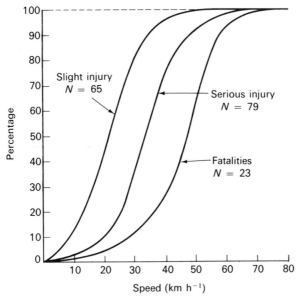

Fig. 3.7 Cumulative impact speed distribution for different injury severities.[3]

minor injuries had resulted from accidents in the 40–48 km h^{-1} (25–30 m.p.h.) speed range. In a sample of 167 children and adults, it was found that 50 per cent of minor injuries occurred at impact speeds below 22·5 km h^{-1} (14 m.p.h.), 50 per cent of serious injuries at speeds less than 33·8 km h^{-1} (21 m.p.h.) and 50 per cent of fatalities at speeds less than 48 km h^{-1} (30 m.p.h.) (Fig. 3.7).

The 50 percentile speed for injury has been assessed as 33·8 km h^{-1} (21 m.p.h.) for injury and death[1] and as 46·7 km h^{-1} (29 m.p.h.)[4] and 43·4 km h^{-1} (27 m.p.h.)[12] for fatalities.

Multiplicity of injury

The findings in all studies confirm that multiplicity of injury is a characteristic of road accident trauma. There are differences in the results, however, due to variations in samples and in the extent of the analyses.

A sample of pedestrian accidents in Birmingham, England, showed that, for all severities of injuries, there was an average of 2·7 injuries per person but that the number fell to 2·15 when minor injuries were excluded.[6] A similar figure for all severities of injury was found in Adelaide, Australia.[19] A study of non-fatal hospital in-patients in Brisbane, Australia, in which only non-minor injuries were considered, noted 1·61 injuries per person; when fatalities were included in this study, the average injuries per person rose to 2·46.[10]

Fatally injured pedestrians generally sustain more injuries than do non-fatalities. Jamieson and Tait[10] reported that there was an average of 3·57 serious and fatal injuries per fatality; they had divided the body into eight regions. Using seven body regions, Huelke and Davis[9] arrived at a comparable incidence of 2·75 injuries. Others have used six body regions and have noted 2·67[25] and 2·3[22] serious and fatal injuries per fatality. The average number drops considerably when only fatal injuries are considered; 1·29[22] and 1·57[9] fatal injuries per fatality have been reported.

The multiplicity of pedestrian injuries is hardly surprising considering the nature of the contact between the pedestrian and the vehicle and the subsequent pedestrian-to-ground impacts. As would be expected, the number of injuries sustained rises with increasing impact speed. In one study, 1·63 injuries per pedestrian were found in the 0–16 km h^{-1} (0–10 m.p.h.) speed range, the incidence rising to 2·43 injuries in the 82–96·5 km h^{-1} (51–60 m.p.h.) speed range.[5]

Time to die

The time to die is greatly influenced by the multiplicity of injury. The percentage of New York fatalities dying within 2 hours of the accident rose from 28 per cent when there were injuries to two or less body areas to 84 per cent when five or more body areas were involved. There was survival for longer than 24 hours in 49 per cent of the cases in which

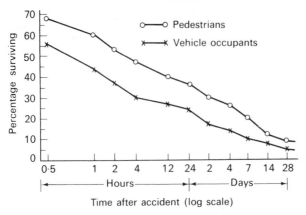

Fig. 3.8   Survival times of fatally injured pedestrians and vehicle occupants.[23]

two or less body areas were injured and in only 3 per cent of the latter category.[13] Solheim obtained similar results in Norway.[25]

Sevitt[23] reported that pedestrians take longer to die than do other fatally injured road users; 32 per cent of fatally injured pedestrians died within half an hour of their accident as opposed to 44 per cent of vehicle occupants (Fig. 3.8). He also found that 20 per cent of fatally injured pedestrians survived longer than 1 week as compared with only 10 per cent of vehicle occupants. These variations are due to differences in the age distributions of the different road users and in the nature and number of injuries sustained. Pedestrians received an average of 1·3 fatal injuries and vehicle occupants received 1·5 fatal injuries per person. The influence of the type of injury sustained was shown in an earlier paper;[22] death occurred in less than 24 hours in 52·8 per cent of those sustaining fatal head injuries but the corresponding figures for fatalities from chest and abdominal trauma were 76 per cent and 83 per cent respectively.

Patterns of injury

Even allowing for differences in the definitions of injury and in the samples used, reported studies generally agree on the relative frequencies with which body areas are injured.

When all severities of injury are considered, the legs show the most frequent injuries, occurring in approximately 85 per cent of pedestrians (Table 3.3). The head, with between 50 and 80 per cent of injuries, is the next most affected area. This is hardly surprising considering the dynamics of pedestrian accidents; the legs are always involved when a pedestrian is struck by the front of a car but there is not necessarily a head contact with the vehicle or with the ground. The arms are generally found to be the third most frequently injured area, followed by the pelvis and then the chest or abdomen. Injuries to the neck and spine are relatively infrequent in overall terms.

Table 3.3 Distribution of injuries: all severities of injury

	Fisher and Hall[5]	Robertson et al.[20]	Jamieson et al.[11]	Ashton[2]
Number	4134	63	51	166
Head	48	} 76·2	64·7	80·1
Neck	5			3
Spine	4			★
Chest	3	22·2	13·7	15·7
Abdomen	1·5	15·9	27·4	15·1
Pelvis	13	17·5†	25·5	
Arms	24	50·8	35·3 L	42·2
			43·1 R	
Legs	86	87·3	70·6 L	84·9‡
			72·5 R	

★ Spine included with neck, chest or abdomen.
† Includes spine.
‡ Includes pelvis.
L, left; R, right.

It is perhaps more important to take account only of the more severe injuries. When minor injuries are excluded from the analyses, the head emerges as the body area most often injured; between 57 and 72 per cent of casualties sustained injury to the head but only 38–57 per cent received severe leg injuries (the variation depending on the study). Injuries to the chest and abdomen occur in less than 10 per cent of the cases at this level of injury severity (Table 3.4).

When the sample is limited to fatalities, and only non-minor injuries

Table 3.4 Distribution of injuries: non-minor injuries

	Gogler[8]	Jamieson and Tait[10]	Mackay[14]	Ashton[2]
Number	1149	113	139	102
Head	} 66·6	} 56·6	72	} 71·6
Face			13	
Neck	} 2·2	} 2·5	3	1
Spine				★
Chest	8·1	5·7	7	9·8
Abdomen	6	} 14	7	10·8
Pelvis	5·6		20	
Arms	14·7	14	16	16·7
Legs	38·3	14·6 U	62	56·9†
		17·5 L		

★ Spine included with neck, chest or abdomen.
† Includes pelvis.
U, upper leg; L, lower leg.

Table 3.5   Distribution of injuries: fatalities—serious and fatal injuries

	Jamieson and Tait[10]	Sevitt[22]	McCarroll et al.[13]	Huelke and Davis[9]	Solheim[25]
Number	186	125	200	231	168
Head	84·9	63	61	61	72
Neck	} 34·9	10	9·5	33	} 16·1
Spine		7	1·5		
Chest	63·9	38	50	44	53·6
Abdomen	} 60·5	14	42	28	24·4
Pelvis		36	46	39	25·6
Arms	23·3	14	19	14	19
Legs	23·3 U 44·2 L	48	54	58	33

U, upper leg; L, lower leg.

are considered, the incidence of chest and abdominal injuries increases to between 38 and 64 per cent for chest injuries and to between 14 and 42 per cent for abdominal injuries (Table 3.5). Injuries to the head are about as frequent, with an occurrence of between 61 and 85 per cent.

Causes of death

It has already been noted that fatally injured pedestrians normally receive multiple injuries. The question arises as to which injuries are responsible for the death.

Huelke and Davis[9] found that 54 per cent of the pedestrians died as a result of one fatal injury, 33 per cent from two, 11 per cent from three and 3 per cent from four fatal injuries. In 12 per cent of the cases, however, death was due not directly to the injuries but rather to complications. Pneumonia, pulmonary emboli or oedema, peritonitis, brain necrosis, renal thrombi or gangrene were listed separately or in combination as a cause of death. Persons over 58 years old account for 88 per cent of those dying from complications. Solheim[25] also found that 12 per cent of fatally injured pedestrians died from complications; 45 per cent of these died from infections. Sevitt[22] reported that respiratory infection caused or contributed to death in 30 per cent of a sample of 125 fatally injured pedestrians. The susceptibility of elderly pedestrians to death from complications associated with relatively modest injuries is a striking general characteristic of trauma in this age group.[19,22]

Head injuries are the most frequent cause of death. Solheim found that 47 per cent of cases died from head injuries alone and 55 per cent from head and other injuries;[25] comparable results from an American study are shown in Table 3.6. Both reports agree that thoracic injuries were the second leading cause of death, being solitary in 14 per cent and 9 per cent respectively; when both solitary and combined injuries

Table 3.6 Location of fatal injuries in 187 pedestrians[9]

Location	No. of cases	Percentage with area injured	Percentage injured with one fatal injury
Head	103	55·1	54·4
Neck	73	39·0	34·2
Chest	78	41·7	20·5
Abdomen	37	19·8	8·1
Pelvis	9	4·8	0·0

were considered, the relative frequencies became 27 per cent and 42 per cent. Fatal neck injuries occurred alone in 14 per cent and were associated with other fatal injuries in 39 per cent of American cases.

Head injuries

Head injuries result from both vehicle and road contacts. A recent study of 171 children and adults struck by cars indicated that the injured pedestrian was more likely to sustain a serious head injury from vehicle contact than from road contact. Of the head injuries derived from contact with the ground, 65 per cent were minor and 11 per cent were critical or fatal; this contrasts with vehicle-induced injuries in which the corresponding figures were 38 per cent and 22 per cent.[2]

When the causes of injury for a given level of severity are considered, it is found that the incidence from ground contact decreases with increasing severity of injury; 68 per cent of minor injuries were caused by the ground, the incidence decreasing to 38 per cent for fatal injuries. This confirms an earlier study which showed that the majority of serious trauma comes from vehicle contacts.[15]

There is a strong relationship between speed and vehicle-induced head injuries—the higher the impact speed, the more severe is the head injury. Ground-induced injury, however, does not show this tendency.

The severity of the injury sustained from contact with the vehicle is greatly influenced by the area of contact; two-thirds of the head contacts on the bonnet caused minor or no injury while two-thirds of the contacts on the windscreen frame resulted in critical or fatal injuries. The windscreen frame is a particularly hazardous structure, being responsible for 80 per cent of the fatal or critical head injuries caused by vehicle contact.

Leg injuries

Serious injuries to the ankle and foot are rare. Injuries to the foot normally result from it being run over by a wheel. Ankle injuries occur when the foot angulates under the bumper following a leg contact by a low bumper at high speed. Lower leg fractures, however, are common and result from either angulation or rotation of the leg or from both.

Table 3.7   Distribution of leg injuries TRRL
study of 149 serious and fatally injured pedestrians[26]

	Cause of injury		
	Vehicle	*Road*	*Both*
Hip and pelvis	46	8	54
Thigh (femur)	41	8	49
Knee	5	2	7
Lower leg	82	8	90

Fractures from rotational (or torsional) forces are spiral in nature and involve the weakest part of the leg. They usually occur at the smallest cross-section and are at different levels in the tibia and fibula. Spiral fractures are caused when the pedestrian contacts the front corner or side of the vehicle and is spun around a vertical axis. Combined angulation and rotation, which is probably more frequent than pure torsion, still results in spiral fractures as the bone is weaker in torsion than in bending.

Pure bending, which occurs when the pedestrian is struck squarely by the front of a vehicle, results in either transverse or oblique fractures and these are the most common lower leg fractures sustained by pedestrians. The fracture is normally at the point of loading; the location of the fracture is thus determined usually by the relative positions of the bumper and the leg. Loading of the shaft of the tibia and fibula causes simple fractures while loading of the tibial head or proximal parts of the shaft is more likely to result in comminuted fractures.

Knee injuries can be divided into two types—those involving damage to the ligaments and fractures of the tibial and femoral condyles including the patella. Injuries to the knee do not occur frequently (Table 3.7). Fractures result from direct contact and ligament injuries from abduction of the tibia upon the femur; typically, the lower leg will angulate under the bumper as the upper leg and torso wrap around the front of the vehicle (Fig. 3.9).

Femoral fractures can also result from torsion or bending but, in

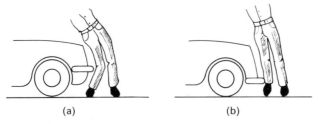

(a)   (b)

Fig. 3.9   Mechanism of lower leg injury: (*a*) injury to knee; (*b*) injury to ankle.

pedestrian accidents, are normally caused by the latter. Angulation of the femur over the leading edge of the bonnet is the most common cause of injury in adults while the bumper is frequently responsible for femoral fractures in children.

Pelvic injuries are caused by contact with the leading edge and occur both independently and in conjunction with femoral injury. Injuries to the acetabulum result from a direct blow at or just below the head of the femur; injuries to the pubic rami, for example, do not necessarily occur on the same side of the pelvis as that impacted, the fracture occurring at the weakest part of the pelvic ring for a given pattern of loading. Although pelvic injuries can also result from ground contact, they are less frequent than are those due to vehicle impacts.

It will be apparent that the location of the bumper and leading edges of the bonnet greatly influence the injuries sustained. Figure 3.10 shows that 65 per cent of pedestrians who were seriously or fatally injured by being struck by the front of the car would sustain a direct knee contact if all vehicles had a bumper with a depth of 5 cm (2 in), the top of which was 50 cm (20 in) above the ground. If, however, all vehicles had a bumper of depth 10 cm (4 in), the top of which was 35 cm (14 in) above the ground, only 30 per cent would be struck on the knee. The data given in Fig. 3.10 allow for the ranging stature of the population at risk. If it is accepted that damage to the knee joint presents a more serious clinical problem than does fracture of the tibia or fibula, then the information gives some guidance to the vehicle designer as to the correct position for the bumper. So far, current vehicle design has not considered this problem at all.

Indeed, the overall relationship of vehicle exterior shape to pedestrian trauma represents one of the major areas of biomechanical research at the present time. Enough evidence exists to suggest that, in

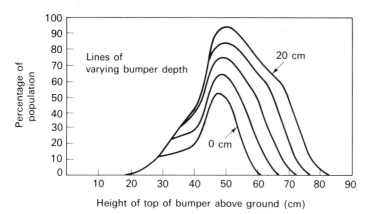

Fig. 3.10 Percentage of involved population (serious and fatal injury) sustaining a direct knee contact from a bumper of given dimensions. Note that the effect of varying bumper depth is shown by considering bumpers of depth 0, 5, 10, 15 and 20 cm.

practice, different car profiles do present different risks of injury. Perhaps the clearest study was undertaken by McLean,[17] who compared two groups of pedestrians, the first being struck by Volkswagens and the second by Cadillacs. The samples were standardized as far as possible with regard to other relevant variables. He concluded that there would be a 30 per cent reduction in pedestrian fatalities in the United States if all cars which struck pedestrians had Volkswagen fronts.

At present, however, neither experimental studies nor field accident investigation projects are sufficiently far advanced for the ideal vehicle exterior to be specified. What may appear to be an optimum design in terms of contour and resilience for one impact speed and one particular height of pedestrian may well produce particularly unfavourable impact conditions in different circumstances.

In addition, the pedestrian population at risk undoubtedly has a great range of values for tolerance to any given injury. There is also some evidence to suggest that children are struck by vehicles which are travelling slower than are those which strike adult pedestrians. McLean and Mackay[18] showed that the segments of the body of children were injured less severely and less frequently than was the case in adults and that the mean estimated impact speed for child collisions was 29 km h^{-1} (18 m.p.h.) compared with 39 km h^{-1} (24 m.p.h.) for adults.

Thus, the production of the least injurious vehicle exterior to suit all circumstances requires a better insight into the circumstances of collisions and into the precise mechanisms of injury than we have at present. Hopefully in the future these problems will receive the attention which they deserve.

References

1. Appel, H., Sturtz, G. and Gotzen, L. (1975). Influence of impact speed and vehicle parameter on injuries to children and adults in pedestrian accidents. *Proc. 2nd Conf. Biomechanics of Serious Trauma*, p. 83. Lyon: IRCOBI.
2. Ashton, S. J. (1975). The cause and nature of head injuries sustained by pedestrians. *Proc. 2nd Conf. Biomechanics of Serious Trauma*, p. 101. Lyon: IRCOBI.
3. Ashton, S. J., Hayes, H. R. M. and Mackay, G. M. (1974). Child pedestrian injuries. *Proc. Conf. Biomechanics of Trauma in Children*, p. 159. Lyon: IRCOBI.
4. Department of the Environment (1974). *Road Accidents in Great Britain 1973*. London: HMSO.
5. Fisher, A. J. and Hall, R. R. (1972). The influence of car frontal design on pedestrian trauma. *Accid. Anal. Prev.* **4**, 47.
6. Fonseka, C. P. de (1969). *Causes and Effects of Road Accidents*. Vol. 4. *The Injuries to Road Users*. University of Birmingham, Department of Transportation and Environmental Planning, Report No. 33.
7. Gissane, W., Bull, J. and Roberts B. (1970). Sequelae of road injuries. *Injury* **1**, 195.

8. Gogler, E. (1974). Road accidents. Series Chirurgica Geigy (No. 5), p. 27.
9. Huelke, D. F. and Davis, R. A. (1969). *A Study of Pedestrian Fatalities in Wayne County, Michigan*, HSRI Report, Bio-9. Ann Arbor: University of Michigan.
10. Jamieson, K. G. and Tait, I. A. (1968). *Report of a General Survey: Traffic Injury in Brisbane*. National Health and Medical Research Council, Spec. Rep. No. 13, Canberra.
11. Jamieson, K. G., Duggan, A. W., Tweddell, J., Pope, L. I. and Zvirbulis, V. E. (1971). *Traffic Crashes in Brisbane*. Australian Road Research Board, Spec. Rep. No. 2.
12. Kamiyama, S. and Schmidt, G. (1970). Beziehungen zwischen Aufprallgeschwindigkeit, Fahrzeugbeschädigungen, Frakturen und 'Wurfweite' bei 50 tödlichen Fussgänger-PKW-Unfällen. *Z. Rechtsmed.* **67**, 282.
13. McCarroll, J. R., Braunstein, P. W., Cooper, W., Helpern, M., Seremetis, M., Wade, P. A. and Weinberg, S. B. (1962). Fatal pedestrian automotive accidents. *J. Amer. med. Ass.* **180**, 127.
14. Mackay, G. M. (1969). Some features of traffic accidents. *Brit. med. J.* **4**, 799.
15. Mackay, G. M. (1971). The other road users. *Proc. 13th Conf. Amer. Assoc. Auto. Med.*, p. 321. Ann Arbor: University of Michigan Press.
16. Mackay, G. M. (1974). Field studies of traffic accidents in Europe. *Proc. 4th Experimental Safety Vehicle Conf.*, p. 601. Washington DC: Dept. of Transportation.
17. McLean, A. J. (1972). Car shape and pedestrian injury. *Proc. Symp. Road Safety*. Canberra: Dept. of Transport.
18. McLean, A. J. and Mackay, G. M. (1970). The Exterior Collision. In: *Compendium on Automobile Safety*, p. 1214. New York: Society of Automotive Engineers.
19. Robertson, J. S. and Tonge, J. I. (1968). Duration of survival time in traffic accident fatalities. *Med. J. Aust.* **2**, 571.
20. Robertson, J. S., McLean, A. J. and Ryan, G. A. (1966). *Traffic Accidents in Adelaide, South Australia*. Australian Road Research Board, Spec. Rep. No. 1.
21. Ryan, G. A. and McLean, A. J. (1966). Pedestrian survival. *Proc. 9th Stapp Conf.*, p. 321. Minneapolis: University of Minnesota Press.
22. Sevitt, S. (1968). Fatal road accidents. Injuries, complications, and causes of death in 250 subjects. *Brit. J. Surg.* **55**, 481.
23. Sevitt, S. (1973). Fatal road accidents in Birmingham: time to death and their cause. *Injury* **4**, 281.
24. Smeed, R. J. (1968). Aspects of pedestrian safety. *J. Transp. Econ. Policy* **2**, 1.
25. Solheim, K. (1964). Pedestrian deaths in Oslo traffic accidents. *Brit. med. J.* **1**, 81.
26. Transport and Road Research Laboratory (1974). *Pedestrian Injuries*, No. 4, April. London: Dept. of the Environment.

4

The aircraft accident as an example of a major disaster

Major disasters with many fatalities arise in several different circumstances and will present in various ways. Thus, the victims of a flood will show little in the way of violent injury; those involved in a hotel fire are likely to be severely incinerated; railway casualties may be subjected to much trauma but are unlikely to be burned. Aircraft accidents provide examples of all these modes of deaths and are, therefore, an especially useful model of the mass disaster situation. The investigation of aircraft accidents is statutory (Civil Aviation (Investigation of Accidents) Regulations 1969—made under Civil Aviation Act 1968) and the medical element of the Inquiry has been particularly well documented.[19] For these reasons, aircraft disasters have been selected for special consideration but it is to be hoped that the description which follows could be adapted to other forms of major accident.

Types of aircraft accident

At one time, aircraft accidents tended to be of the 'all or nothing' type. Although this still holds to some extent, accidents with both survivors and fatalities do now occur fairly often; the results of 23 consecutive fatal commercial and 2 troop-carrying accidents are shown in Table 4.1.

Wholly fatal accidents may be of the disintegrative type; these are generally associated with structural failure in the air or with flying into high ground. A further group of accidents are attributable to emergencies occurring between 150 and 600 m (500 and 2000 ft)—the classic take-off catastrophe; while these will result in severe crash forces, they are unlikely to cause fragmentation of bodies and patterns of injury are discernible (Fig. 4.1). Accidents resulting from an error of judgement on landing—the categories of overshoot or undershoot—are, however,

Table 4.1 Twenty-five Accidents of Potential disaster type

Wholly fatal	18
Minority of survivors	5
Majority of survivors	2

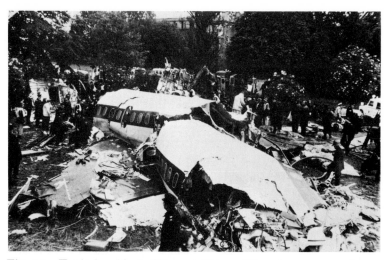

Fig. 4.1 Typical accident of 'deep stall' type. There is very severe damage but this is short of disintegration. Cadavers are likely to be relatively intact and patterns of injury will be discernible. (Reproduced by courtesy of Chief Inspector of Accidents, Department of Trade.)

likely to be survivable. Death may be due either to relatively localized injury or to trapping within the aircraft structure; it is in this last group that death from burning is so frequent. Fire and survivability are inter-dependent. Fire was a major feature in 7 out of 23 fatal accidents involving laden commercial passenger aircraft which were investigated. There were a significant number of deaths due to burning in 6 of those 7; there were survivors in 5 of those accidents associated with burning but in only 1 of the other 16 (Table 4.2).

Injuries sustained in aircraft accidents

The practical importance of the recognition of common injuries occurring in major accidents lies in its application to disaster planning;[17] it is

Table 4.2 Survival in 23 consecutive accidents to airliners

	Total	Fire a major feature
Accidents	23	7
Disintegrative injury	13	0
Less severe injury	10	7
With survivors	6	5
Significant number of deaths due to burning	—	6

possible to establish priorities only by knowing what is likely. Since survivable aircraft accidents are likely to occur at airports, they will be closely associated with major cities; those responsible for the provision of an emergency programme are, therefore, stimulated by the high quality of the services at their disposal and by the very real possibility of the contingency occurring.

It is apparent from what has been said that burns are likely to be a major problem in survivors from aircraft accidents. Modern aircraft fuels burn with a savage intensity—thermal injuries in both survivors and fatalities are therefore likely to be very severe. Apart from this question of degree, the management of burned casualties from aircraft accidents does not differ materially from that in other situations; the subject is covered in Chapter 7.

Survivors will otherwise fall within two main categories—those who are fortuitously thrown from the aircraft and those who are trapped within the hull but are rescued before fire takes hold. Injuries in the former category are caused by the primary crash forces, by impact with other structures during ejection and by secondary impact with the ground. They are therefore likely to be severe and multiple but are unpredictable and are generally those of acute acceleration and deceleration which have been described in Chapters 1 and 2. Injuries in the latter group, however, will have been directly responsible for preventing voluntary egress from the crash environment; they are therefore of fundamental importance in aircraft accident pathology. Violent injuries to the head, the spine and the legs are among those of greatest significance.

Leg injuries

The importance of leg injuries in association with the failure of seat mountings was emphasized in the serious accident at Stockport in 1967[2] in which widespread fractures of the tibia and fibula were thought to be due to the presence of a horizontal bar at the rear of the seat in front. This incapacitating lesion, which will occur when there is seat displacement irrespective of a forward or rearward orientation, can be prevented by suitable design modifications. In more recent accidents, however, the more typical leg injuries have been found to involve fractures of the femur. These fractures occur particularly often in crashes involving aircraft of the rear-engine, high tail-plane configuration which are characterized by unusually high vertical forces. It is assumed that the fractures are caused on the front bar of the seat as the torso penetrates the seat pan; this mechanism is generally mirrored in deformity of the seat structure and of its front legs (Fig. 4.2).

Thoracic spine fracture

Fracture of the thoracic spine can be regarded as the injury most specific to aircraft accidents. The common site is in the upper half, and its frequent association with sternal injury indicates that it is of flexion type. It has been shown in light aircraft that the spinal injury is

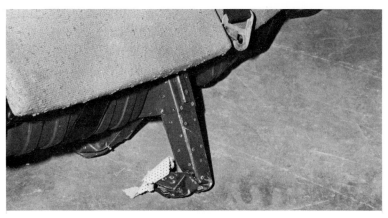

Fig. 4.2 Crushing deformity of the legs of a rearward-facing passenger seat subjected to severe vertical deceleration forces.

markedly modified by the provision of a shoulder harness—even if this gives way during the crash—and passenger-carrying aircraft studies clearly indicate that the lesion is related to the severity of the accident. The incidence ranged from 78 per cent in passengers killed in disasters due to inflight structural failure, through 13 per cent at Stockport to 5 per cent in an undershoot involving a jet aircraft. The distribution of spinal fracture as a whole is related to the precise conditions of the accident. In an accident resulting from a stall at approximately 360 m (1200 ft) thoracic spinal fracture was present in 13 per cent of fatalities but extension fracture of the cervical spine occurred in 50 per cent. The spinal lesions were associated with severe craniofacial injuries and were due to impaction of the head on the seat in front while the flailing body was subjected to severe vertical loads.

Craniofacial injuries
Craniofacial injuries are extremely common, the major feature being the high incidence of middle third maxillary fractures due to striking the seat back in front of the passenger. Fracture of the base of the skull is to be anticipated in accidents involving severe vertical forces; the lesion is often of the classical ring type surrounding the foramen magnum and may well be the primary, if not the only, cause of death.

Over all, death in aircraft accidents is most usually due to multiple injury of extreme degree. Individual causes of death do, however, appear if accidents of disintegrative type are excluded. Burning has already been discussed. Rupture of the heart or aorta is almost as common and is caused in two main ways—either the heart is compressed between sternum and spine during acute flexion (Fig. 4.3) or the mobile

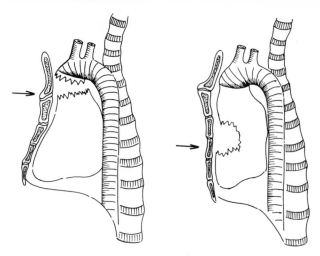

Fig. 4.3   Mechanism of crush injury to the heart. Depending on the precise application of force, the heart is either squeezed from its attachment to the aorta or it is burst like a 'paper bag'. (From Mason, J. K. (1978), *Forensic Medicine for Lawyers*, Bristol; Wright, by permission of the Publishers.)

heart is torn from the static aorta during whole body deceleration in the vertical plane. The frequent occurrence of endocardial or endovascular tears suggests that raised internal pressure, due to violent compression of the legs and abdomen, may be an additional factor; such partial thickness lesions may predispose to delayed cardiovascular rupture. The occurrence of thoracic and abdominal injuries in aviation as a whole has been discussed elsewhere.[14]

The medical investigation of aircraft accidents

All investigation is an exercise in prevention. It is this aspect of accident pathology which makes the work so satisfying to the forensic pathologist whose contribution to the saving of lives follows two main lines. These are, first, the prevention of accidents through identification of and, hopefully, elimination of the cause of the individual disaster and, secondly, the prevention of fatal accidents by identifying fatal injuries and thus indicating specific needs for improved safety features. The intense, multidisciplined investigative effort applied to aircraft accidents highlights this aspect of the pathology of violence; despite, or perhaps because of, their relatively small numbers (Table 2.1) these accidents provide exceptionally useful experience.

The pattern of injuries

The pattern of injuries has been described above as an aid to patient management and treatment. The autopsy findings can, however, be directed not only to therapy and preventive medicine but also to the diagnosis of the type of an individual accident. The prevention of

Table 4.3 Patterns of passenger injury in two accidents occurring short of the runway

Nature of accident	*Case 1* Known undershoot	*Case 2* Possible fatal hijacking
Fatalities examined	48	63
Proportions of asphyxial deaths	69%	68%
Lap belt injuries	20%	14%
Femoral fractures	43%	60%
Diagnosis	Undershoot	Undershoot

injuries in vehicular accidents has been discussed in Chapter 2. The diagnosis of the accident may be made direct from the autopsy findings or from comparison with other accidents of known type.

Two examples of comparative accident investigation are shown in Tables 4.3 and 4.4. Case 1 was a known undershoot involving a rear-engined high tail-plane jet aircraft. The nature of Case 2 was in doubt —it was either a case of hijacking or it was a simple undershoot. The correspondence of injury pattern is not absolute—largely due to great differences in conditions for rescue—but it is sufficient to suggest strongly that the two accidents were not dissimilar in nature. Case 3 was a known structural failure in the air in which all the passengers were in the compartment at impact with the ground. Case 4 occurred over the sea and the aircraft was not recovered; the type of accident required diagnosis. Case 5 was a known catastrophe at altitude which also occurred over the sea. The evidence that Case 4 was of a 'crash' type rather than similar to Case 5 is overwhelming.

Table 4.4 Patterns of passenger injury in an accident of uncertain type compared with two accidents of known aetiology

Nature of accident	*Case 3* Crash into ground	*Case 4* Uncertain	*Case 5* Break up at altitude
Severe injury	100%	100%	45%
Minimal external injury	Nil	Nil	25%
Head injury	91%	100%	72%
Tibial/fibular lesions	98%	100%	20%
Typical seat head/leg impact injuries	89%	100%	Nil
Lap belt injuries	85%	60%	Nil
Evidence of O_2 lack	Nil	Nil	25%
Diagnosis		Crash into water	

Table 4.5　Sabotage in passenger aircraft, 1949–74: 35 cases excluding hijacking

Accidents with fatalities	17	*Location of bomb*	
Total fatal casualties	653	Passenger cabin	8
		Baggage compartment	9
Airlines		Toilet	10
Western European	6	Wheel well	2
North American	11	Flight deck	1
South and Central		Unknown	4
American	6		
Asian	7	Sabotage by shooting	1
Middle Eastern	4		
African	1		

Case 5 was an example of direct diagnosis through autopsy examination of the passengers. In practice, this is largely devoted to proving or excluding sabotage in the air—the occurrence of which is shown in Table 4.5; the frequency is such as to suggest that an unexplained disaster at altitude should be positively suspected of being due to sabotage until the contrary is proved. Much may therefore depend upon the pathologist's findings, particularly if the explosion took place over water.

Most aircraft accidents produce something of a uniform pattern of fatal injuries; the discovery of a discordance may well indicate an unusual situation. The suspicion of sabotage is reinforced if the anomalous findings can be rationalized as to the location of major damage (Fig. 4.4); search must then be made for a specific target victim. It may be possible to identify such a casualty visually if, say, the accident occurred over water or the subject was thrown from the air-

INJURY & SEATING

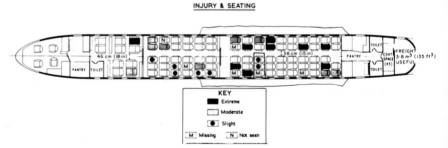

Fig. 4.4　Pattern of injuries related to seating as known in a proportion of the occupants of an aircraft lost over the sea. There were very good reasons for supposing that the slightly injured group (circled) shown in the rear compartment would have moved to the forward compartment during the final phase of the flight. If this be so, it will be seen that no one in the forward compartment was extremely injured while no one in the rear was slightly injured. There is a strong suspicion of some catastrophe arising in the rear compartment.

craft before being subjected to the very destructive forces of a crash on land. More often, however, discovery is based on routine X-ray of all the human remains. Any metallic fragments so discovered—other than those which are clearly derived from the aircraft structure—must then be removed and preserved for metallurgical examination.

It cannot be over-emphasized that the solution to such cases depends upon a co-ordinated effort by all parties to the investigation—the pathologist cannot work in isolation; this principle has been well established in the medical literature.[6, 16]

Toxicological causes of aircraft accidents
Toxicological causes of aircraft accidents or, indeed, of any vehicular accident can be looked on as being due either to accidental inhalation or to deliberate ingestion of toxic substances. Neither of these is common in commercial aviation but the former has provided one remarkable example of co-operative investigation.

In this accident, reported by Stevens,[19] a fully laden aircraft diverted from its intended path, overflew its port of arrival and crashed into a mountainside. Carboxyhaemoglobin to the extent of 19·9 per cent in the captain, 11·0 per cent in the first officer and 6·3 per cent in the second officer was discovered in the muscle remnants of the crew and, as a result, a special search for and examination was made of the cockpit heater. It was concluded[3] that the accident was due to carbon monoxide poisoning of the crew and that the most likely source of the gas was a leak at a joint between the heater exhaust pipe and the main exhaust pipe from the engine; improved maintenance schedules were immediately issued.

This case illustrates points of great importance in the interpretation of findings in accidental death. First, it is to be emphasized that the mere discovery of abnormalities—whether they be of chemical or pathological type—does not necessarily imply a causative relationship with the accident; the *common* cause of a raised carboxyhaemoglobin discovered in fatalities from vehicular accidents is survival in the post-crash fire, while there is no doubt that heavy smoking can produce a 'natural artefact' of up to 8–10 per cent carboxyhaemoglobin saturation of the blood.[18] The values obtained in Stevens' case were not so high as to be immediately suspect of causing a decrement in performance but the synergistic effect of adverse physiological factors must be taken into account in every vehicular accident; environmental hypoxia is the obvious co-factor in the instance under discussion but, in others, the summative effects of hypoglycaemia, fatigue, etc. would need consideration.[9] Perhaps the most important lesson lies in the field of methodology. Techniques which are effective when dealing with high concentrations of the substance sought in specimens of good quality may be quite inadequate when related to lesser amounts in, say, putrefied post-mortem material. Suicidal concentrations of carboxyhaemoglobin will not be discovered as causes of accidents, particularly those involving aircraft, because a crash will be precipitated at relatively low levels; specimens derived from severely traumatized bodies may also be technically difficult to handle. Sophisticated techniques are, therefore, needed; the subject has been well reviewed by Blackmore.[1]

United Kingdom experience has been that alcohol or other drugs are neither causative nor contributory to major commercial aircraft accidents. This is not, however, true of light private aviation in which many accidents, on a world-wide basis, appear to be associated with the drinking of alcohol. It is thought that blood ethanol levels should be estimated in the operator of any vehicle involved in an accident irrespective of the probability of a positive result; at least, a negative result will serve to allay public anxiety while, very occasionally, a cause may be discovered for an apparently inexplicable disaster. Current interest, highlighted by the widely publicized Moorgate train accident, centres upon the artefactual production of ethanol in the dead body; the problem is not yet solved. Variable findings appear both in practice and in experimental work but it seems now agreed that post-mortem production of alcohol can occur[7] and is particularly likely to do so in the badly mutilated body. The interpretation of post-mortem results must, therefore, be cautious; experience has shown that a dual analysis of blood and of urine, which is resistant to putrefaction, is very desirable. The medicolegal importance of the finding in relation to liability and to negligence scarcely needs emphasis.

Disease as a cause of aircraft accidents
The cause of a serious aircraft accident *must* be discovered if similar future disasters are to be prevented; the role of the pathologist in eliminating or incriminating disease is pre-eminent in this class of accident. Moreover, it is doubtful if there is any other occupation in which such intense effort as is applied to airline pilots is made to ensure physical fitness; the autopsy in such a death therefore offers a unique opportunity to assess the efficiency of supervisory methods.

Occasional cases have been reported in which an aircraft accident has been attributed to unusual disease conditions; epilepsy and upper respiratory tract infections are examples, the latter indicating how minor pathology may assume major significance in the hostile environment of the air. Such conditions, while indicating the need for microscopic examination of the tissues of aircrew killed in all types of aircraft accident, are generally problems of private aviation and are of no significance in commercial flying; the latter is dominated by considerations of coronary disease as a cause of accidents and it is in this context that disease will be discussed.

Any disease discovered in a pilot killed in an aircraft accident may be causative of, contributory to or merely incidental to the accident. This interpretation is complicated by the fact that trauma is often superimposed—and is also interposed—on the natural process. Thus, in the case of coronary disease, the chances of finding a recent infarct—or evidence of acute coronary *heart* disease—are negligible because the pain of an ischaemic episode will be sufficient of itself to cause a crash;

Table 4.6 Occurrence of coronary artery disease in
United Kingdom aviators

Grade of disease*	Military		Civilians		Total	
	No.	% of group	No.	% of group	No.	% of total
0	114	40	38	34	152	38
1	103	36	48	43	151	38
2	46	16	16	14	62	15·5
3	23	8	10	9	33	8·5
Mean age	27·6		34·9		29·7	

* Grade 0, normal arteries; Grade 1, less than 50% restriction of the lumen; Grade 2, 50% or more restriction; Grade 3, degenerative changes. Note that the evaluation is maximal—the degree given is the worst disease found at any one point in the coronary arterial tree.

death will be due to trauma and the role of disease in precipitating that death must be interpreted on the basis of the precursor condition—that is, coronary *artery* disease. As has been described elsewhere,[14] the conclusion that the accident was due to disease can be reached only in terms of probability—from near certainty to possibility—and this must take into consideration the occurrence of the asymptomatic precursor in the population, the circumstantial evidence surrounding the accident and the quality of the pathology discovered.

The extent of the precursor condition in the flying population is indicated in Table 4.6. Perhaps this is of less importance as regards interpretation than in relation to the screening of aircrew for fitness; the results indicate that routine methods currently in use will often not reveal uncomplicated restrictive disease of the coronary vessels; it is, therefore, possible for a highly selected aircrew-man to have a 'coronary attack' while at the controls.

The quality of the pathology will depend largely on evidence of activity of the lesion. The presence of adventitial infiltration by inflammatory cells, first described by Gerlis,[10] has been found to be a useful indicator of significant disease as, of course, is associated myocardial fibrosis. Ultimately, however, the finding of a true acute change in the vessel must provide the highest quality evidence. In the nature of things, this is likely to be of the intramural haemorrhagic type and it is here that the superimposition of trauma assumes its greatest significance. The problem is illustrated in Fig. 4.5.

The value of the circumstantial evidence and the problems introduced by the factors discussed above were all well illustrated in the Trident disaster of 1972.[5] The cause of the accident, a matter of error by the crew, was never in doubt; the main area of concern related to the reasons for failure to recover from that error. It was concluded as probable that at least a contributory cause lay in the captain sustaining a 'coronary attack' at a critical point in the flight. Table 4.7 shows the

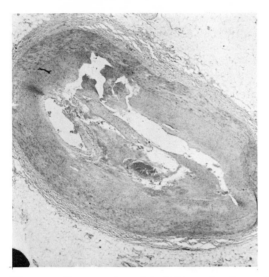

Fig. 4.5   Cross-section of the left anterior descending coronary vessel from a pilot aged 43. The circumstantial evidence strongly indicated that death was due to natural disease but, at autopsy, the heart was found to be severely damaged. The diagnostic dilemma is apparent. (From Mason, J. K. (1963) *Med. Sci. Law* **3,** 194.)

number of commercial accidents, in not all of which were passengers being carried, that have been attributed as being probably associated with heart disease in the crew—the occurrence is quite remarkably small. On the other hand, Hemming[12] has drawn attention to the rather high proportion of airline pilots among those persons who have died from coronary disease while flying in a private capacity. This, together with the fact that the great majority of commercial accidents caused by disease have occurred at a phase of flight when both pilots are heavily engaged, suggests that double crewing rather than intensive selection is the main safety factor as regards disease-associated accidents in commercial airline operations. Indeed, were it possible to exclude all those with some demonstrable restriction of the coronary vasculature, the result might be more dangerous in that only young, inexperienced pilots would be available as captains and first officers.

Legal implications of the cause of death in passengers
Confronted with multiple fatalities, many of whom are extensively mutilated, it is tempting to ascribe death to multiple injuries on the basis of an external examination. Such practice has minimal effectiveness in preventive medicine. There are, however, additional reasons of legal importance for ascertaining the precise cause of death and for distinguishing those injuries which were part of the lethal process from those which were inflicted post mortem.

A search for a natural cause of death must be made in fairness to those responsible for the settlement of life insurance policies which are

Table 4.7 Accidents to commercial aircraft probably associated with coronary disease in the aircrew[15]

Year	Aircraft type	Country of occurrence	No. of persons killed	Phase of flight
1961	DC4	Australia	2	Night approach
1962	Lockheed 1049	USA (California)	3	Instrument landing approach
1966	Lockheed 188C	USA (Oklahoma)	83	Approach
1966	DC4	Colombia	56	Minutes after take-off
1966	CV 440	Norway	1	Approach
1972	Trident 1	United Kingdom	118	Take-off
1974	Piper 31-350*	United Kingdom	8	Shortly after take-off

* Single crew only.

limited to, or increased as a result of, accidental death. Closely linked with this is the need for an assessment of the physical state or life expectancy of the victim; this may well affect the level of payment of compensation.

Because air travel is so much a family affair, the solution of 'commorientes', or simultaneous death, is a most important feature under this heading; what was at one time an esoteric legal distinction has become a recurring practical problem.[13] All countries have laws which govern the disposal of estates in the event that the precise succession between close relatives cannot be established. These differ from one jurisdiction to another. That which holds in England and Wales effectively states that, in the event of two persons dying apparently at the same time, the younger will be deemed to have survived the elder; this is almost directly opposed to the rules obtaining in the United States of America which have it that, in similar circumstances, neither person survived the other.* These details are of little significance to the pathologist. What is of paramount importance is that, under all jurisdictions, the presumptions in law are rebuttable by evidence; since this evidence must be almost entirely pathological, an unusual and serious responsibility devolves on the pathologist attending a major fatal disaster.

The primary indication as to survival must lie in the cause of death—a person who has died from burning must be assumed to have survived another who has died from cardiovascular rupture sustained in the same accident, always provided that delayed rupture can be eliminated. Any type of asphyxial death could be similarly interpreted but the distinction of death due to burning from post-mortem incineration depends upon the discovery of products of combustion within the

* Scots law follows the English pattern but adopts the US rule in the case of husband and wife, thus avoiding the major inequities inherent in the English law.

respiratory or alimentary tracts and upon the concentration of carbon monoxide in the blood. The latter is, therefore, an essential part of the autopsy examination of a person accidentally burned. It must be emphasized that only the absence of (or normal concentration of) and the presence of excess carboxyhaemoglobin can be used comparatively as measures of the agonal periods; relative differences in concentration, which depend upon many extraneous factors, cannot be so used. The presence of pulmonary bone marrow embolism can also be accepted as objective evidence of survival following fracture; again, however, the degree of embolism cannot be used comparatively, while the difficulty of discovering emboli which are present in small numbers somewhat vitiates the value of a negative finding. The subject is referred to in greater detail in Chapter 20.

Identification in a major disaster
Virtually every aspect of the major aircraft accident so far discussed has been dependent upon accurate identification of the fatal casualties. Identification in the mass presents special problems but these are not uniform. As pointed out in Chapter 8, much depends on how well known is the list of potential casualties; from this aspect, an aircraft accident provides a much easier task than does, say, a railway disaster. Identification in the former will, however, be complicated by severe mutilation and/or burning even to the extent of uncertainty as to the precise number of bodies present; the author has been involved in the investigation of one accident where it had to be assumed that no less than 23 bodies had been totally destroyed in the crash and conflagration which followed. Specific complications in aircraft accidents derive from the facts that the casualties will be of varying nationalities, that some at least are likely to be far from their native land and that the accident will probably occur a long way from the operator's base.

Whatever the nature of the disaster, the sheer volume of the task dictates the acceptance of far more circumstantial evidence of identification than might, perhaps, be allowed in the case of a single unknown body. Since the pioneer work of Stevens and Tarlton,[21] the following major categories of identification techniques have been used extensively in United Kingdom practice.

1. *Documents.* All airline passengers are well documented but documents are destroyed by fire and are virtually useless in the case of women who become separated from their handbags. Interchange of tickets is a problem which seems to be increasing and is a real danger to accurate identification.

2. *Clothing.* Since few clothes are carried in air travel, relatives can often state with certainty the likely clothing of the casualties. The world-wide use of chain-store clothing is a feature which limits the usefulness of the method.

3. *Jewellery.* Most jewellery is fire resistant and much has personal characteristics. It would be far more valuable as a means of identifica-

tion were it not for the frequent amputations which occur in aircraft accidents.

4. *Medical findings.* The medical findings, particularly related to previous surgery, are often of value when separating a few cadavers. Occasionally, the finding of a prosthesis, which can be compared with X-rays taken in life, leads to definitive identification. The confirmatory identifying value of medical evidence is sufficient of itself to indicate the need for internal autopsy.

5. *Tattoos.* These are common and are easily recognized if photographs are shown to relatives. They are often present deeper in the dermis than is superficial charring of the skin and can be visualized by scrubbing. However, many tattoos are of very standard pattern and should be interpreted with care.

6. *X-rays.* Identification by X-ray is often extremely useful and has the merit that the same process is being used as part of the accident investigation. Possessions may be visualized in charred remains, prostheses may be revealed and distinctive bony or other radio-opaque changes can be compared with pictures taken in life. Comparative dental X-rays are as personalized as are fingerprints.

7. *Dental identification.* This is of such importance as to deserve a separate section (below).

8. *Exclusion.* In the circumstances of an airline accident, in which the passenger manifest can be accepted as accurate with relatively minor reservations, exclusion methods can be used; the rationale has been described by Stevens.[19] The dangers of the method, particularly as related to the possibility of stowing-away or changing tickets, scarcely needs emphasis.

9. *Visual.* Visual identification is regarded as the standard method by many police forces but has very serious drawbacks in the major disaster situation. Very many victims of aircraft accidents are frankly unrecognizable while, short of this, the injury sustained often produces surprising artefactual changes in appearance. It is almost inhumane in many instances to expose relatives to the sight of mass disaster victims and, if this has to be done, the impulse to make an identification and escape is often so intense that serious mistakes can be made (Fig. 4.6). Our experience has been that it is preferable to make an identification by other means and then to present the relatives with a choice of, say, three bodies prepared in the laying-out room.

The role of the dentist at the major disaster
The author believes that the dental officer can play an important role in accident investigation through an analysis of faciomaxillary injuries. His most important role, however, lies in identification. The teeth are fire-resistant, which the fingers are not; the permutations of possible alterations, restorations, removals and replacements of teeth are such that, ultimately, a dental record is almost as individual as are the fingerprints; the very great majority of persons in the United Kingdom have their dental state recorded and readily available, in contrast to their

fingerprints which are held only in the case of merchant seamen and convicted criminals. Dental identification is, however, of major significance even in the United States where fingerprint recording is commonplace.

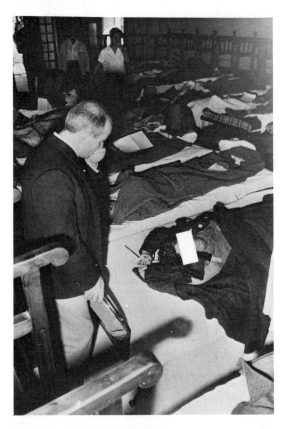

Fig. 4.6   Laying-out in the mass. In such intensely emotional circumstances, one observer made no less than three incorrect visual identifications on successive days.

The basis of dental identification in the mass is the comparison of findings in the bodies with the records of missing persons—that is, in an aircraft accident, those on the passenger manifest. The more work performed on the teeth—and the more unusual it is—the more personalized is the dental record; as indicated above, X-rays are of greatest value in this context. Any other abnormalities of the soft or bony parts of the mouth can also be used as points of positive identification. It is, however, emphasized that, in the context of an aircraft accident, absolute identification is not required; the most that is needed is a definite indication that a given cadaver is that of a person known to be among the dead. Dental evidence can therefore be of value when only a few comparatively common restorations or extractions are encountered, while even minimal conservation may be useful in an 'exclusion' capacity; it is these features which make the method so ideal in the disaster situation yet somewhat disappointing in the usual run of police work.

Even so, the contribution of the dentist in a mass disaster is dependent upon certain prerequisites:

1. There must be *some* conservative work among the casualties, it being virtually impossible to distinguish between a number of perfectly normal mouths. The more developed the countries of origin of the casualties, the more there will be for the dentist to observe.

2. Records of the in vivo state must be available. The more advanced the medical services, the better will these records be.

3. A method of obtaining records rapidly from far distances must be available if the bodies are to be disposed of in reasonable time. This dictates the use of the Telex and of a code which is easily transmitted, easily translated and easily documented.

In practice, it is seldom that the records of treatment exactly correspond to the post-mortem findings. 'Compatible inconsistencies', mainly deriving from undocumented treatment, have to be accepted; in very exceptional circumstances, an 'incompatible inconsistency', which would usually exclude identification, has to be interpreted as a transcription error. For a full exposition of the techniques used in dental identification, the reader is referred to the many excellent review articles available.[8, 11, 19]

The medical organization for a major disaster

Space does not permit a discussion of disaster plans involving survivors—such plans must, in any event, be individually tailored to the local circumstances. Experience has shown, however, that the organization for processing the dead bodies can be reasonably standardized; even so, the resources of the pathology services will be severely stretched. The first priority is the provision of mortuary facilities. The 'take-over' of permanent buildings is generally inadvisable—few organizations can tolerate disruption of routine work for several days. The author's preference is for tented accommodation, though that most normally provided—and equally effective—is a disused hangar, warehouse or other large space. The essentials are ease of access, adequate space and privacy; ideally, areas for reception, post-mortem examination, laying out and encoffining should be contiguous.

From what has been said, it is apparent that the two main features of a large aircraft accident—investigation of the cause and identification of the casualties—are interdependent and any attempt to separate the two functions will be to the detriment of both. It follows that the medical and police enquiries must be closely co-ordinated through an identification secretariat and that the recording forms used must incorporate

observations made for both purposes.* It is the function of the combined secretariat to compare the observations recorded on these forms
with details of the missing persons transcribed on to comparable 'information' forms. A useful design of forms which has the approval of the
International Civil Aviation Organization, together with the *modus
operandi* of the identification secretariat, has been described elsewhere.[20]

In practice, some sort of production line approach to post-mortem
examination has to be adopted. How many lines are used depends on
the number of consultant pathologists and, here, a compromise must be
reached between speed on the one hand and, on the other hand, the
retention of an overall view of the injury pattern by a single observer. It
is, in this respect, important that cadavers are not preselected on, say,
the basis of easy identification; an erroneous subjective impression of
the type of accident is easily generated in this way. Each cadaver is
given a number at the accident site which it retains until identification.
Each body is dealt with in the order in which it is presented at the
mortuary area, the exception being that isolated limbs and the like are
considered last. It would, however, be proper to examine the flight deck
crew selectively and with particular thoroughness should they be easily
identifiable.

Once the system is in motion, a cadaver is undressed and unjewelled
at one table where an external examination is also made by the doctor;
the findings, which may all be of importance both to the investigation
and to identification, are recorded together. In the event that sabotage
has not been eliminated as a possible cause of the accident, the cadavers
are then passed for radiology—during inevitable periods of inactivity,
the radiologist can examine such fragments as do not constitute recognizable corpses. The remains are then examined by internal autopsy
and, at the same time, the dental officer conducts his own investigation.
The cadaver may then be passed to the funeral directors for preparation
for viewing or for encoffining. The latter should certainly be temporary
until identification has been accepted; ideally, it should remain so until
all the bodies have been identified and it is most strongly advised that
none should be released for burial—and certainly not for cremation—
until this has been achieved.

Meantime, the senior pathologist should be in frequent and regular
communication with the Inspector of Accidents. Each may then be able
to eliminate certain lines of inquiry or to suggest fresh approaches to
the other; unnecessary effort is thus avoided and loss of evidence is
reduced to a minimum.

This method of investigation, which has been responsible for the
solution of many complex accidents, is colloquially known as 'the

* Recommendation 4.5.6, Annex 13 to the Convention on International Civil Aviation[4]
states: 'The State conducting the Inquiry should recognize the interdependence of the
investigation itself and the identification of victims and should ensure co-ordination
between the judicial authority and the Investigator-in-Charge.'

Group System'. It seems fitting to conclude this chapter with the official international definition of this concept:[4]

'The primary purpose of Group function is to establish the facts pertinent to an accident by making use of the specialized knowledge of the participating individuals. It also ensures that undue emphasis is not placed on any single aspect of the accident to the neglect of other aspects which might be significant and that, whenever it is possible to establish a particular point by means of several methods, all those methods have been resorted to and coordination of results has been ensured.'

References

1. Blackmore, D. J. (1970). The determination of carbon monoxide in blood and tissue. *Analyst* **95**, 439.
2. Board of Trade (1968). *Report of the Public Inquiry into the Causes and Circumstances of the Accident to Canadair C4 G-ALHG which Occurred at Stockport, Cheshire on 4th June 1967*, CAP 302. London: HMSO.
3. Board of Trade (1969). *Report on the Accident to Skymaster DC4 G-APYX near Mount Canigou, Pyrenees Orientales on 3rd June 1967*, CAP 312. London: HMSO.
4. Convention on International Civil Aviation (1973). *Aircraft Accident Inquiry*, 3rd edn. Attachment B to Annex 13. Montreal: International Civil Aviation Organization.
5. Department of Trade and Industry (1973). *Trident 1 G-ARPI. Report of the Public Inquiry into the Causes and Circumstances of the Accident near Staines on 18 June 1972*, Civil Aircraft Accident Report 4/73. London: HMSO.
6. Dille, J. R. and Hasbrook, A. H. (1966). Injuries due to explosion, decompression and impact of a jet transport. *Aerospace Med.* **37**, 5.
7. Editorial Comment (1975). Post-mortem alcohol. *Lancet* **i**, 1229.
8. Ford, M. A. and Ashley, K. F. (1973). The role of the forensic dentist in aircraft accidents. In: *Aerospace Pathology*, Chap. 8. Eds. J. K. Mason and W. J. Reals. Chicago: College of American Pathologists Foundation.
9. Franks, W. R. (1959). The summation of some physiological factors leading to incidents in the air. In: *Medical Aspects of Flight Safety*, Chap. 4. Eds. E. Evrard, P. Bergeret and P. M. van Wulfften Palthe. Oxford: Pergamon Press.
10. Gerlis, L. M. (1956). The significance of adventitial infiltrations in coronary atherosclerosis. *Brit. Heart J.* **18**, 166.
11. Haines, D. H. (1973). Mass disaster identification. In: *Forensic Dentistry*, Chap. 8. Eds. J. M. Cameron and B. G. Sims. Edinburgh and London: Churchill Livingstone.
12. Hemming, F. O. (1970). In-flight coronary occlusions: a short series of cases. *Aerospace Med.* **41**, 773.

13. Martin, P. and Mason, J. K. (1969). Commorientes: some legal and medical observations. *New Law J.* **119**, 325.
14. Mason, J. K. (1973). Injuries sustained in fatal aircraft accidents. *Brit. J. Hosp. Med.* **9**, 645.
15. Mason, J. K. (1974). Disease of aircrew as a cause of aircraft accidents. *Community Hlth* **6**, 62.
16. Mason, J. K. and Tarlton, S. W. (1969). Medical investigation of the loss of the Comet 4B aircraft, 1967. *Lancet* **i**, 431.
17. Ministry of Health (1954). *Medical Arrangements for Dealing with Major Accidents*, HM (54)51. London: HMSO.
18. Russell, M. A. H., Wilson, C., Patel, U. A., Cole, P. V. and Feyerabend, C. (1973). Comparison of effect on tobacco consumption and carbon monoxide absorption of changing to high and low nicotine cigarettes. *Brit. med. J.* **4**, 512.
19. Stevens, P. J. (1970). *Fatal Civil Aircraft Accidents*. Bristol: Wright.
20. Stevens, P. J. (1973). Investigation of mass disaster. In: *Modern Trends in Forensic Medicine—3*, Chap. 8. Ed. A. K. Mant. London and Boston, Mass: Butterworths.
21. Stevens, P. J. and Tarlton, S. W. (1963). Identification of mass casualties: experience in 4 civil air disasters. *Med. Sci. Law* **3**, 154.

5

Violence and civil disturbance

Civil disturbance is no new feature in the world but the reinforcement of ordinary rioters with sophisticated terrorists and the use of modern weapons has given present-day civil disturbance an uglier countenance. The motives have also changed. Whereas, in the past, rioting was on a relatively local scale and concerning a correctable grievance, much of the civil disturbance nowadays is about political ideology and is organized by people dedicated to a cause and willing to go to any lengths of terrorism to support it. These terrorists have international connections through which they can develop their method of operation. Since their crimes are 'political', it is not difficult to find asylum in countries which accept them and refuse to grant warrants of extradition. Even within the frontiers of their terrorist activities, the terrorists often have the sympathy, if not active support, of sections of the community. This frustrates the efforts of the security forces in their endeavours to uproot them. It turns citizens against each other. Rumours circulate and inflame feelings. Allegations are made by one faction against the other. The security forces, in trying to keep the peace impartially, come under attack from all sides.

Injuries sustained in times of civil unrest have to be assessed against this background. The injuries themselves are usually easy enough to recognize and describe. What matters is how they are caused and what light this sheds on the incident. It is with this aspect in mind that this chapter has been written.

Civil disturbance usually escalates; it is uncommon for it to explode with ferocious intensity. When a near-war situation, with shootings and explosions, overtakes an area it has usually started somewhere with a crowd throwing stones. Thus, it helps to organize thought on the subject by considering the injuries associated with each stage of the escalating violence.

Injury by stones and truncheons

Unsophisticated rioting usually concerns a crowd confronting the security forces, be they police or army or a mixture of both. The crowd hurls bricks, stones and other missiles which come conveniently to hand. The security forces retaliate with truncheons. Those in the crowd might all be ordinary rioters but often there are professional agitators among them, usually towards the middle or the back, who incite the rest to press forward but who will disappear when the action is joined. People on both sides get hurt in the melee. They are struck by truncheons, bricks, stones and bottles. Some are kicked. Many are injured in falling. They sustain bruises, abrasions and lacerations of a non-specific character, a relatively large proportion of serious injuries being to the head and neck. Sometimes there are fractures of the skull or facial bones. Rather surprisingly, fractures of the main limb bones are infrequent.[16,17] These injuries are no different from those sustained in accidents; they are due to blunt force and they usually give no clue to the agent responsible. Just occasionally, an abrasion or petechial bruise will reproduce the texture of the brick or stone, more rarely the outline of a missile with a particular shape.

Confrontations of this kind often lead to allegations that the security forces hurt an innocent bystander or that they were irresponsibly violent to the demonstrators. Doctors examining these wounds must be prepared for this. Later questions which might be asked include: could the wound have been caused by a truncheon or rifle butt? or how violent was the blow? A doctor needs considerable experience of wounds before he can give authoritative answers. Not only does he need to assess the actual injury but also its situation, the kind of victim and other possible causes for the injury. He must guard particularly against being persuaded, by his own prejudices or by other people, to give a more dogmatic opinion concerning the cause of the injury than the evidence warrants.

Ways of controlling rioters have occupied the minds of security forces throughout the world. They have sought a method of temporarily repelling a violent mob without causing serious injury. It must be capable of quick application by individuals without too sophisticated apparatus and without harming innocent people in the vicinity. No method is ideal. If the force is effective in halting rioters, it is likely to have some harmful effects and, once in a while, due to unusual circumstances, these may become serious and perhaps end in death. It is a matter of finding an acceptable balance between the general good and the calculated risk. One of the popular methods of riot control is the use of sensory irritant agents, particularly *o*-chlorobenzylidenemalononitrile (CS) and dibenzoxazepine (CR).

Injury by sensory irritant agents

Irritant chemicals have been used for many years to quell violent groups of people and individuals. The agent 1-chloracetophenone, otherwise known as CN or 'tear gas', is well known. It can be incorporated in grenades and it is available in the United States as a 1 per cent solution in a hand-held pressurized canister for personal protection. Chemical Mace is such a device and the solution emerges as a jet which can be aimed over distances of about 3 m (10 ft) at the face. Some pen guns contain the chemical as a micropulverized powder which is ejected by the propellant as a mist. It causes immediate intense pain in the eyes, tight closure of the eyelids and a copious flow of tears, these symptoms lasting for about 15 minutes. The eyes redden within minutes and the inflammatory reaction increases for an hour or two. It does not resolve for about three days and the eye may be damaged. There are reports of permanent eye damage when personal protection devices have been fired into the face at too close a range or when a grenade has exploded while being examined.[8, 11] On the skin, CN causes stinging and a feeling of heat, often with reddening, over a period of an hour or so. It may produce contact dermatitis.[13] There may be stinging in the nose and, if it gains the mouth, pain and profuse salivation may persist for about 15 minutes. Occasional deaths have been reported after exposure to abnormally high concentrations.[19]

In 1958, *o*-chlorobenzylidenemalononitrile, otherwise known as CS, was introduced as a riot-control device to replace CN. It is a white crystalline solid, ten times more potent an irritant than CN but significantly less toxic. Experimental work has shown that CS is least severe and persistent in smoke form; its immediate irritative effects act as a rapid sensory warning which compels the victim to seek fresh air and so limit exposure. Greater irritant effects are produced by solid CS and these become most intense with CS solutions in a concentration of 1 per cent or more.[4]

The usual method of using CS is to fire a cylindrical cartridge or grenade, 3·8 cm (1·5 in) diameter, containing the irritant from a riot gun or Very pistol. It emerges with a muzzle velocity of about 80 m s^{-1}. The container contains a pyrotechnic mixture and when it lands it gives off large quantities of smoke composed of suspended particles for up to 20 seconds. A later development is to use a rubber grenade, containing slow-burning pellets of CS, which bursts on the ground and scatters the pellets over a wide area thus producing smoke from many separate sources. With all grenades there is a danger of striking someone and causing a bruise or, at close range, a lacerated wound. However, the healing of such a wound or a burn is not adversely affected by the presence of CS.[1]

CS has a pungent, pepper-like odour. In concentrations of the order of 5 mg m^{-3}, it causes an intense burning sensation in the eyes, tight closure of the eyelids due to spasm and a copious flow of tears. Inhalation results in sneezing, soreness or a gripping pain in the chest with salivation, coughing and difficulty in breathing. The exposed skin stings, particularly if it is moist, and it may become red for a day or two. By contrast, the face is usually abnormally pale. If the person is exposed to very high concentrations, as when trapped in a confined space, the skin may blister if moist and there may be nausea and vomiting. Under ordinary circumstances, however, the victim, though incapacitated enough to stop rioting, is able to effect his escape into the fresh air where he recovers dramatically and completely in about 15 minutes without the need for treatment. Those who suffer from asthma, chronic bronchitis and emphysema may experience an acute attack though this is not different from the exacerbations normally encountered in these conditions.

The effect of CS gas on civilians in a riot area was investigated in detail by a committee of experts under the chairmanship of Sir Harold Himsworth following the use of about 1100 cartridges of CS by the police during two days of rioting in Londonderry in 1969. They went into the matter extremely carefully and their first report published in 1969,[14] and their second in 1971,[15] confirm the safety of CS as an anti-riot agent.

Dibenzoxazepine, or CR, is another highly irritant chemical which can be used for riot control. It is a yellow crystalline solid about six to eight times more potent than CS though less toxic.[2] Although only sparingly soluble, it is stable in solution and, so, active for a longer time than CS. It can be used as an aerosol or in solution when it can be directed at groups of rioters or fairly accurately at individuals. Solutions as weak as 0·000 06 per cent are effective, causing the usual irritant symptoms in the eye, nose, mouth and on the skin.[3] The eye may remain red for up to 6 hours. Erythema of the skin is intense and corresponds exactly to the area of contamination.

Injury by rubber bullets

Another device used for riot control is the baton round, popularly known as the rubber bullet. It looks like a small black shell, about 15 cm (6 in) in length and 3·5 cm (1·4 in) diameter, with a tapered blunt tip. It is of hard rubber, just dentable on pressure and slightly flexible, weighing about 160 g (6 oz). It slides into a metal cartridge case which has a small charge of powder in the base. It is fired from a riot gun or Very pistol and the muzzle velocity of the round should be about 70 m s^{-1} (230 ft/sec). However, its discharge from the barrel is inefficient so that the muzzle velocity varies considerably; its poor aerodynamic characteristics make it unstable in flight and it soon tumbles.

The bullet is fired at a range of 20–40 m (65–130 ft). When it strikes, it is like a hefty kick and it can cause a painful bruise which is rectangular if the baton strikes side on and circular if it strikes base on. Two or three batons fired at a mob are usually effective in dispersing it temporarily.

The disadvantage of the missile is its inaccuracy. It is difficult to hit a target of 2 m (6·5 ft) diameter at a range of 18 m (59 ft) and it is impossible to strike a particular rioter in a crowd. Aiming at the legs will not avoid hitting the head occasionally and aiming at a rioter will not avoid hitting a small boy nearby. It is not surprising, therefore, that a rubber baton causes serious injury every now and again. Much depends on the part of the body which is struck. Impact with the head is the most serious and can result in fractures of the skull and facial bones and injury to the eyes. Impact with the trunk can cause bruising of the lungs with haemoptysis,[18] and laceration of the abdominal viscera has been recorded although it is infrequent.[12] Impact with the limbs is not serious.

Rubber baton rounds have been used during the civil disturbances in Northern Ireland. Over one period of about two years, 33 000 rounds were fired; Millar et al.[12] collected data on 90 people who attended hospitals for treatment of rubber baton injuries during this time. One boy aged 11 years, who was struck on the head at a range of 3 metres, sustained serious comminuted fractures and died 54 hours later. Another victim may have died in the Republic of Ireland from a chest injury. Of the rest, 40 people required admission to hospital: 32 with head and neck injury, 7 with chest injury and 1 with injury to the abdomen. Eye injuries were seen in 24 patients and the injury was bilateral in 4 patients. Most of the 49 injured who were treated as outpatients had sustained bruises of varying severity. The only fracture of a long bone was in a finger, crushed between a baton round and a wall, although, since the report was published, a person with fractured tibia and fibula alleged that he had been struck by a rubber bullet.

The rubber baton round has now been replaced by a shorter round having an outer layer of plastic and not being tapered. It does not tumble as readily and it can be fired with greater accuracy.

Injury by petrol bombs

The home-made petrol bomb is not infrequently used by a rioting mob; it is one degree of sophistication beyond the throwing of bricks and stones. A small container is filled with petrol and sealed with a rag bung which is lit just before the bomb is thrown. Many thousands of such bombs were used in the earlier stages of the civil disturbances in Northern Ireland; they were made from glass milk bottles. These bombs were expected to break when they struck a hard surface and splash burning petrol around. Some were hurled into premises and started fires in which people sometimes got burned and occasionally died. One woman travelling in a bus was seriously burned when a petrol bomb was thrown through the window and landed in her lap; she died in hospital from intercurrent bronchopneumonia 7 weeks later. Most of the petrol bombs were used in the open and, remarkably, they caused very little injury. Of about 1800 persons with civil disturbance injuries who were treated in a large Belfast hospital during 1969–71, when petrol bombs were popular, only 9 persons were injured by them and only 6 had to be admitted. There was no really serious disability.[17]

Injury by bullets

Rioting takes on a serious aspect when guns are brought out. At first the shooting is probably by a few gunmen belonging to a terrorist organization which is more sophisticated and sinister than are the simple rioters it hides behind and encourages. Eventually there is the likelihood of the organization appearing in strength as a form of 'liberation' army when gun battles are joined with the security forces. The ordinary rioter then disappears from the scene.

The bullet wounds sustained during these gun battles are usually inflicted at considerable range and number no more than one or two to each victim. There is little problem in differentiating the entrance from the exit wound. The entrance wound is usually a neat round hole, 3–9 mm diameter, often with funnel-shaped margins, surrounded by a fairly even zone of red or cream abrasion (Fig. 5.1). This abrasion will be eccentric if the bullet has penetrated at an angle. The exit hole is usually larger, more irregular in shape, sometimes stellate, sometimes linear, with eversion of the marginal tissue. Its margins may bear some irregular abrasion but this will not encircle the hole as it does at the entrance site.

There are times when differentiation is difficult, however. Sometimes the entrance hole has no obvious abrasion collar; this is more likely where the tissues are soft and yielding as in parts of the neck, the breast, loin and buttocks. Also, in these situations, the entrance hole from a 7–9 mm bullet may be unusually small, no more than 3 mm diameter. Such a hole occurring on or between the buttocks is easily overlooked. The typical abrasion collar is often lacking when the bullet passes into the skin very obliquely. Then there is a shelving abrasion leading to the hole but something similar is seen when a bullet comes out through the skin very obliquely. Eversion of the marginal tissues, though common at the exit site, is not specific enough to be relied on to solve a problem of differentiation; it can also occur at the entrance site. Of more help is the dark soiling of the margins of the entrance hole by dirt or grease on the bullet or by contact traces from the overlying clothing. Sometimes the entrance hole is larger than the exit hole; this can occur when the bullet strikes over bone and the

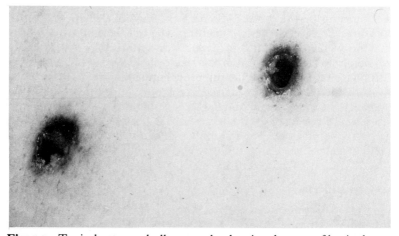

Fig. 5.1　Typical entrance bullet wounds, showing the zone of bruised abrasion around the holes. The abrasion around the wound on the left of the picture is eccentric, indicating that the bullet pierced the skin obliquely.

margins of the hole are split radially. The exit wound is sometimes due to a secondary missile such as a spicule of bone, the bullet remaining in the body. A similar event arises when the bullet jacket detaches from the core and only one piece makes its exit.

The more one gains experience of bullet wounds, the more one encounters wounds which are impossible to classify as entrance or exit from their appearance alone. Nevertheless, when there are only a few wounds on the body, it is usually not difficult, having assessed all the features, to pick out the entrance wounds and pair them up with the wounds of exit.

Bullets fired in terrorist situations are often of many different calibres since the terrorists obtain their weapons from different sources. The entrance hole of the 0·45 calibre bullet as fired from hand guns and the Thompson submachine gun are usually large enough and with such an obvious abrasion collar as to indicate a bullet of that calibre. The wounds caused by the 0·22 bullet and the bullet of 0·223 calibre as used in the Armalite rifle are often small enough to indicate a calibre of this low order but care should be taken in expressing an opinion when the entrance hole is in a soft part of the body such as the buttock. In these situations, a very small entrance wound often results from a bullet of medium size. Between these two extremes, it is hazardous to express any opinion on the calibre of the bullet from the size of the entrance hole. Nor is it possible to say from the appearance of an entrance wound whether the bullet was fired from a rifle or a pistol but, whenever there is a large ragged exit wound, the bullet was travelling with the high velocity of a rifle bullet.

Low and high velocity bullets are best differentiated by the internal injury they cause. The damage done by a bullet inside the body is a function of the energy it surrenders to the tissues and this, in turn, depends on the difference between its entrance and exit velocities. Bullets from revolvers and Thompson submachine guns, having low initial energies, make a simple lacerated track and the bullet is frequently arrested in the body, particularly if it strikes bone. The rifle bullet is likely to pass through the body but it usually surrenders considerable energy and causes much more destruction around its track with considerable laceration of organs such as the heart and liver. There is extensive comminution if it strikes bone. Most damage occurs when the bullet is arrested in the tissues, a common event with the Armalite bullet of 0·223 calibre. Although this has one of the highest velocities, it is less stable and less robust than, say, the NATO 7·62 mm bullet, the jacket frequently separating from the core. The fragments have little mass but their arrest in the tissues is associated with severe injury. Between these extremes of revolver and rifle velocities, say between 365 and 670 m s^{-1} (1200–2200 ft/sec), it is difficult to distinguish bullets of different velocities by their damaging effects.

A surgeon needs to be told whether a patient was shot by a hand pistol or rifle, for this will influence his treatment. Since bullets from hand pistols cause little damage around the lacerated track, the track need only be cleansed by the pull-through method and the skin wounds sutured about 5 days later. On the other hand, the serious damage to tissue for some distance round the track of a rifle bullet necessitates surgical opening of the whole track and excision of the devitalized tissue.

Gun battles between terrorists and the security forces are only one aspect of civil disorder. There are also shootings between the various factions, often sudden strikes by small groups armed with machine guns. The victims have numerous bullet wounds sustained at relatively close quarters, and the difficulties of pairing entrance and exit wounds increase as more bullets perforate a body. The entrance wounds are not necessarily all on the same aspect of the body because the victim might turn during the burst of firing and they can be found on, say, both the front and back of the body. If he were erect when the firing started, the first bullets would probably pass through the body more or less horizontally, but the bullet tracks will decline towards the feet if the firing continues as the victim slumps. The tracks may incline towards the head if he is fired on when lying on the ground. The result is a scattering of entrance sites and a criss-crossing of tracks which it can be practically impossible to unravel. A similar situation may arise when a person is fired at by two or more terrorists.

Assassination
Gun battles and strikes by murder gangs account for many of those shot in times of civil disorder. Other shootings are deliberate assassinations. There are many reasons for them. The organization may have to eliminate an important enemy. It might be routine action against any member of the opposition group or of the security forces who falls into its hands. It might be necessary to murder someone as a show of strength or to increase the hold over a community. It is a way of teaching a lesson to those who will not submit to intimidation and the method of disciplining their own members and dealing with informers. Some of those assassinated are gunned down in their homes or in the streets and the injuries are no different from those already described. Others, however, are assassinated in some quiet place after being kidnapped, and their wounds are often distinctive. These victims are usually shot in the back of the head or neck and the bullet wound shows the features of a close range; the skin around the wound is soiled by smoke and sometimes bears punctate abrasions due to the impact of particles in the discharge, features which are more likely when a revolver has been used than when the weapon was a semi-automatic pistol (Fig. 5.2). These features are lacking when the muzzle has been pressed against the skin but the subcutaneous tissues are then soiled and there may also be a trace of soiling on the skull bone and dura around the entrance hole. The surface features of smoke soiling and particulate abrasion also tend to be eliminated if the discharge passes through the hair or through a bag or coat put over the head as a hood. Many assassins do not rely on one single shot, and fire a second or third shot

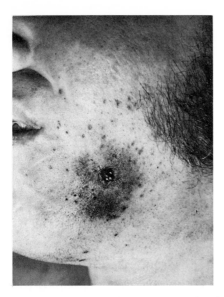

Fig. 5.2 A victim of terrorist assassination. This bullet wound was inflicted at close range and the skin around the entrance hole is heavily soiled by the soot in the discharge gases. Particulate matter in the discharge has produced numerous punctate abrasions over a wider area. Obvious discharge effects such as this are typical of revolvers.

into the side of the head as a *coup de grâce*. These can be in any position. They are usually inflicted at a greater range, probably 0·3–0·6 m (1–2 ft), and there is little or no discharge soiling or punctate abrasion.

Torture
The victim may be beaten up, perhaps during interrogation, before being shot. The wrists and ankles may bear the pale and purple streaky marks of a ligature. There may be extensive bruises and abrasions of the face, black eyes, fractures of the nasal bones, displaced teeth and fractures of the jaws with injuries of comparable severity elsewhere on the body. It may not be possible to say with what the victim had been struck but, at other times, there are indications of the kind of object. Kicking with a boot, for instance, can cause linear lacerations, perhaps 2·5–5 cm (1–2 in) long, often with a shelving margin. They are more easily caused over bone and are particularly common beneath the chin and on the sides of the head and neck. Beating with a broom handle causes long bruises consisting of a central pale area outlined by confluent purple petechial haemorrhages. Some victims display signs of overt torture. Burning with a cigarette produces a discrete, circular, yellow-brown burn. Incisions and stab wounds are inflicted by knives. Hot metal may be used to brand the victim with a symbol or a word. Injuries of all these types may be so extensive that death by shooting must have come as a welcome relief.

A specific method of disciplining erring members of a terrorist organization, short of shooting them dead, is to inflict a bullet wound which incapacitates but does not kill. In Northern Ireland this is referred to as 'knee-capping' but this is usually a misnomer. Sometimes the victim is shot through the knee cap and knee joint and such an injury leaves a permanent disability. More often, however, the bullet goes through the fleshy part of the lower thigh. It may do serious damage to the vascular supply but, in many instances, the injury is confined to muscle and it heals quickly.

When a simple lesson needs to be taught, the person may be 'tarred and feathered'. He is tied to a tree or lamp-post and tar, bitumen or paint is poured over him before material such as earth or grit is added. He may have first been beaten up and so bear bruises, abrasions and lacerations. Women have often had their hair cut off.

Allegations, rumours and alibis

One of the main reasons for subjecting a shot victim to a careful post-mortem examination is to glean information which may be helpful in confirming or refuting allegations which are the inevitable corollary of civil disturbance. It is a specific gambit of a dissident group to make accusatory allegations. No matter how far-fetched they are, they get immediate world-wide coverage by the press and television. It is important to make the allegations as soon after the event as possible; it will be some little time before the authorities can glean hard and fast evidence to refute them and, by that time, the damage is done. When such refutations are made they receive less prominent publicity. However, this problem is one for the authorities and not the doctor. The pathologist must be aware of the political climate in which he works but his duty lies only in the collection of impartial evidence. When it is used is, fortunately, not his concern.

If a person is killed accidentally during a gun battle between terrorists and the security forces, it is not unusual for the sympathizers of the terrorists to claim that the person was shot deliberately by the other side. The pathologist must attempt to test the validity of the accusations.

If an accidental bullet wound is due to a direct hit, the wound cannot be differentiated from one deliberately inflicted. However, many accidental wounds are ricochets and these have definite characteristics. The entrance hole is definitely rectangular if the bullet goes in sideways. There is a scatter of punctate abrasions and small entry wounds if it has fragmented. These wounds vary in size and most are smaller than those made by bullets. They may be grouped irregularly round a ragged hole, 1–3 cm (0·4–1·2 in) diameter, where the largest fragment of the bullet penetrated. Injuries of this type are seen when bullets strike near to a victim lying on the ground and, if the person is lying there because he has been shot, it will be possible to demonstrate the initial bullet wound and the ricochet injuries received subsequently. Sometimes the ricochet injuries are those responsible for death.

Other accidents might be inferred when the bullet has first gone through a partition. In this case the deformity or instability of the bullet often produces an unusually large entrance wound and there are often punctate abrasions and puncture lacerations in the surrounding skin due to the impact of particles of the partition substance, be it plaster, metal or glass, scattered by the missile (Fig. 5.3). Some of these particles may be found embedded in the skin.

In some shootings it may be important to determine from which side the bullet came. The direction of a bullet through the body is then helpful. This can be ascertained by pairing the entrance and exit wounds but if this should prove difficult, an X-ray is useful because bone fragments will be seen scattered along the track in the direction of the bullet's flight when the bullet has traversed a rib, shoulder blade, spine or pelvis. When a bullet goes through the thicker part of the skull, the naked-eye examination is usually conclusive. The direction of transit is indicated by the bevelling of the margins of the holes at the entrance and exit sites, but great caution must be used in giving an opinion on the situation of the gunman because of the considerable mobility of the head. Thus, a bullet striking above the right ear could conceivably have come from the left of the trunk if the victim were looking back over his left shoulder. However, when a soldier was hit by a single bullet in the right temple while driving a vehicle along a main city road, it seemed reasonable to conclude that the bullet was in fact fired from the area to his right. Sometimes the vault of the skull is shattered and the hole made by the bullet is not apparent at the post-mortem examination. If the pieces of bone are carefully collected, cleaned and glued together the hole can usually be reconstituted and the information it gives often repays the effort.

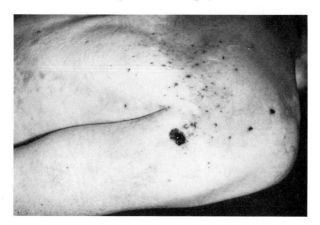

Fig. 5.3 This victim was shot while he sat in the driving seat of a car. The bullet went through the side window and its instability or deformation accounts for the entrance wound being somewhat larger than usual. Fragments of glass scattered by the bullet pierced the clothing and produced numerous punctate abrasions in the adjacent skin.

The most useful evidence of who fired the bullet often comes from the bullet itself. The security forces are armed with a limited range of weapons and use only a few types of ammunition. Terrorists, on the other hand, use a large range of ammunition, some of it from foreign countries, and the recovery of non-official bullets from the body is prima facie proof that the security forces were not involved in the fatality. Finding a bullet in the body is not as easy as many people imagine. A successful search, as with other aspects of the post-mortem examination, requires a good technique.

Post-mortem technique
Each pathologist develops his own post-mortem routine as he gains experience in a particular type of death and the author has found the following suitable for civil disturbance cases.

1. Arrange the clothed body neatly on the post-mortem table and photograph, from each side if necessary. It is useful for record purposes to take one photograph with a card on the body stating the victim's name and any other important particulars.

2. Remove the clothing garment by garment, listing each in turn and describing the position of bullet holes. Take care not to turn a garment inside out as it is removed. Be alert for bullets falling from the clothing. The direction of the torn fibres around a bullet hole will often indicate whether it is entrance or exit. Dry the clothing in air and transmit it in plastic bags to the laboratory for more careful study.

3. Photograph the unclothed body again if there are blood stains or dirt marks of significance.

4. Clean the body with sponges or wet towels, taking care not to remove any discharge soiling around the bullet wounds. Dry with towelling.

5. Measure the crown–heel length.

6. Describe the normal external features: sex, apparent age, build, rigor, hypostasis, eyes, ears, nose, mouth, scars, tattoos, deformities, etc.

7. Describe the injuries other than the bullet wounds.

8. Describe the bullet wounds. Start with the body supine or prone according to the major distribution of the wounds. Measure the distance of each wound both from the heel and from a nearer reference point. Describe each wound in detail. If two wounds are obviously entrance and exit and a pair, describe them consecutively. This helps to fix attention on the remaining problem wounds. It is permissible to probe the track of a wound to assess its direction provided this is done carefully.

9. Photograph this aspect of the body full-length. Then photograph the wounds in groups as necessary and then each one individually in close-up. Keep the main axes of each photograph in the longitudinal and transverse planes of the body. When a wound is in a hairy part of the body, cut the hairs away close to the skin and then pluck out the hairs

immediately around the wound one by one with forceps. This is quicker than it sounds. It gives a clear wound area with no shadows. Do not scrape hairs away with a razor; this can damage the skin.

10. Turn the body over and describe and photograph the bullet wounds on the other side.

11. Review the bullet wounds. Try to pair up entrance and exit wounds and determine which entrance wounds have no exit. Then list what needs to be confirmed or solved by X-ray and internal examination.

12. X-ray the body when necessary.

13. Carry out an internal examination. Sometimes it is necessary to dissect the track of a bullet through the subcutaneous tissue and muscle. Proceed carefully with humility because at times the pathologist is completely lost before he has proceeded more than an inch. It helps to insert a probe first and to be guided by it but sometimes the probe follows a false track and leads the pathologist astray. Then, the more one dissects, the more the true track is obscured. Do not hope to feel the bullet easily just because it is metallic. It needs only to be enveloped by 1·3 cm (0·5 in) of tissue to be impalpable. If a bullet is not quickly found by dissection and palpation, it is best to stop mangling the tissues further and take an X-ray. It saves time in the end.

Injury due to explosions

The use of bombs by terrorists is at present the height of their sophistication. They use them to destroy specific targets such as government buildings or premises owned by a member of the opposition group. They use them indiscriminately without warning to terrorize the community at large. They use them as booby traps against picked individuals or any members of the security forces who can be lured into the trap. The explosive varies. It might be commercial gelignite or a home-made explosive such as a sugar–sodium chlorate mixture. The bomb may be made up in a parcel or bag and carried into the premises to be attacked, packed into iron piping or gas cylinders of one kind or another or packed into a vehicle which can be parked outside its target. Detonation might be through a length of time fuse, by delayed chemical action or by an electrical circuit. Some bombs with timing devices and anti-handling mechanisms are very complex. Nevertheless, they are much less efficient than those of military type and, in spite of the large amount of explosive mixture many of them contain, the severe damage they cause is relatively localized. Their explosion is accompanied by blast, flame and fragments, and the victims include those who were the specific target, others who are accidentally involved in the explosion, bomb disposal men who have an unlucky day and sometimes the terrorists themselves during the process of manufacture, transport or arming of the bomb.

The injuries caused by terrorist bombs fall into six categories.

1. *Complete disruption*

The times when someone is literally blown to bits are few. The victim has to be in contact with the bomb, either carrying it or sitting with it. Then pieces of the body fly in all directions for distances up to 200 m (220 yd). They are collected by members of the security forces and other helpers over the following day or two and as they accumulate at the mortuary they will be found to consist mainly of pieces of scalp and skin, portions of spine and pelvis, parts of limbs and lumps of muscle. Most of the internal organs are usually missing. Pieces of skull, too, are rarely found.

2. *Explosive injury*

Most victims are not so close to the bomb and the body, though badly injured, remains largely in one piece. Those within a metre of the explosion can have parts of limbs blown off and sustain severe mangling of other areas of the body with breaching of the head and trunk cavities. Outside this range the body is less severely mutilated, the characteristic injury being a triad of punctate bruises, abrasions and small puncture lacerations (Fig. 5.4). The bruises and abrasions are circular and about 2–10 mm in diameter. They may be so numerous as to be confluent and give the skin a purple discoloration. The puncture lacerations are more sparse and are larger, up to about 3 cm (1·2 in) diameter; some of them have fragments of metal, wood or clothing sticking out of them. Equally distinctive and diagnostic, though of little concern medically, is a dirt tattooing of exposed areas of skin. It does not occur on all bodies but, when present, it gives the area a dark-brown colour.

3. *Injury by separate fragments*

The triad of small bruises, abrasions and puncture lacerations is to be

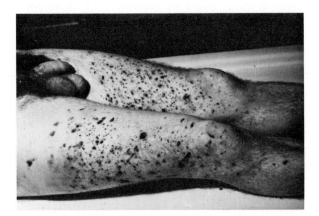

Fig. 5.4   The characteristic small bruises, abrasions and puncture lacerations caused by terrorist bomb explosions.

seen on a victim peppered with minute fragments from the bomb, its container and the surroundings. He has to be within a few metres of the bomb to be struck by such a concentration of debris. Beyond this distance, the peppering kind of injury disappears although serious injury and death can arise from the impact of larger separate fragments, usually of metal. Experience of injury by these objects illustrates the force with which they strike. A small fragment of sheet metal, perhaps only 1 cm (0·4 in) diameter, will penetrate a thick skull, edge-on, as if through butter and so cleanly that the metal cannot be again passed through the hole at the post-mortem examination. A blunt 12·7 cm (5 in) nail, which could not be hammered through a skull without causing localized comminution, will be found projecting through a neat round hole. In one victim, a ragged piece of sheet metal transfixed a plastic upper denture without breaking it. Another victim had the right loin transfixed by some malleable wire 20 cm (8 in) long. These cases also underline how big a part bad luck plays in the fatality. One man was talking to a friend when a car bomb exploded 150 m (165 yd) further up a street; his chest was perforated by a solitary fragment of metal. He died within seconds and was the only casualty. Similar incidents are by no means rare.

4. *Injury by falling masonry*
Those caught inside buildings which are demolished by an explosion are buried under the rubble. They sustain bruises, abrasions, lacerations and fractures of a non-specific kind. Some die from the injuries and some from crush asphyxia. These injuries need to be separated from those due directly to the explosion. Apart from being soiled by dirt, plaster dust, wood debris and possibly oil, they do not differ from the injuries on accident victims with which pathologists are familiar.

5. *Burns*
Those very near to the seat of the explosion might have their hair, eyebrows and eyelashes singed and sustain a superficial burn on some part of the exposed skin. The explosion itself will do no more than this and, since these people are likely to be badly—perhaps fatally—injured, the burns they sustain have interest only in so far as they indicate that the victim was in the immediate vicinity of the bomb. When there are burns of medical importance, they have been sustained after the explosion from the clothing or surroundings which have been set alight. The one exception arises when a bomb factory explodes and sets light to the chemicals lying about. There is a momentary flame of high intensity and those in the room can have their outer clothing burnt off and sustain flash burns of uniform thickness over extensive areas of the body surface. However, tight clothing, such as a brassiere or trunks or a tight waistband, protects the underlying skin.

6. *Blast*
An explosion gives rise to a narrow wave of very high pressure which

advances concentrically from the seat of the explosion at about the speed of sound. The pressure is exceptionally high at the front of the wave but it decreases towards the back and becomes a slight negative pressure, or suction, before the wave is complete. Such a wave will temporarily engulf a person as it moves past him. At about 9 m (30 ft) from a 32 kg (70 lb) charge, the pressure component will last for about 5 ms and the suction component for about 30 ms. It is the impact of the steep pressure front of the wave which can knock a person over. However, the peak pressure of the wave falls rapidly, almost exponentially, as the wave gets more distant from the explosion and whereas a 32 kg (70 lb) charge can produce a pressure of 759 kPa (110 p.s.i.) above the normal atmospheric pressure, at 4.3 m (14 ft), the overpressure has dropped to 103 kPa (15 p.s.i.) at 9 m (30 ft).[22] It is said that the air overpressure must be in the region of 690 kPa (100 p.s.i.) before human beings are endangered.[5]

Blast is said to exert its effects, not by travelling along the trachea and bronchi, but by passing directly through the body wall.[21] It passes through solid, relatively homogeneous, tissues such as muscle and liver without doing much damage, but air-containing organs such as the lung are vulnerable due to a number of mechanisms,[20] the most important probably being the shredding effect at the tissue–air interface as the shock wave crosses it and the shearing movements of different parts of the tissue. In the lung, the result is patchy intra-alveolar haemorrhage which might be severe enough to cause serious, even fatal, respiratory embarrassment. If the victim survives for a while, a neutrophilic inflammatory reaction may arise and progress to bronchopneumonia. The haemorrhages can be anywhere in the lung but they sometimes extend outwards from the hilum. Just occasionally, the hilar tissue is lacerated and contains a blood-filled cavity or a bronchus is lacerated or the mucosa of the trachea contains petechial haemorrhages. These kinds of injury throw doubt on the argument that blast never acts through the air passages.

Blast damage to the lungs received considerable attention during the Second World War when aerial bombs became ever bigger. Blast damage in a relatively pure form was often seen when bombs of 910 kg (2000 lb) size and greater affected people in underground shelters and the like. By contrast, blast damage to the lungs due to terrorist activity is not usually important because the explosive charge is relatively small, it is inefficiently packed and it explodes in unconfined spaces. With terrorist bombs, the victim of blast lung has to be so near to the explosion that he is likely to be injured fatally in other ways. Even when pulmonary haemorrhage is found, it need not necessarily have been due to blast. It can be simply bruising of the lungs caused by a blow on the chest or upper abdomen. Post-mortem autolysis as a result of the aspiration of stomach fluid into the air passages also causes pulmonary haemorrhages.

The ear is the organ most vulnerable to blast, and most people in the near vicinity of an explosion are likely to be affected. Damage varies from only a slight reddening of the tympanic membrane, through bruising and perforation of the membrane to damage of the cochlea which might occur even when the tympanic membrane remains intact. Rupture of the eardrum can occur at overpressures as low as 34 kPa (5 p.s.i.) and 50 per cent of eardrums are likely to be ruptured at overpressures of 103 kPa (15 p.s.i.).[7] However, it is a well known fact that the ear damage sustained in any explosion varies considerably and, sometimes capriciously, from person to person. The principal symptom is deafness, usually complete just after the explosion and associated with tinnitus, but some recovery usually occurs during the next few hours.[9]

As with shooting during civil disturbance, explosions are associated with allegations, rumours and alibis which the forensic pathologist can often support or refute once the post-mortem examinations have been concluded. He must also turn his attention to other problems which arise in the circumstances of terrorist activity.

Identification
Many of the victims can be identified by visual inspection yet care has to be taken because the relatives, harassed by the event and the sight of the body, will often identify it more on a basis of inference than on any critical assessment of physical features. Mistakes have been made by relatives when there are a number of bodies, each badly injured and heavily soiled by blood and dirt. Difficulty is to be expected when the head is mutilated out of all recognition. Then help can sometimes be obtained from a remnant of clothing of distinctive colour or pattern (Fig. 5.5), although this too can be misleading when its appearance has been radically changed by impregnation with plaster dust and grit. In some cases it might be necessary to chart the teeth, record tattoos and search for scars. The fingerprints should be taken by the police routinely in every case.

Cause of death
When a dead body is recovered from the rubble, there is a *prima facie* inference that death was due to the explosion. Careful investigation sometimes shows this simple view to be wrong. It is likely to be right when the body bears the typical small bruises, abrasions and puncture lacerations or has parts of limbs blown off or has areas of the body mangled. Such injuries indicate that the victim was directly exposed to the bomb and not too far from it. There is usually enough internal injury to account for death. Sometimes, however, the victim bears the ordinary kinds of abrasion and laceration with fractures typical of death under falling masonry. Occasionally there are signs of crush asphyxia. Burns have usually been sustained after death. Just now and again, one of the dead victims is remarkably little injured, certainly not in a way to account for death, and then the pathologist has to invoke 'shock' or 'lethal reflexes'. Little is known about it. Experiments with animals have shown that an explosion can cause slowing of the heart which might

stop altogether and remain so. The breathing, too, can be arrested, but the respirations usually start again after a minute or two albeit irregularly.[10] Human victims who survive can be profoundly shocked and lethargic with a low blood pressure and it would be reasonable to infer that those who react most severely might die. Another possible cause of rapid death after an explosion without severe injury is systemic air embolism. Air has been found in lethal quantities in the arteries of animals killed by blast and it is thought to have entered the circulation through the veins of the blast-damaged lungs.[6,20]

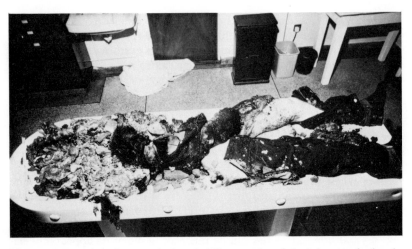

Fig. 5.5   A victim of a terrorist bomb. The severity of the injury to the head and trunk indicate that he must have been very close to the bomb, perhaps carrying it. It was in fact a booby-trapped transistor radio which he was inspecting. There will be obvious difficulty in identification of such a body. The hair might help and also the remnants of clothing.

It must not be forgotten that a person found dead after a terrorist explosion might have died from shooting. It is not uncommon for terrorists about to plant a bomb, to fire indiscriminately into the room to reduce resistance and ease their escape. A person might be fatally injured and left lying on the floor as the others flee in panic. Also, anyone trying to resist the planting of a bomb in his premises might be shot dead by a terrorist and then injured in the subsequent explosion.

Bullets in bodies injured by explosions are best detected by X-rays after the body has been unravelled, undressed and cleaned up. The X-ray films will also reveal any metallic fragments of the bomb mechanism and these are of interest to the forensic scientists. Not all mortuaries have X-ray facilities, however, and these bodies are not in a state which appeals to those working in a hospital X-ray department. Taking X-rays of the body may be a necessity in theory but, in practice, may have to be dispensed with.

Circumstances of the death

The pathologist always finds it rewarding to be able to reconstruct what happened at the time of death, and he can frequently give useful opinions following explosion. This stems from two facts. First, the force of the explosion is very directional and when all the injuries are assessed it is often possible to state the particular stance of a victim at the time and his position in relation to the bomb. Secondly, explosive force declines very rapidly and only people quite near to a bomb are badly mutilated. This knowledge applied to the pattern and severity of the injuries on the victims can do much to confirm or refute allegations, alibis and rumours.

In times of civil strife it is always the other side who is at fault and terrorists are often made out to be innocent victims when they are blown up by their own bombs. If a bomb goes off prematurely while being manufactured or loaded into a vehicle and a terrorist is killed, his family and confederates will insist that he was just passing in the street at the time. Sometimes a bomb will explode while being transported in a car; then the terrorists blown out of the car will be said to have been innocent bystanders. If their car was near another which is also damaged, the other car will be incriminated as having housed the bomb. When a bomb goes off as it is being planted in premises full of people and a number of people are killed, it is important to distinguish those with the bomb from the innocent victims. When a booby-trap bomb kills people, it might be helpful to the investigation to know the position of the victims relative to the bomb at the time.

Experience with terrorist bombs has shown that, when a person is very badly mutilated or has parts of limbs blown off, he has been adjacent to the bomb, perhaps carrying it, standing or sitting next to it or interfering with its mechanism. A person as badly injured as this could not have been passing by, even 3 m (10 ft) away. Beyond 0·6–1 m (2–3 ft) from the bomb, the injuries usually consist of bruises, abrasions and puncture lacerations distributed on the area of the body facing the bomb. Some of the abrasions and lacerations at the periphery of the area are linear and may show an obvious radiation from the seat of the explosion. Thus, it is usually possible to say whether the bomb was to the front, back, left or right side of the victim and when there are a number of victims, their relative positions can often be determined. Explosions at ground level obviously cause most injury to the lower limbs (Fig. 5.6). When someone is bending down over a bomb when it goes off, there is mangling of the face, upper chest, lower abdomen and lower legs while the hands and forearms are probably blown off. Folding in of the upper abdomen protects it. It is not too difficult to work out other likely patterns of injury on, for instance, a person sitting on his heels or kneeling in front of a bomb.

How many bodies?

Although this question is one of the first to be asked, it cannot be answered until the medical examinations are concluded. Most of the

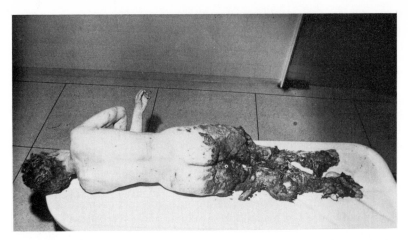

Fig. 5.6 A victim of a terrorist bomb. The severe injuries, limited to the lower limbs, indicate that the bomb went off close to the feet as he stood erect.

victims of terrorist bombs can be counted and the need to ask the question at all arises only because occasionally a person is sufficiently close to a bomb to be completely disintegrated. Evidence of his involvement will come to light only if the scraps of human remains collected from the area are carefully examined with this question in mind.

First, any limb pieces must be apportioned to the bodies. Should there be any trunk portions, these are fitted together and any remaining limb pieces matched up, by inference if necessary. This work does not usually produce any surprises. Interest centres around pieces of soft tissue which are usually mangled and dirt soiled. Each piece must be washed under running water and examined. On one occasion, a piece of scalp was found bearing hair of a different colour from that of the other victims. At another time, there was a ruptured eyeball which was not from one of the other dead bodies. On yet another occasion it was a penis which indicated an extra victim. When a bomb blew up while being loaded into a car, four identifiable bodies were recovered, numerous body parts and a mound of small bits of soft tissue weighing 21 kg (47 lb). Careful examination of this revealed two prostate glands and two uterine cervices—positive evidence of four other victims.

Conclusion

The violence of civil disturbance stems from conflict between factions and no matter which group is thought to have the just cause, none remains entirely blameless of negligent or criminal acts. Doctors who examine the injured for medicolegal purposes and pathologists who examine the dead are usually acting in an official capacity instructed by, and perhaps paid by, a department of the government. Having such a connection, the doctor or pathologist might be said to be biased. To maintain credibility and retain respect, these doctors must do all in their power to maintain strict impartiality. Their work must be thorough and confined within the limits of their knowledge and experience. Their reports must be fair and unemotive, unaffected in any way by pressure from whatever quarter and devoid of bias arising from personal prejudice. The findings must be submitted through the recognized official channels only to those entitled to receive them. Finally, care must be taken to ensure that those parts of the reports which are eventually used in evidence tell not only the truth but the whole truth.

References

1. Ballantyne, B. and Johnston, W. G. (1974). *o*-Chlorobenzylidene malononitrile (CS) and the healing of cutaneous lesions. *Med. Sci. Law* **14**, 93.
2. Ballantyne, B. and Swanston, D. W. (1974). The irritant effects of dilute solutions of dibenzoxazepine (CR) on the eye and tongue. *Acta pharmacol. toxicol.* **35**, 412.
3. Ballantyne, B., Beswick, F. W. and Price Thomas, D. (1973). The presentation and management of individuals contaminated with solutions of Dibenzoxazepine (CR). *Med. Sci. Law* **13**, 265.
4. Ballantyne, B., Gazzard, M. F., Swanston, D. W. and Williams, P. (1974). The ophthalmic toxicology of *o*-chlorobenzylidene malononitrile (CS). *Arch. Toxicol.* **32**, 149.
5. Bernal, J. D. (1941). The physics of air raids. *Nature (Lond.)* **147**, 594.
6. Clemedson, C.-J. and Hultman, H. I. (1954). Air embolism and the cause of death in blast injury. *Milit. Surg.* **114**, 424.
7. Hirsch, F. G. (1968). Effects of overpressure on the ear—a review. *Ann. N.Y. Acad. Sci.* **152**, 147.
8. Hoffmann, D. H. (1967). Eye burns caused by tear gas. *Brit. J. Ophthal.* **51**, 265.
9. Kerr, A. G. and Byrne, J. E. T. (1975). Concussive effects of bomb blast on the ear. *J. Laryng.* **89**, 131.
10. Krohn, P. L., Whitteridge, D. and Zuckerman, S. (1942). Physiological effects of blast. *Lancet* **i**, 252.
11. Levine, R. A. and Stahl, C. J. (1968). Eye injury caused by tear gas weapons. *Amer. J. Ophthal.* **65**, 497.
12. Millar, R., Rutherford, W. H., Johnston, S. and Malhotra, V. J. (1975). Injuries caused by rubber bullets: a report on 90 patients. *Brit. J. Surg.* **62**, 480.
13. Penneys, N. S., Israel, R. M. and Indgin, S. M. (1969). Contact dermatitis due to 1-chloroacetophenone and Chemical Mace. *New Engl. J. Med.* **281**, 413.
14. *Report of the Enquiry into the Medical and Toxicological Aspects of CS (Orthochlorobenzylidene Malononitrile)* (1969). Part I. Cmnd 4173. London: HMSO.
15. *Report of the Enquiry into the Medical and Toxicological Aspects of*

CS (*Orthochlorobenzylidene Malononitrile*) (1971). Part II. Cmnd 4775. London: HMSO.

16. Rutherford, W. H. (1970). Medical consequences of the riots in Belfast in 1969. *Brit. J. Hosp. Med.* **4**, 641.

17. Rutherford, W. H. (1974). The injuries of civil disorder. *Community Hlth* **6**, 14.

18. Shaw, J. (1972). Pulmonary contusion in children due to rubber bullet injuries. *Brit. med. J.* **4**, 764.

19. Stein, A. A. and Kirwan, W. E. (1964). Chloracetophenone (tear gas) poisoning: a clinico-pathologic report. *J. forensic Sci.* **9**, 374.

20. White, C. S. and Richmond, D. R. (1960). Blast biology. In: *Clinical Cardiopulmonary Physiology*, 2nd edn., Chap. 63. Ed. B. L. Gordon. New York: Grune and Stratton.

21. Zuckerman, S. (1940). Experimental study of blast injuries to the lungs. *Lancet* **ii**, 219.

22. Zuckerman, S. (1941). Discussion on the problem of blast injuries. *Proc. roy. Soc. Med.* **34**, 171.

6

Modern war wounds

'War, which has been a bane to man since his earliest days, has always been characterized by the presence of those who attempt to devise more and more effective ways to maim and destroy the enemy, of others who strive to develop the means to protect their comrades from the implements of the foe, and of still others on both sides who devote themselves to improving techniques for the care and repair of the unfortunates who are the casualties of war. These three facets of war are interdependent, and one group cannot achieve the best results without the advice and assistance of the others. The thread which binds and correlates their activities is the science and application of the principles of wound ballistics.'

LTG Leonard D. Heaton[6]
The Surgeon-General,
United States Army

Introduction

The pathology of violent acts on the battlefield can frequently result in wounds similar to those caused in civilian life by high-speed transportation injuries, industrial accidents and acts of aggression found in urban violence. Nevertheless, man's inhumanity to man is most obvious during the time of armed conflict between nations or other large collections of armed troops because of the magnitude of the involvement. History is replete with the development of more sophisticated weaponry in modern time. Because recent events are the best known and understood, some might believe that modern weapons cause the worst wounds. However, historically, there is a vast documentation of the development of various types of weapons during the past several thousand years; all of these had the potential of causing devastating wounds, the vivid descriptions of which are quite impressive, even to the present-day surgeon. Many facts must be considered in forming the proper perspective regarding modern-day war wounds. Today, when the tremendous destructive powers of the atomic and hydrogen bombs are well known and there is an increasing knowledge of such potential weapons as those which utilize laser beams, fuel air explosions and high-frequency sound, battles are still fought in many areas of the world with an assortment of primitive devices. In a brief review of the effects of modern weapons, it becomes necessary to emphasize the unique aspects of fighting in many regions where adversaries still rely on anti-personnel weapons including home-made booby traps. During hostilities in the Republic of Vietnam in the 1960s, at a time when both sides utilized rockets, artillery, and even the most sophisticated electronic weapons such as surface-to-air missiles, the use of primitive weapons was still very evident. At the Second Surgical Hospital (MA) in the Central Highlands of the Republic of Vietnam, 324 soldiers with 342 punji stick* wounds were treated.[37] Frequently, the loss of active duty time was very similar to that from many minor missile wounds.

Only through a better understanding of the wounding power of various missiles can surgeons provide the best treatment possible for those who are unfortunate enough to be wounded. A basic understanding that there is a difference between high-velocity and low-velocity gunshot wounds is of paramount importance. Recently, the concern regarding weapons which may have indiscriminate effects on those wounded or cause what is considered to be inhumane suffering has stimulated international exchange among the nations of the world, including those with different political and ideological ideas.[20] An observation considered pertinent by many is that the most sophisticated conventional weapons are being used presently in fighting even in the more remote parts of the world. This has increased the challenge to the medical profession in managing resultant wounds, particularly as the medical support which is available is frequently not given equal attention to that of providing weapons.

A relatively new dimension has been introduced in this century in the management of war wounds. Medical treatment of those injured has been vastly improved and this has been aided by rapid evacuation of the wounded. Abdominal wounds were usually fatal before the beginning of this century. The situation has changed drastically if one contrasts the carts that picked up the dying after the battle of Waterloo with the helicopter evacuation of American wounded in South-east Asia, the latter often occurring within minutes after wounding. It should be recognized, nevertheless, that not all armies, even today, have the medical evacuation and medical care support which is available to the American forces. Also, there is only minimal documentation of the types of medical support which wounded guerrilla fighters have received in various parts of the world. Yet, despite all of these ramifications, it is safe to state that tremendous advances have been made in the medical care of war wounded. To cite the battle of Waterloo again, the major method of treatment for extremity wounds was amputation and it was reported that some wounded with even minor extremity wounds were frequently so treated. Although mortality figures have been kept with accuracy only within recent wars, it is clear that amputations have been markedly reduced to approximately 2 per cent of those wounded in battle who reached definitive surgical centres. There has been con-

* Punji sticks are fire-hardened, pointed pieces of bamboo, often contaminated with excreta, placed in the ground so as to impale persons who walk or fall on to them.

siderable support for a world medical force to ensure that all injured have received comparable medical care. This latter subject, however, is well beyond the scope of this review.

Historical

Since the days of Ambrose Paré, who is often considered the father of military surgery, there have been a myriad of reports regarding the experience of surgeons treating combat wounded. The names of Roger Bacon, Bernal Diaz, John Randy and Theodor Billroth are just a few of the many other physicians easily recognized by their interest in wounds caused by missiles. It is beyond the scope of this limited review to provide a detailed analysis of the many documents and references that are available but additional source material can be found in Amato and Rich,[1] Beyer,[6] DeMuth,[8] Finck,[11] Heaton,[12] Neel,[14] and Shepard and Rich.[36] Specific areas of interest in managing gunshot wounds, in the treatment of specific organ injuries, such as vascular trauma, and in the evacuation of wounded have received intensive interest and produced important results.

Types of wounds

The purpose of this presentation is to emphasize modern war wounds. Appropriately, representative material comes from the personal experience of the author who has had a responsibility for managing combat casualties, both at the front-line surgical hospital and in the rear echelon medical centre, during the past 15 years. A particularly intense effort was made to document valid statistics regarding the management of combat forces who sustained missile wounds in South-east Asia.

A preliminary report from the Central Highlands of the Republic of Vietnam outlined the experience at a surgical hospital in managing 1196 patients (Table 6.1). It is significant that less than half—43·6 per cent sustained missile wounds. Unique to the time and place, one-fifth of the injured soldiers sustained punji stick wounds. Because the hospital was designated as a surgical hospital, only 8 per cent of the

Table 6.1 Admission categories of 1196 cases at the Second Surgical Hospital[32]

1966	Missile	Trauma	Punji	Surgery	Medicine
January	45	33	5	13	13
February	106	36	24	26	13
March	70	47	93	32	35
April	76	46	83	33	23
May	224	33	38	37	12
Totals	521	195	243	141	96
Percentage	43·6	16·3	20·3	11·8	8·0

Table 6.2   Second Surgical Hospital
(MA), 2048 admissions[15]

		(%)
Missile wounds	750	36·6
Punji sticks	324	15·8
Trauma	446	21·8
Surgical	361	17·6
Medical	167	8·2

patients were treated for medical problems, usually malaria. At the completion of this review, a total of 2048 patients had been managed and there was no significant change from the original report (Table 6.2). Missile wounds accounted for 36·6 per cent of the hospital admissions—750 patients. The punji stick wounds remained a formidable problem involving 324 wounds, or 15·8 per cent of the total.

Thorough documentation of the details of wounding in all patients sustaining missile wounds was carried out at the Second Surgical Hospital (MA) during a 9-month period from January 1966 through September 1966. A total of 750 patients sustaining missile wounds were included in this study. Over 500 bullets and fragments were removed. Nevertheless, even with adequate debridement, nearly two-thirds of the patients sustaining penetrating missile wounds still had retained fragments or bullet fragments after treatment. The necessity for careful debridement was emphasized by removal of many pieces of clothing and equipment (Fig. 6.1) from the wounds. Foreign material such as this carried into the wound appeared to potentiate the development of a wound infection in contrast to the inert metallic fragments. It was possible to obtain support from experts in the area of explosive ordnance, small arms and military intelligence which provided an opportunity to obtain the high degree of accuracy needed to identify specific wounding agents. This was important from the medical standpoint. Obviously, the military tactician also found this material to be of interest.

Two major groups of missile wounds exist for classification: (1) bullet wounds from small arms; and (2) fragments from exploding artillery

Table 6.3   Missile wounds at the
Second Surgical Hospital, 1966[15]

		(%)
Gunshot	321	42·1
Fragment	435	57·1
Arrows and unknown	6	0·8

Twelve patients had wounds from
more than one source.

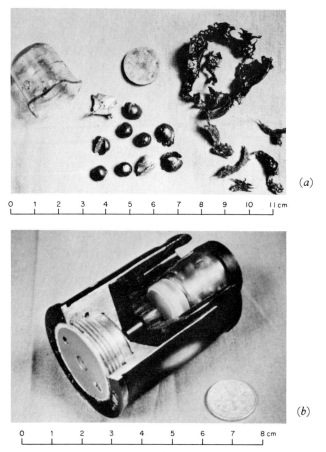

```
0   1   2   3   4   5   6   7   8   9   10   11 cm
```

(a)

```
0   1   2   3   4   5   6   7   8 cm
```

(b)

Fig. 6.1 (a) Adequate wound debridement is mandatory in modern war wounds. This is emphasized by material above removed from a wound, which includes plastic material, wadding and clothing, in addition to the metallic pellets. The risk of infection is increased if such foreign material is not removed. (b) A cutaway of the offending round fired from a hand-held rifle.

rounds, mortars, mines, rockets and grenades. In the missile study cited,[15] just over half of the wounds were caused by fragments from the various exploding devices: 435, or 57·1 per cent (Table 6.3). Identification of these offending missiles was often suggested by appearance on roentgenograms (Fig. 6.2). In many combat situations, the percentage of patients sustaining fragment wounds may approach 80–90 per cent.

Despite the relative infrequency of bullet wounds compared to fragment wounds, the difference between high-velocity and low-velocity bullet wounds emphasizes a major aspect of the importance of wound ballistics. An understanding of the wounding power of missiles is important to the surgeon in providing the best care possible for the patients. Figure 6.3 demonstrates the minimal tissue damage caused by

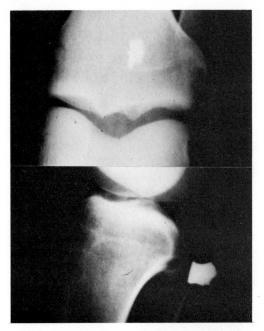

Fig. 6.2   Anteroposterior and lateral roentgenograms of the knee demonstrate an irregular metallic foreign body in the area of the neurovascular bundle in the popliteal fossa. This type of wound from a fragment from an exploding mortar round causes a wound which requires debridement and exploration of the neurovascular bundle to determine the extent of the trauma.

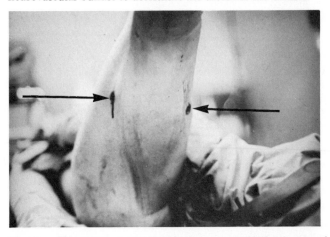

Fig. 6.3   The two arrows identify the entrance and exit wounds of a 0.45 calibre gunshot wound of the posterior thigh. The entrance and exit wounds of this low velocity missile were of a similar size, measuring about 1.5 cm (approx. 0.5 in) in diameter. Minimal soft tissue destruction required minimal debridement, contrasted with many high velocity wounds with more massive tissue destruction and subsequent larger debridement.[15]

a low-velocity bullet wound. This is contrasted by Fig. 6.4, where there is massive tissue destruction associated with the high-velocity bullet wound. This is a graphic demonstration to stress the two extremes, but the situation as a whole is not quite so simple. Table 6.4 provides an equation important to anyone with an interest in missile wounding. The impact kinetic energy of the missile equals the weight of the missile times the velocity (squared) divided by the gravitational force. It is

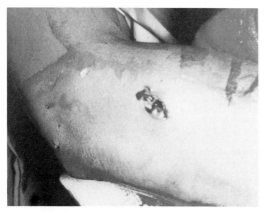

(a)

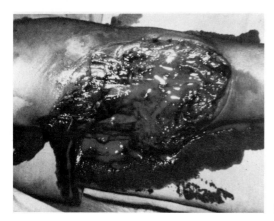

(b)

Fig. 6.4 *(a)* The entrance wound from an M-16 bullet fired from approximately 10 m (30 ft) is visualized on the lateral aspect of the right forearm just below the elbow. There is minimal soft tissue destruction that is obvious at the entrance, which measured about 1·5 cm (approx. 0·5 in) in diameter. *(b)* The exit wound, in marked contrast, emphasizes the massive soft tissue destruction of a high velocity missile with an exit wound measuring approximately 8 × 10 cm (4 × 5 in) on the volar aspect of the forearm. The challenge to the surgeon with additional debridement and reconstruction emphasizes the increased problems frequently found with high velocity missile wounds compared to low velocity missile wounds.[10]

Table 6.4

$$E = \frac{Wv^2}{2g}$$

E = Impact kinetic energy
W = Weight of the missile
v^2 = Squared impact velocity of missile
$2g$ = Gravitation acceleration

obvious that the velocity of the missile is very important. Nevertheless, the weight of the missile also plays an important role. There is an additional important factor not shown in this table which involves the tissue struck by the missile. An example is the greater resilience of the air-filled lung tissue contrasted with the more solid liver. The latter may demonstrate a larger wound than the former. Table 6.5 provides

Table 6.5 Muzzle velocity

	$m\ s^{-1}$	ft/sec
0·22 calibre (short)	275	900
0·380 calibre	282	925
0·45 calibre	259	850
Carbine (0·30 calibre)	600	1970
0·30 calibre (7·62 mm)	730–853	2400–2800
0·223 calibre (5·56 mm)	990	3250

some details for the type of missiles that are fired from small arms in many parts of the world. The lower velocity 0·45 calibre bullet caused the wound shown in Fig. 6.3, and the higher velocity 0·223 calibre bullet caused the wound shown in Fig. 6.4.

Table 6.6 demonstrates the regional distribution of wounds which might be anticipated in the management of combat casualties. Of prime

Table 6.6 Regional wound distribution in 750 patients at the Second Surgical Hospital, 1966[15]

		(%)
Lower extremities	430	36·5
Upper extremities	317	26·9
Head and neck	123	10·4
Chest	107	9·1
Abdomen	67	5·7
Flank, back, genitalia	134	11·4
Totals	1178	100

Table 6.7
Regional distribution of 342
punji stick wounds in 324
patients in the Second
Surgical Hospital, 1966[37]

Foot	38
Ankle	22
Leg	206
Knee	26
Thigh	29
Scrotum	1
Buttocks	2
Hand	12
Arm	5
Palate	1
	342
Double wounds	14
Triple wounds	2
Total patients	324

importance is the fact that approximately two-thirds of the wounds are found in the extremities. Many patients with wounds of the head and torso do not survive long enough to reach a definitive surgical centre. Specific types of weaponry may be associated with a varied wound distribution. This is emphasized in Table 6.7, where it is shown that the vast majority of the punji stick wounds occurred, as might be anticipated, in the lower extremities.

Resuscitation, general care of the wounded patient and management

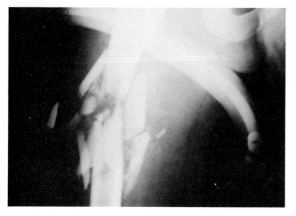

Fig. 6.5 The 7·62 mm bullet seen on the left on the above roentgenogram was responsible for the markedly comminuted femoral fracture. The metallic ring at the top of the picture is part of the external immobilization device utilized to provide stability of the fracture.

of specific injuries cannot be covered in this short review. Additional material, however, can be obtained from the references cited in this chapter. The main concern should be to salvage life. When this is threatened by serious injury to a limb, primary amputation may be indicated. Removal of a lacerated spleen may be life-saving to prevent exsanguinating haemorrhage. Primary repair of lacerated nerves is usually not performed in the combat zone. Figure 6.5 shows a markedly comminuted right femoral fracture caused by high-velocity 7·62 mm

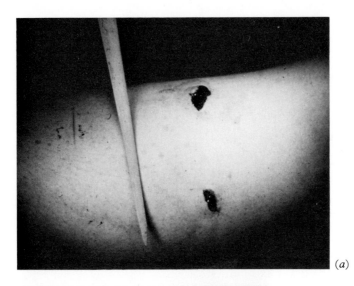

(a)

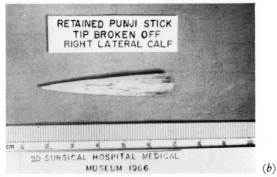

(b)

Fig. 6.6   During the hostilities in the Republic of South Vietnam in the late 1960s, a somewhat unique aspect in the fighting occurred. At a time when both sides were armed with sophisticated modern weapons, the primitive punji stick, as seen above, created extremity wounds which disabled soldiers frequently as long as many minor missile wounds. (a) An example of a punji stick and resulting wound. (b) Retained fragments of punji stick tip, broken off in right lateral calf. Such fragments from punji sticks can cause infection associated with the foreign body.[15]

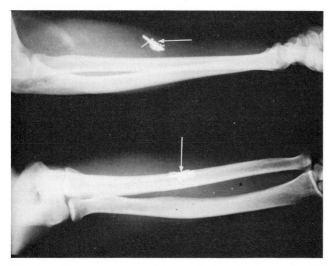

Fig. 6.7 Roentgenograms show a coiled spring (arrows) which was one of many miscellaneous missiles in a home-made booby trap which was detonated by a trip wire. Frequently, guerrilla warfare in this century has utilized any available metal fragments and an assortment of small missiles of various compositions in booby traps.

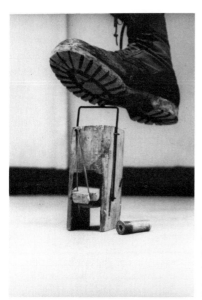

Fig. 6.8 In modern-day guerrilla warfare fought in many areas throughout the world, home-made booby traps emphasize the ingenuity of utilizing many simple and easily available materials to create a devastating weapon. In the above simulated demonstration, a soldier's foot is about to depress the trip mechanism made from a wire coat-hanger. In actual practice, this would release a rubber-band and subsequently allow a nail in a small piece of wood to act as a detonator against the primer of a shotgun shell or a bullet.[15] (See also Fig. 6.9.)

bullet, which can also be seen on the roentgenogram. External immobilization of fractures is usually practised in combat wounded in preference to attempting to obtain immobilization of fractures by internal fixation devices. The repair of vascular injuries has been one of the most important aspects of modern war surgery. There has been a marked improvement of the amputation rate when repair of injured arteries—as opposed to ligation—has been performed.

There are many unusual occurrences and unique aspects associated with the management of modern war wounds. Figure 6.6 is an example of the primitive punji stick wound. Figure 6.7 demonstrates the type of missile that may come from home-made ordnance. Figure 6.8 emphasizes the ingenuity in guerrilla warfare for manufacturing simple devices which can inflict injury. An example of the massive tissue destruction that can occur from this primititive type of weaponry is shown in Fig. 6.9.

Management of wounded and results obtained

As previously mentioned, there is no intent in this review to provide even an outline for the management of war wounds. An attempt is made to provide examples of some of the type of injuries which can occur.

Even efforts to establish outstanding medical support can flounder

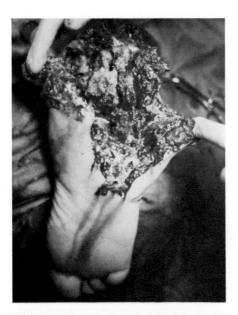

Fig. 6.9 Massive destruction of the heel is obvious in the above photograph. This soldier stepped on an anti-personnel device consisting of a home-made booby trap similar to that shown in Fig. 6.13.[15]

Table 6.8 Missile wounds in 750 patients at the Second Surgical Hospital, 1966[15]

Operative mortality	1·2%
Deaths:	
at Second Surgical	7
after evacuation	2

without logistical support. This is highlighted by the evacuation of wounded. In the unique situation in South-east Asia, where helicopter evacuation was available, it was not unusual to have severely injured patients under treatment at a definitive surgical centre earlier than that possible in the civilian circumstances where victims of motor vehicle accidents may have to travel by land conveyances over a period of several hours.

Table 6.8 documents the results of management of 750 patients sustaining missile wounds in South-east Asia. The mortality rate was 1·2 per cent; 61 per cent—445—of the survivors were returned to active duty within the theatre of operation.

Comment

Armed confrontation exists in some part of the world nearly every day. Even in the civilian life, criminals and belligerents continue to effect wounds similar to those seen on the battlefield. This stresses the need for a comprehensive understanding of the wounding power of missiles. Only through this approach can the physician provide the best care possible for those who have the misfortune of sustaining missile injury.

Other than the representative types of wounds which have been demonstrated, there is very minimal documentation and minimal scientific data regarding wounds from some of the newer types of weaponry such as flechettes.* The increased interest in modern war wounds has stimulated educational programmes and conferences with exchange between the developers of weapons and physicians who must care for the resulting wounds. All of this will, hopefully, have a positive effect on reducing the long-term ill effect of the destruction caused by the implements of war.

Protective armour has been utilized for many years with a varying degree of success. At present, protective headgear can reduce some potential types of head wounds. Protective jackets can reduce thoracic injuries from many types of fragments. Currently, however, new development is proceeding in this area and the true role of protective equipment, other than that mentioned above, is not totally known.

* The flechette is a steel dart similar to a small nail, with stabilizing fins on the back; thousands of these can be placed into an explosive device and the flechettes are thrown in all directions upon detonation.

Even the best trained military medical service may be taxed beyond the ability to respond. The ability to handle hundreds of thousands of casualties, which would be produced by known weapons, is nearly beyond comprehension. It would be superficial to attempt to document a plan in this short review. There are a number of studies currently under way in an effort to computerize the expected type of wounds and the anticipated method of management. Obviously, in mass casualty situations, neither essential time nor limited supplies can be provided for those who fall in the 'expectant' category. Effort would have to be expended to assist those who have the highest probability of survival.

At a time when most would rather discuss the prohibition of all weapons of war, we must recognize the fallibility of mankind. Unfortunately, it appears that the management of modern war wounds will remain a topic of interest by necessity.

References

1. Amato, J. J. and Rich, N. M. (1972). Temporary cavity effect in blood vessel injury by high velocity missiles. *J. cardiovasc. Surg.* **13**, 147.

2. Amato, J. J., Billy, L. J. and Rich, N. M. (1974). High velocity missile injury: an experimental study of the retentive forces of tissue. *Amer. J. Surg.* **127**, 454.

3. Amato, J. J., Billy, L. J., Gruber, R. P., Lawson, N. S. and Rich, N. M. (1970). Vascular injuries: an experimental study of high and low velocity missile wounds. *Arch. Surg.* **101**, 167.

4. Amato, J. J., Rich, N. M., Billy, L. J., Gruber, R. P. and Lawson, N. S. (1971). High velocity arterial injury: a study of the mechanism of injury. *J. Trauma* **11**, 412.

5. Amato, J. J., Billy, L. J., Gruber, R. P. and Rich, N. M. (1974). Temporary cavitation in high velocity pulmonary missile injury. *Ann. thorac. Surg.* **18**, 565.

6. Beyer, J. C. (Ed.) (1962). *Wound Ballistics*. Office of the Surgeon-General. Washington, DC: Department of the Army.

7. Billy, L. J., Amato, J. J. and Rich, N. M. (1971). Aortic injuries in Vietnam. *Surgery* **70**, 385.

8. DeMuth, W. E. Jr. (1969). Bullet velocity as applied to military rifle wounding capacity. *J. Trauma* **9**, 27.

9. DeMuth, W. E. Jr. and Smith, J. M. (1966). High velocity bullet wounds of muscle and bone: the basis of rational early treatment. *J. Trauma* **6**, 744.

10. Dimond, F. C. Jr. and Rich, N. M. (1967). M-16 rifle wounds in Vietnam. *J. Trauma* **7**, 619.

11. Finck, P. A. (1965). Ballistics and forensic pathologic aspects of missile wounds. *Milit. Med.* **130**, 545.

12. Heaton, L. D., Hughes, C. W., Rosegay, H., Fisher, G. W. and Feighny, R. E. (1966). Military surgical practices of the United

States Army in Vietnam. In: *Current Problems in Surgery*. Chicago: Year Book Medical Publishers.

13. Levin, P. M., Rich, N. M. and Hutton, J. E. Jr. (1971). Collateral circulation in arterial injuries. *Arch. Surg.* **102**, 392.

14. Neel, S. (1973). *Vietnam Studies: Medical Support of the U.S. Army in Vietnam, 1965–1970*. Washington, DC: US Government Printing Office.

15. Rich, N. M. (1968). Vietnam missile wounds evaluated in 750 patients. *Milit. Med.* **133**, 9.

16. Rich, N. M. (1968). Wounding power of various ammunition. *Resp. Physiol.* **14**, 72.

17. Rich, N. M. (1969). Evaluation of missile wounds at the Second Surgical Hospital (MA) in Vietnam. *Plastic and Maxillofacial Trauma Symposium*, Chap. 2. Ed. N. G. Georgiade. St Louis: C. V. Mosby.

18. Rich, N. M. (1970). Vascular trauma in Vietnam. *J. cardiovasc. Surg.* **11**, 368.

19. Rich, N. M. (1973). Traumatismo en vasos. *Clin. Chir.* **7**, 1367.

20. Rich, N. M. (1975). Weapons and wounds (editorial). *J. Trauma* **15**, 464.

21. Rich, N. M. and Dimond, F. C. Jr. (1967). Shrapnel—a misnomer. *Milit. Med.* **132**, 470.

22. Rich, N. M. and Hughes, C. W. (1969). Vietnam vascular registry: a preliminary report. *Surgery* **65**, 218.

23. Rich, N. M. and Hughes, C. W. (translation by Rignault, D. and Moine, D.) (1970). Statistiques sur les plaies vascularies au Vietnam (4500 Cas). *Soc. Med-Chir.* **9**, 805.

24. Rich, N. M. and Hughes, C. W. (translation by Rignault, D. and Moine, D.) (1971). Rapport sur les plaies vascularies au Vietnam. *Rev. Cps Santé Armées* **12**, 673.

25. Rich, N. M., Amato, J. J. and Billy, L. J. (1971). Arterial thrombosis secondary to temporary cavitation. *Surg. Digest* **6**, 12.

26. Rich, N. M., Baugh, J. H. and Hughes, C. W. (1970). Acute arterial injuries in Vietnam: 1,000 cases. *J. Trauma* **10**, 359.

27. Rich, N. M., Baugh, J. H. and Hughes, C. W. (1970). Significance of complications associated with vascular repairs performed in Vietnam. *Arch. Surg.* **100**, 646.

28. Rich, N. M., Clarke, J. S. and Baugh, J. H. (1969). Successful repair of a traumatic aneurysm of the abdominal aorta. *Surgery* **66**, 492.

29. Rich, N. M., Hobson, R. W. II and Collins, G. J. (1975). Traumatic arteriovenous fistulas and false aneurysms: a review of 558 lesions. *Surgery* **78**, 817.

30. Rich, N. M., Hobson, R. W. II, Wright, C. B. and Fedde, C. W. (1976). Repair of lower extremity venous trauma: a more aggressive approach required. *J. Trauma* **14**, 639.

31. Rich, N. M., Hughes, C. W. and Baugh, J. H. (1970). Management of venous injuries. *Ann. Surg.* **171**, 724.

32. Rich, N. M., Johnson, E. V. and Dimond, F. C. Jr. (1967). Wounding power of missiles used in the Republic of Vietnam. *J. Amer. med. Ass.* **199**, 157.

33. Rich, N. M., Manion, W. C. and Hughes, C. W. (1969). Surgical and pathological evaluation of vascular injuries in Vietnam. *J. Trauma* **9**, 279.

34. Rich, N. M., Metz, C. W., Hutton, J. E. Jr., Baugh, J. H. and Hughes, C. W. (1971). Internal versus external fixation of fractures with concomitant vascular injuries in Vietnam. *J. Trauma* **11**, 463d.

35. Scott, R. (1974). *Projectile Trauma: An Enquiry into Bullet Wounds*. Porton Down: Royal Army Medical Corps.

36. Shepard, G. H. and Rich, N. M. (1972). Treatment of the soft tissue war wound by the American military surgeon: a historical review. *Milit. Med.* **137**, 264.

37. Shepard, G. H., Rich, N. M. and Dimond, F. C. Jr. (1967). Punji stick wounds: experience with 342 wounds in 324 patients in Vietnam. *Ann. Surg.* **166**, 902.

38. Whelan, T. J. Jr. (Ed) (1975). *Emergency War Surgery*, First United States Revision, NATO Handbook. Washington, DC: US Government Printing Office.

39. Whelan, T. J. Jr., Burkhalter, W. E. and Gomez, A. (1968). Management of war wounds. In: *Advances in Surgery*, Vol. 3. Ed. C. E. Welch. Chicago: Year Book Medical Publishers.

7

Injury by burning

Burns and scalds are common injuries. They may vary from minor and insignificant accidents to the most severe injuries that man can experience. The burn injury evokes many pathophysiological responses and much of our knowledge of the body's response to injury in general stems from research into the metabolic and biochemical changes associated with burns.

In the last 10 years the numbers dying from burns and scalds in England and Wales have declined by about 20 per cent. The Registrar-General's statistics show that 492 died from thermal burns in 1975. On the other hand, fire departments report 900 deaths in conflagrations. The difference is attributable to many of the latter dying from asphyxia or from the inhalation of poisonous fumes rather than from the effect of the flames.

Incidence and causation of burns

The total numbers who are burned and require hospital treatment can only be guessed. Burn injuries are not notifiable and statistics are sparse.[25] Figures have been deduced from relating the numbers of burns cases admitted to a burn unit to the mortality in that group and scaling up for the mortality over the whole country. It is suggested that 10 000 burns a year require admission to hospital and their average stay will be 5–6 weeks.[32] Figures as high as 100 000 have been estimated for the numbers seeking treatment in accident departments.

Most hospital statistics show an equal number of admissions of children (under 10 years) and adults. Very young infants, who have not begun to walk, sustain burns as a result of carelessness on the part of the parent or those caring for them. Toddlers, in the age group 1–3 years, are exploring their environment continuously and may injure themselves. Nevertheless, these domestic 'accidents' can be anticipated and are preventable. Scalding is by far the commonest cause of injury. It may result from upsetting a kettle, saucepan or teapot by reaching up for the handle or pulling on a table-cloth, or a toddler may be unable to turn off a hot tap while standing in a bath (Fig. 7.1). Other burns are due to contact with an electric fire bar or from a coal or gas fire—always a source of fascination to the young. Scalding is less common in older children but burns are frequently more severe from the ignition of

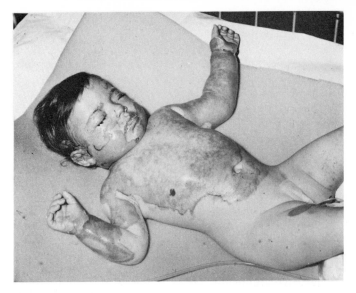

Fig. 7.1   Scalds in an infant.

clothing upon contact with a heat source or from playing with matches, bonfires or fireworks.

A very small group of children sustain burns as a form of deliberately inflicted injury. There are certain circumstances when suspicion of non-accidental injury should be aroused in examining a burned or scalded child.[18] The history may vary or be contradictory or it may be inconsistent with the lesion; thus, a child reaching up overturning a saucepan will invariably sustain scalds of the submental region and axillae but not if the arms are by the side. Circular burns on the buttocks, or 'dip' scalds of hands and feet, with well-defined margins, cigarette burns, repeated burn accidents and burns associated with bruises or fractures all arouse suspicion. A radiographic skeletal survey is indicated in such cases. Of non-accidental injuries to children, 10 per cent involve some form of localized burn or scald.[12] The subject is discussed further in Chapter 13.

Legislation has gone some way to reduce the incidence of preventable burns. The Children Act of 1908 aimed at protecting children from various forms of negligence on the part of those upon whom they are dependent for their welfare and safety. One section of this Act made it an offence for an adult, having custody of a child, to leave it in a room with an open fire insufficiently guarded, if by so doing the child did, in fact, suffer injury. This section is retained in the more recent Children and Young Persons (Amendment) Act 1952. There is legal recognition of the peculiar liability of children to injury by burning and scalding, and a measure of responsibility is placed on those caring for them. When death or serious injury occurs the circumstances are investigated and charges may result.

The first attempts to enact legislation to *prevent* such injuries were those made under the Heating Appliances (Fireguards) Act 1952, requiring that a guard be fitted to all domestic heating appliances. This applies now to coal, gas and electric fires and oil stoves. However, the regulations are still sufficiently lax to permit large enough spaces between the wires of the guard for a toddler to insert his hand and to grip the bars of an electric fire. Fireproof clothing and fire-resistant materials are encouraged but proofing is an added expense for the manufacturer (particularly in the case of cheap imports from overseas) and the impregnating chemical may wash out in time. From 1964, the Children's Nightwear Regulations (SI 1153) prohibited manufacturers from using inflammable materials. Fortunately, fashions have changed and nightdresses have given way in popularity to pyjamas and dresses to jeans. Of deaths from burning, 90 per cent are associated with clothing catching alight.

Legislation restricting the sale of fireworks to children under the age of 16 has been enacted and manufacturers no longer produce 'thunderflashes'. There continues to be public demand for yet further restriction on their distribution and use by younger children.

Between the ages of 15 and 64 years, men are burned slightly more frequently than women mainly because of the greater risk of industrial injury to those at work. Two-thirds of males injured are burned at work but only one-tenth of the females. Nevertheless, domestic accidents still account for the majority of burns in the whole group. Highly inflammable plastics and synthetic polymers are increasingly used in the home: the polyurethanes are widely used as foams for upholstery, mattresses and the backing of carpets; the rigid polyurethanes, polyvinyl chlorides and phenol formaldehyde are the raw materials of much modern furniture. A blaze spreads with horrific speed when these materials are involved. Efforts are being made to reduce the fire risks by incorporating chemical fire retardants but some additives are themselves toxic, even in minute traces.

Fire brigades were called to 23 160 fires in vehicles in 1973, including 900 in motor-cycles; 237 road casualties sustained burns, but only 46 were fatal. In most cases the victim was rendered unconscious and was trapped in the vehicle.

Epileptics are one particular section of the population at risk; 10 per cent of the total admissions to burns units are so afflicted. Burns arise during a fit from falling into a fire or causing a conflagration by overturning a light or heater. The burns may be particularly deep and involve the head or hands. Since loss of consciousness accompanies the attack, there is no attempt to escape from the flames.

Persons aged over 65 years are another group at risk and suffer injury from accidents in the home. The ratio of women to men in this age group is 1·7:1, yet three times as many women are burned as men, primarily because of the nature of the clothing which accidentally catches alight. The other causes are fainting attacks or blackouts near a heat source, smoking in bed and scalds from leaking hot-water bottles.

Table 7.1 analyses a series of 1105 burns treated in Mount Vernon Hospital, Northwood, during the period 1954–59 and in Pinderfields Hospital, Wakefield, in the years 1966–69; the main differences in causation of burns in the various age groups are summarized.[33]

The figures for Europe and the United States are comparable. About 80 per cent of burns are domestic accidents. Clothing burns are the commonest cause of death. Various accounts of causation of burns in the less developed countries have been given by Antia[2] in Bombay, Tempest[43] in Nigeria and Mabrouk[26] in Egypt. In all cases children are at risk from open fires required for cooking and from fires in simple houses of non-brick construction. Paraffin stoves are also commonly used for cooking in these countries and explosions may cause severe burns. In countries such as India the sari type of clothing may accidentally catch fire. Migration of thousands of families from the country to cities and the fundamental change in their environment increases the risk of burns from unfamiliar cooking appliances for which inadequate instructions are available or cannot be read by the illiterate.

Table 7.1   The causation of burns in different age groups

Type of accident	Children, 0–14 (%)	Adult, 15–64 (%)	Elderly, 65 + (%)
Scald	42	8	13
Flame burn	28	30	43
Epileptic attack or blackout	1	13	42
Other (chemical, electrical, flash, contact)	29	49	2

Reproduced by kind permission of the authors and publishers.[33]

There is considerable scope for prevention of burns in all countries in all parts of the world, which the World Health Organization and the International Society for Burn Injuries are now studying.

Burns in war

High explosive bombs are unlikely to cause burns unless the explosion occurs in a confined space. An urban terrorist bomb of 13·5 kg (30 lb) may produce a fireball up to 18 m (60 ft) across. This is immediately dissipated in the open air but, in a confined space with solid walls, the heat is reflected on to the victims and also raises the air temperature. Partial-thickness flash burns may result.

In warfare, injury from incendiary attacks from the air with conventional weapons has produced devastation comparable with the two attacks with nuclear weapons on Hiroshima and Nagasaki. At Hamburg in 1943, hundreds of tons of incendiary bombs (together with high explosive 'block-busters') caused a fire-storm destroying 60 per cent of the city and killing at least 65 000 persons. A second fire-storm destroyed Dresden in February 1945, engulfing 21 km² (8 square miles) of the centre of the city in flame and causing an estimated mortality of 135 000; 70 per cent of casualties probably succumbed to asphyxia or carbon monoxide poisoning rather than to fire.[22] The atomic attack on Hiroshima destroyed a city and 80 000 people. Death was caused by the terrific heat at the centre of the explosion and the secondary fires started over a wide area, from the concussion and destruction of buildings and from exposure to gamma-radiation. The development of nuclear weapons can escalate these horrors.

Burning in aircraft accidents is rare except in the destruction of an aircraft which ignites on impact. Injury to the limbs may prevent even the slightly injured from escaping the flames. Tank crews are particularly at risk from severe burns. Anti-tank missiles penetrating steel cladding produce fires of intense heat in the enclosed space. The results are severe soft tissue wounds, extensive burns and pulmonary injury. Of the total injured in the 1973 Yom Kippur War, 10 per cent were burn casualties.[5]

Napalm has been developed as a particularly effective weapon against military targets. Petrol, which is volatile, burns in one relatively large, harmless flash. It is modified by mixing with additives which change its flow properties. It is thus cohesive but also adhesive, sticking to surfaces as burning gobbets. Rubber was used in 1935 but, in 1942, an aluminium soap obtained from coconut oil, naphthenic acid and oleic acid produced a particularly effective thickener. 'Napalm' (a name derived from aluminium naphthenate and palmitate) is now a generic term for all types of thickened hydrocarbons used as incendiary agents. These include synthetic polymers such as polyurethane or polystyrene, and may be modified further by mixing in other materials such as aluminium powder or metal carbonyls. White phosphorus or magnesium are usually added to ignite these oil-based incendiaries. As weapons they produce very high temperatures on burning, well in excess of 1000°C (1832°F), and, since they are adhesive, targets ignite easily. The effect on individuals is devastating. The full-thickness burns are usually extensive (over 25 per cent of the body surface), the phosphorus present causes toxic injury and the adhesive properties make the material impossible to remove. In closed spaces the available oxygen is used up and death may follow from carbon monoxide poisoning or asphyxia. The inhalation of hot gases may cause asphyxia from obstruction of the air passages or destruction of the alveoli.

Phosphorus burns as encountered on the battlefield or in industry may cause death even if only 12–15 per cent of the body surface is involved.[40] Burning phosphorus causes a lesion which progresses until either all the phosphorus is consumed or the area of the lesion is deprived of oxygen, e.g. by immersion in cold water. Pain is severe. The wound is necrotic and yellowish, smells of garlic and glows in the dark. Apart from the actual burn, there is primary renal damage from specific toxic injury, with glomerular and tubular necrosis causing oliguria and early death from renal failure. Liver damage may occur later. It is suggested that inorganic phosphorus enters the bloodstream and is the cause of these toxic changes.[23] For decades it has been advocated that copper sulphate is the optimum substance for the therapy of burns due to organic phosphorus; it produces an inert shell of cupric phosphide over the surface. This reaction may be effective but it may also result in copper toxicity, manifested primarily by the massive haemolysis of red cells and subsequent acute renal failure.[11, 40]

Burns mortality

Although the incidence of burns can only be estimated, the mortality is accurately known and is recorded in the UK in the Registrar-General's statistical review. There has been a slight fall in deaths over the last 10 years, primarily due to a decline in the deaths of children and young adults. This is probably associated, in part, with the control of gram-negative septicaemia by topical antibiotics and also with some success in campaigning for prevention.

Statistical methods must be used to assess the efficiency of the treatment of burns. Mortality is the index of therapy most amenable to analysis and interpretation and is least liable to subjective error.

The simplest method is to calculate the case mortality in relation to the two factors most likely to determine the death of patients—their age and the size of the burn. This can be done as scatter diagrams showing survivors and those who die plotted against age and the percentage full-thickness burn. Figure 7.2 shows the curve of mortality in patients

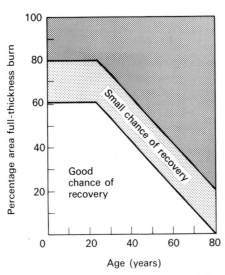

Fig. 7.2 A simplified form of 'probability' chart showing how the chances of recovery vary with age and with the area of the burn. (Reproduced by kind permission of the authors and publishers.[34])

treated at a large and active Burns Centre in the UK (Mount Vernon Hospital, Northwood). Not one of the patients whose co-ordinates met in the dark stippled area survived.[34]

This method, while giving a satisfactory rule of thumb assessment of a given patient's chance of surviving (and hence some comfort to relatives or to counsel), is a gross over-simplification. Very small numbers of patients are being considered in certain age groups. The clinical outcome in these small groups may vary and the resulting sampling errors make accurate comparison with other units impossible. Bull and Fisher[8] utilized probit analysis to construct a grid of mortality probabilities for various combinations of age and surface area involved. A revised grid was published[7] in 1971 and should be used for assessing modern results. However, it is based on only 122 deaths in 1922 patients admitted to the Birmingham Accident Hospital in the period 1965–70. Comparable figures from Massachusetts General Hospital[4] differ significantly since, once again, the curves are being constructed from minimal data exaggerating random effects (Fig. 7.3).

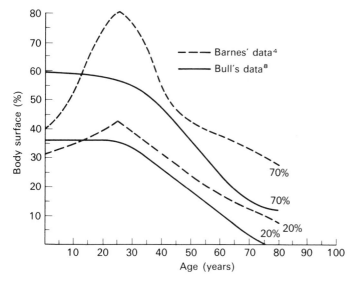

Fig. 7.3 Iso-mortality contours for various ages and percentage of area burned.

A mortality square can be prepared comparing the expected mortality from probit figures with the actual mortality relating to the numbers treated in any age group and area burned in any given burns unit. Changes in management and therapy can thus be assessed and also the theoretical prognosis for any individual patient. Recently, more precise statistical methods have been used to determine which characteristics of burns most significantly affect their prognosis.[29] Again, mortality is the end-point being investigated and such data as the patient's age, sex, extent of burn and whether or not he is prone to *Pseudomonas* infection are recorded to determine which significantly affect prognosis. These statistics are then subjected to discriminant function analysis.* Once the relevant factors have been identified, then the efficacy of treatment regimes can be assessed and management analyses or work load and material provision calculated.

The pathology of the shock phase

Immediately following burning, a series of pathological changes will occur, and an untreated patient will pass into a state of shock. A greater or less depth of skin may be destroyed but deeper layers, although still viable, are severely affected by the heat. The capillaries become widely dilated and, as the permeability of the walls increases, fluid is rapidly lost from the plasma into the extracellular space, causing gross oedema and a loss of circulating blood volume. At the same time, there is further fluid loss or blister formation if the surface of the burn is moist. The rate of loss of fluid is rapid for some hours but slows over the following 2–3 days, when reabsorption of oedema fluid occurs. This lost circulating blood volume must be replaced by intravenous transfusion if the area burned is greater than 15 per cent of the body surface in an adult or 10 per cent in a child. Transfusion may be with plasma, dextran or saline. Full-thickness burns may not cause oligaemia in the lean, elderly patient since interstitial oedema may be minimal. These patients may survive for days without intravenous fluids, succumbing eventually to infection.

Extensively burned patients now usually survive this period of resuscitation and their general condition will improve clinically. The pathophysiological factors which give rise to grave circulatory and metabolic disorders in the first 3–4 days post-burning cannot be identified precisely histologically or in terms of cellular physiology. Only the biochemical or physical effects of the injury can be described.

Occasionally, even in apparently well-treated patients, cellular membrane changes may cause abnormalities in the intracellular electrolytes, which cannot be deduced from examination of the plasma electrolytes. These changes have been referred to as the 'sick cell syndrome' by Allison et al.[1] and are associated with loss of intracellular potassium and its replacement by abnormal levels of sodium. Tissue hypoxia should be corrected and the administration of insulin and glucose may help the restoration of normal cell membranes.

Red cells may be destroyed at the burn site in deep burns or be

---

* This essentially represents an attempt to determine from which of two distinct populations an observation or event has originated. A value will be derived by analysis of past experience and, in an individual case, the value will be calculated and related to it. If it is greater, the patient belongs to one group; if less, to another—in this case, survivor or victim. Multiple factors can be taken into account and compounded and data are treated in a continuous manner without clustering exaggerating random effects.

rendered abnormally fragile and filtered out in the reticuloendothelial system. However, an additional red cell loss continues for unknown reasons and may require early transfusion of whole blood.[31]

Renal failure, which is discussed in detail in Chapter 19, may follow delay in instituting treatment for shock. Three types of renal failure are describe in burns:

1. Acute renal failure during the initial shock phase is invariably fatal and is associated with very severe burns, probably themselves likely to prove lethal. Urine output falls below 35 ml per hour in spite of adequate fluid replacement.[39]

2. Uraemia without anuria is typically a later phenomenon at the end of the shock phase or some days later and has been described by Sevitt.[38] Necrosis of the distal convoluted tubules is described but, though the prognosis is grave, dialysis may be successful.

3. Kidney failure with haemoglobinuria follows rapid destruction of red cells and only occurs if the concentration of plasma haemoglobin is over 1·2 g/litre. The precise part these factors play in renal failure is doubtful since it is not easy to eliminate others which may be equally relevant.

The symptoms of the shock phase relate to the extent of the area burned rather than to the depth of burning. Formulae for determining the transfusion rate rely on the 'rule of nines' for assessing the surface area burned in adults[44] (Fig. 7.4) and on the weight of the patient. The surface area covered by any patient's hand with fingers extended and closed equals 1 per cent of the body surface.

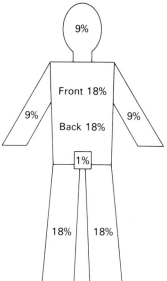

Fig. 7.4 'Rule of nines' for determining surface area in adults.[44]

Subsequently, monitoring the physical signs, the urine output, the central venous pressure and the changes in capillary haemoglobin or haematocrit level enables the physician to adjust the rate of transfusion to the patient's needs more precisely.

The local severity of the burn varies from simple erythema and blistering (as in sunburn) to deep charring down to muscle and bone, depending on the injurious agent. Different classifications have been proposed at different times and in different countries. Numerical degrees of burning (i.e. 'first' or 'second' degree burning, etc.) can be misleading and descriptive assessment of the depth of skin destruction is to be preferred, i.e.

Partial-thickness skin loss
{ superficial
  deep

Whole-thickness skin loss

In the first, although the epidermis is completely destroyed, epithelial elements remain in the hair follicles, sebaceous and sweat glands and re-epithelialization can eventually occur from these centres. The time required will vary with superficial or deep loss from 2 to 6 weeks. In the former case, the regenerating epithelium will be elastic, supple and appear normal whereas, in the latter, there may be extensive hypertrophic scarring which may cause deformity and disfigurement. Deeper partial-thickness burns, which are treated by exposure, dry out and deteriorate further since the exposed dermis may be damaged or destroyed by the continued desiccating process. Blisters, early homograft-

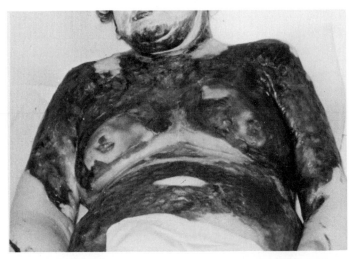

Fig. 7.5 Deep, full-thickness burn eschar in an elderly woman, resulting from ignition of clothing.

ing or tangential excision and grafting may avoid this;[16, 17] the more rapid healing thus achieved may limit scarring and disfigurement.

In whole-thickness burns *all* the epithelial elements of the skin are destroyed. The area of destroyed skin becomes hard, black and dry (Fig. 7.5), and fibroblasts and actively dividing capillaries gradually create a layer of granulation tissue in the living tissue adjacent to the dead skin or eschar. Autolytic enzymes in this layer eventually—in weeks or months—loosen the slough which comes away, exposing the granulating surface. Healing can only occur from the edges and in untreated cases may still not be complete months or years later. Collagen is found in the granulating tissue which becomes scar tissue and creates gross deformity by contraction. Skin grafting not only speeds healing but also reduces deformity by limiting scar formation.

The depth of a burn will depend on the temperature and the exposure time. Water above 60°C which is in contact with skin for 10 seconds will cause partial thickness skin loss and, above 70°C, will result in full thickness skin loss.[6] Hence, water will produce scalds at well below boiling point although blood flow may cool the skin (the temperature of bath water averages 36–42°C). The temperature of the skin/object interface should not exceed 42°C if any object is to be handled comfortably or is to be in contact with the skin for any appreciable time. The skin proteins coagulate and full thickness burns result if the deepest layers of the skin reach a temperature of 45°C. It follows that cold water is unlikely to be effective as a first-aid measure to prevent burn injury unless it is applied within seconds of contact.

Burn wound infection

Burns are open wounds and are thus liable to invasion by bacteria. Infection of the wounds is still the most difficult problem to overcome in treatment; it is now the major contributory factor causing death and remains so in spite of the development of new and more effective antibiotics. For a short period post-burning, the surface of the wound is generally sterile. Within 48 hours, bacteria reach the surface of the burn and colonize the depths of the necrotic eschar. The source of these bacteria includes not only organisms from the patient's natural bacterial flora (skin or bowel) but also the hands and respiratory tracts of those in attendance, the other patients in the vicinity and the ward environment.

Having colonized the eschar, bacteria multiply and invade the underlying living tissues, producing local infection or generalized septicaemia. The raw, moist granulation tissue may be likened to a gigantic agar plate which is actively supporting the growth and multiplication of bacteria. Keeping the eschar dry and cool limits bacterial growth but does not prevent it. Early removal of slough and the use of autogenous or homologous skin grafts helps to prevent infection. Indeed, this may be the only hope of survival in the elderly, even with relatively small burns; their immunological competence may be very low and they are thus particularly susceptible to infection. In addition, burns units demonstrate the proven principles of isolation to prevent cross-infection and utilize non-touch techniques, protective clothing, gloves and the rigid control of the circulating air for the same purpose.

The degree of invasion may range from microscopic foci of bacteria adjacent to the eschar to diffuse bacterial infiltration of all the soft tissues with generalized septicaemia. In examination of pseudomonal burn wound sepsis, involvement of 2000 cm^3 (122 in^3) of previously viable subcutaneous tissues has been found, a magnitude of infection which is equal to seven times the volume of tissue involved in massive diffuse bilateral pyelonephritis.[41]

The clinical pictures associated with burn wound sepsis caused by gram-positive, gram-negative and yeast organisms differ in several respects.[24] In patients with *Staphylococcus pyogenes* invasive sepsis there is extensive liquid suppuration of the subcutaneous fat with an insidious course over 2–6 days. They may be severely disorientated and hyperpyrexial with considerable gastrointestinal ileus. Hypotension followed by oliguria is frequent and the white cell count is raised.

The picture associated with *Ps. aeruginosa* invasive infection is characterized by black patchy necrosis or gangrene of the granulations, which is usually seen within a period of 12–36 hours of death. The clinical course is very rapid but usually free from disorientation; the temperature is seldom raised and the leucocyte count may fall below 3000/mm^3.

Invasive infection with *Candida albicans* occurs in patients who are extensively burned and debilitated and who have usually been on long courses of broad-spectrum antibiotics. The downhill course is slow but steady. The granulating wounds are dry, flat and yellow-orange in colour. It may well be that pathogenic yeasts, fungi and viruses may become a major problem in the future. Already infection with a bacterium, *Providencia stuartii*, has been reported resistant to all available antibiotics.[35]

At post mortem the microscopic and bacteriological examination of subcutaneous tissue can only be achieved by careful techniques. The examination of cubes of tissue excised and immediately immersed in 100 per cent alcohol and flamed for 5 seconds has been described by Teplitz.[41] Subsequently the cubes are transected and the central portions can be cultivated on a Petri dish; the colonies can be counted and, in addition, a microscopical examination can be made.

The visceral manifestations of septicaemia may be apparent in only 30–50 per cent of patients dying from pseudomonal burn wound sepsis; this correlates well with the frequent sterile blood cultures. On the other hand, staphylococcal septicaemia is associated with extensive metastatic infection and positive blood cultures. Thus, it is the liberation of toxic bacterial products from the site of the primary infection which is fatal in pseudomonal infection whereas, in staphylococcal septicaemia, it is the haematogenous spread of sepsis to the viscera.

Healing may still occur satisfactorily if the body's defences can match

the virulence of the organism. However, infection may delay local healing, particularly if viable epithelial cells are killed, thereby converting
partial- to full-thickness loss. Toxins may be absorbed causing general
symptoms, and bacteria will cause cellulitis and generalized septicaemia.

The β-haemolytic *Streptococcus* was the organism most feared in the
days before penicillin. It is now easily controlled by antibiotics and is
rarely a problem. Once established it effectively destroys surviving
epithelial cells or skin grafts. *Staph. pyogenes* is widely found in the
hospital environment and most burns are colonized. The body's
defences are effective but the organism develops resistance to penicillin
and to newer antibiotics with depressing regularity; these resistant
strains may become endemic in burns wards and will require special
measures to control them. In recent years, the gram-negative *Ps. aeruginosa* has become increasingly troublesome. It produces large
amounts of pus containing toxins which kill surviving epithelial cells
and may cause generalized toxaemia. In addition, the large volume of
exudate may float off skin grafts, complicating or delaying healing.

Much experimental work on the use of 0·5 per cent silver nitrate
solution, mafenide, gentamicin and silver sulphadiazine as topical
antibacterials has resulted in some reduction in the number of fatal
cases of septicaemia in extensive burns, particularly in the 20–40-year-
old age group.[21, 24, 37]

Apart from the evidence of infection, post-mortem examination of
burn fatalities may show evidence of intercurrent disease, particularly
in the elderly. Terminal bronchopneumonia or congestive cardiac
failure may result from the enforced immobility and contribute to the
fatal outcome.

The appearance of burned skin

The appearance of the burned surface in life is a measure of the intensity of the heat stimulus and is not a reliable indicator of the depth of
the burn.[15] Thus, a very high temperature applied for a short time may
scorch the surface while deeper layers survive; by contrast, a scalding
fluid which continues in contact with skin from adherent garments may
produce surprisingly deep burns. Simple erythema is always superficial
and blistering usually so. As the superficial layers are lost, the deeper
layers are pink and viable. However, mottled red and white areas unaffected by pressure cause difficulties in diagnosing depth. The redness is
due to the passage of the red cells from damaged dermal capillaries into
the tissues; the white areas are burned and may later turn red. These
appearances are more likely to be areas of full-thickness loss unless the
skin is particularly thick, as on the back.

Burns which are black or brown and leathery hard, particularly if
black thrombosed veins are visible through them, are obviously deep.
Occasionally, however, pale skin with apparently normal texture but
with no evidence of circulation and loss of elasticity is mistaken for

normal. The appearance is due to prolonged exposure to relatively low temperatures.

The presence of sensation (reaction to pinprick) indicates that a skin area is viable. Absence suggests full-thickness loss although oedema may give misleading results.

The causation of the burn is a useful guide to the anticipated depth of burning. Burns associated with loss of consciousness are invariably deep, as are those associated with flame (e.g. clothing burns); scalds or fat burns are usually of deep partial thickness.

Pulmonary complications of burns

Burns of the air passages can result from the inhalation of flame or hot smoke and have a grave prognosis. The lips and mouth usually show signs of burning and the same changes will be present throughout the respiratory tract. Tracheostomy and humidification of the inspired air is urgently required at the first signs of respiratory distress.

Progressive pulmonary insufficiency[37] complicates thermal injury, as, indeed, it may complicate hypotension from any cause. The only sign of underlying pulmonary injury in an otherwise fit patient after resuscitation is persistent spontaneous hyperventilation that fails to respond to oxygen inhalation. There is later a progressive decrease in the arterial Po_2.

The cause is either disruption or injury of the capillary endothelium of the lung or increased capillary hydrostatic pressure leading to interstitial and alveolar oedema. Fluid accumulation alters the rate of blood flow, the ventilation dynamics of the alveoli and the diffusion characteristics of the capillaries. The condition is reversible with treatment.

Pulmonary complications arise early when there is carbon monoxide inhalation; this often occurs in conflagrations in confined spaces or in incendiary warfare. In addition, fire may produce poisonous fumes which can cause death; thus, burning polyurethane foam (used as upholstery) forms lethal toluene di-isocyanate. Inhalation injuries from the entry of steam or smoke into the lungs, causing tracheobronchitis, are preceded by a period free from symptoms but, later, acute bronchitis supervenes with casts and hypoxia. Mafenide acetate, used as a topical antibiotic, acts as a respiratory stimulant, producing hyperventilation and inhibiting carbonic anhydrase; the pulmonary response to a 40 per cent or more body burn is exaggerated.[36] The late pulmonary complications of thermal injury include bronchopneumonia which may be either haematogenous or airborne. It is very common in the elderly and associated with immobility.

Acute gastric and duodenal ulcers described by Curling[9] are still found as complications of acute burns. They are morphologically identical to acute stress ulcers. The incidence in an American series was 47 per cent although few showed symptoms.[41] The absence of inflammation is characteristic and, almost certainly, the ulcers develop in the terminal stages of the patient's illness. Severe visceral vasoconstriction may also be a factor. The blood loss is seldom obvious or serious enough to warrant transfusion.

Table 7.2 lists the occurrence of the major factors contributing to the cause of death in 88 burn autopsies.[42]

Electrical burns

In the UK the majority of electrical burns are due to contact with the domestic electrical supply at 220–240 volts AC, but burns due to contact with high voltage grid systems (11 000–66 000 volts AC) or to overhead wires on the railway (25 000 volts) are seen in adventurous boys, in attempted suicides and in accidents to engineers.

The true electrical burn is due to the passage of electricity through the tissues between the two points of contact of the current or from one to earth. The severity will depend upon the strength of the current (itself dependent on the voltage and skin resistance—which may be very low if the skin is wet) and the time for which contact is maintained.

The skin component is clearly demarcated corresponding with the area of contact. Deeply, the degree of damage decreases with the square of the distance. The depth is invariably full-thickness, and the area of destruction is seen as a dead-white slough with a rim of bright red capillary injury (Fig. 7.6). Gradually over the weeks, the slough separates and final healing is slow if untreated. In severe burns, tendons and bone can be progressively exposed and thrombosis of main vessels may cause gangrene distally. In high-tension injuries the current enters through the skin and passes up the core of the limb, causing extensive necrosis of all soft tissues. Gangrene from vascular insufficiency may necessitate amputation. If the current passes through vital organs—e.g. the brain or the heart—the systemic effects are more serious, with loss of consciousness or cardiac arrest.

Table 7.2 Major contributing pathogenic factors found in 88 cases of fatal burns injury (US Army Surgical Research Unit, 1961–63)

Pathogenic factor	Occurrence (%)
Sepsis (type not specified)	93
Burn wound sepsis (flora not specified)	74
Burn wound sepsis (Pseudomonas)	39
Infected transfusion site with infected emboli	7
Pulmonary oedema	32
Other mixed pulmonary alteration	20
Bronchopneumonia (grossly significant)	13
Tracheostomy complications	7
Acute tubular necrosis of kidneys	11
Gastroduodenal ulceration	7

Reproduced by kind permission of Dr. Curtis P. Artz.[42]

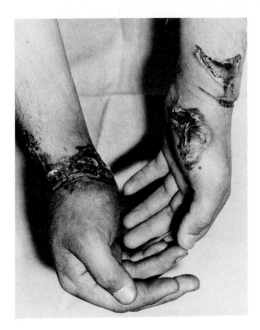

Fig. 7.6 Electrical burns 1 week after injury.

In addition to the passage of the current, burns can occur due to electric flash with or without actual contact. The hand may be covered by a black film of volatilized metal which gives a strange appearance but may not be associated with injury to the underlying skin. Flash or arcing, however, can ignite clothing and cause burns from conflagration.

Contact with the hot elements of the domestic electric fire (which still occurs in toddlers who can insert their hands between the protective grid compulsorily fitted) causes pure heat burns which behave as such and not as true electric current burns. Even a switched-on electric fire which is not red-hot can cause severe burning to the fingers and palm.

Lightning burns are rare although about 150 persons are killed each year in the United States. They can cause both thermal burns and injury to many body systems. A flash of lightning is estimated to release a charge of 20 000 amperes at thousands of millions of volts lasting 30 ms.[13] It may be 6 m (20 ft) in diameter and 1·6 km (1 mile) long. The charge may be conducted by metal objects or trees to living creatures in contact. Surviving cases will generally receive only partial-thickness burns while those who sustain full-thickness skin loss will usually succumb to respiratory or cardiac arrest which, in other cases, will only be temporary. As with all electrical burns, the injury is deepest where the current is concentrated at the entry and exit points.

Many organs can be damaged by lightning blast and the injuries are reviewed by Milward.[27] He describes a case of a patient suffering a 3-

week period of gastric dilatation and obstructive jaundice but recovering.

Burns in oxygen-rich environments

So far, burns at normal atmospheric oxygen levels have been described. In oxygen-rich environments, such as hyperbaric chambers or space capsules, the fire risks are very different:[10]

1. The spark energy required to ignite normal clothing may be as slight as the electrostatic spark from the human frame.
2. The rate of burning is increased fivefold if the air is replaced by oxygen at 101 kPa (1 atm) and flame propagation is equally fast.
3. Conventional flame-proof fabrics, paints or insulating materials burn fiercely when the oxygen concentration exceeds 30–40 per cent.
4. Smothering is ineffective in extinguishing a conflagration in oxygen.

The consequence is a greatly increased risk of severe burn injury and difficulty in providing adequate protection. In oxygen-rich atmospheres, normal denim overalls are consumed in flames in 20 seconds. A total body burn would be received in this time. Protective clothing burns slower; the best protection is a tight, single layer of lightweight open-mesh fabric. Flame-proofing prevents flash-over and a water sprinkler system—from the sides as well as from overhead—would control any conflagration although hidden areas (e.g. the axillae or crutch) would continue to burn. The trigger mechanism for such a spray would have to be effective within 20 seconds to save life.

Chemical burns

The most serious chemical burns will be seen in industry or perhaps in military conflicts. However, domestic and laboratory mishaps or even deliberate criminal assaults, though causing smaller burns, are more frequent and cause many problems.

The injury is due both to thermal and chemical changes in the tissues except that, with phosphorus, the latter predominates. Damage may be deep as the chemical penetrates the soft tissues. Table 7.3 summarizes the pathophysiology of chemical injury.[3]

Treatment aims at rapid neutralization of the agent by dilution with large quantities of water or by a specific antidote if one be known. The skin loss is managed by early debridement and skin grafting if necessary. The scarring following healing may be particularly unsightly with a strong tendency to contracture.

Friction burns

Friction burns occur in road accidents, usually at low speeds and are due to the exposed soft parts being dragged along the rough surface of

Table 7.3　Summary of the effects of chemical burns

Agent	Mechanism of action	Appearance	Texture
Acid burns Sulphuric Nitric Hydrochloric Trichloroacetic Phenol	Exothermic reaction, cellular dehydration and protein precipitation	Grey, yellow, brown or black, depending on duration of exposure	Soft to leathery eschar, depending on duration of exposure
Hydrofluoric	Same as other acids plus liquefaction and decalcification	Erythema with central necrosis	Painful, leathery eschar
Alkali burns Potassium hydroxide Sodium hydroxide Lime	Exothermic reaction, hygroscopic cellular dehydration with saponification of fat and protein precipitation	Erythema with bullae	Painful, 'soapy' or slick eschar
Ammonia	Same as other bases plus laryngeal and pulmonary oedema	Grey, yellow, brown or black; often very deep	Soft to leathery, depending on duration
Phosphorus	Thermal effect, melts at body temperature, runs, ignites at $34°C$ ($93·2°F$), acid effect of H_3PO_4	Grey or blue green, glows in dark	Depressed, leathery eschar
Mustard gas	Vesicant, alkalization effect	Marked erythema with vesicles and bullae	Painful, soft vesicles and bullae
Tear gas	Weak acid effect	Similar to superficial partial thickness flame burn	Soft and wet

Reproduced by kind permission of Dr. Curtis P. Artz.[3]

the road. They are seldom deep but are deeply ingrained with dirt and grit; it is essential to remove this by gentle scrubbing or dermabrasion before healing occurs in order to prevent permanent tattooing of the skin. In industry, contact with moving belts or wheels may cause skin loss, the seriousness depending on the period of close contact.

Burn scars

The major adverse sequelae of healed burns are hypertrophic or keloid scar formation and scar contracture, both of which can cause severe disfigurement and functional disability. The initial result of the healing of burns, with or without skin grafting, may be acceptable but, over the ensuing months, the soft areas of healed epithelium become increasingly livid, indurated and raised above the surrounding normal skin, contracting across flexor surfaces. This contracture always limits the range of movement but may be so severe as to dislocate joints.

Hypertrophic scarring occurs only in the deep partial-thickness burn when the deeper portion of the reticular dermis is injured. In addition, there appears to be a racial or familial predisposition to heavy scarring. The quality of the healed skin is much improved and hypertrophic scarring minimal if the deep dermis is preserved—either by preventing extension of the depth of the burn by controlling infection[21] or by achieving early healing by tangential excision of the superficial coagulated burned areas and immediate split-skin grafting of the exposed zone of stasis and punctate bleeding.[16, 17]

Fortunately, although hypertrophic scarring is common and, indeed, usually to be expected following deep partial burns, the scars gradually become paler, softer and flatter though they remain as permanent blemishes. This improvement will not begin until 6–12 months have elapsed from healing and the scars may irritate excessively during this time (Fig. 7.7).

All free grafts tend to shrink, thin ones more so than thicker or full-thickness grafts. Contractures therefore follow most severe burns when split-skin is required to achieve skin cover and late reconstructive procedures may be necessary (Fig. 7.8).

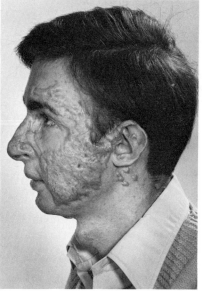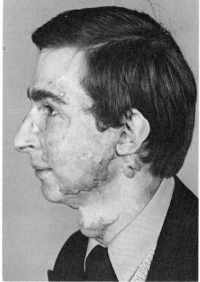

Fig. 7.7 (*a*) Hypertrophic scarring from deep partial thickness burns 6 months after injury. (*b*) The same patient, after 3 years' maturation of scars and intralesional injection of triamcinolone.

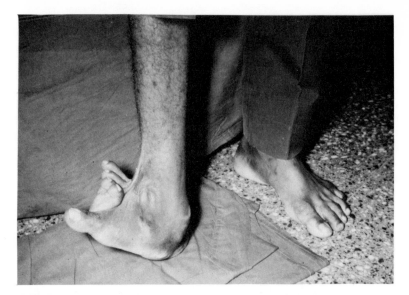

Fig. 7.8   Severe contractures of the foot following the healing of untreated burns in childhood.

Grafts on flexor aspects will shrink more than those on extensor aspects since they are not put on the stretch. Deformity may be limited if surrounding undamaged skin is drawn in to take the place of the shrinking graft. Immobilization and splinting to maintain extension may succeed but must be maintained effectively and continuously for at least 3 months while the graft (which must be of good quality) matures. Children respond to such treatment better than do adults since permanent joint stiffness is less likely. If joint movement is severely limited, the joint capsule may be secondarily contracted and the congruency of the joint surfaces impaired. This sequence of events can be especially crippling in the fingers and hands where immobilization other than in the position of function will aggravate the changes due to scar contraction. Treatment to speed the natural resolution of hypertrophic scars is unsatisfactory. It has been demonstrated that compression bandaging speeds such maturation.[19] Intralesional injection of 0·5 per cent triamcinolone (a form of cortisone) is also advised. Exposure to deep X-rays, though popular in the past, is now considered neither effective nor safe. Excision and resuturing or regrafting of the burns is unlikely to improve the quality of the skin unless the direction of the scars can be improved; it is not advised on purely aesthetic grounds.

Established contractures will require treatment either by redistributing the available skin (e.g. by Z-plasties) or by inserting more skin, usually as free grafts of thicker skin. Pedicle skin from a distance will not contract and may be used over exposed bone or joints and to permit subsequent secondary reconstructive surgery of injured tendons or nerves.

Unstable scars, usually over deep fascia, muscle or bone (particularly when this lies subcutaneously as in the lower limb), will frequently break down following minimal trauma and cause chronic and persisting ulceration. Apart from the morbidity there is the possibility of malignant change taking place in the unstable scar tissue, the so-called Marjolin's ulcer. These are usually squamous cell carcinomata but basal cell lesions also occur after a latent period of several years when chronic ulceration has been neglected. Less commonly, keratoacanthoma has been described in newly healed scars.[28] Such lesions may represent a disorder of wound healing lying between the hypertrophic burn scar and typical burn scar cancer.

True keloid scars, though frequently diagnosed, are rare and very difficult to treat. Essentially they are identical in their early stages to hypertrophic scars but, unlike the latter, they are progressive and tend to involve adjacent undamaged skin (Fig. 7.9). They do not resolve with the passage of time. Although much work has been devoted to the

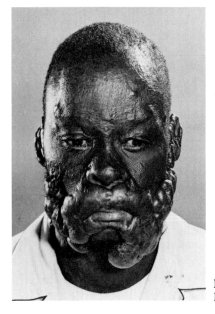

Fig. 7.9 True keloid scarring following burning in a Nigerian.

problem, the essential nature of keloid remains unknown. Simple excision and resuture invariably results not only in recurrence but also in recurrence in a more florid form. There is certainly a racial and familial tendency which may have accounted for the apparent high incidence of keloid scarring in radiation burn victims in Japan.

Gubianni[14] has described a type of fibroblast in a granulating wound in guinea-pigs, characterized by intracellular fibrils, 4–8 nm (40–80 Å units) in diameter, deeply indented nuclei and a rough endoplasmic reticulum. These he has called myofibroblasts and they appear to have a contractile function. Similar cells have been found in burn wounds and in cases of Dupuytren's contracture of the hands. They may account for the centripetal contractile forces at work.

Electron microscopy demonstrates the maturation of scar tissue and shows how the rigid collagen bundles with multiple nodules forming solid mats gradually give way to the loosening of the bundles with the matrices becoming much less dense as the scar softens.[20]

The biochemical changes associated with the maturation of scars still remain a confused mixture of incidental observations.

However well treated burns may be, the social and psychological consequences in determining the final outcome must be recognized. The patient's fear and horror following the accident can lead to despair when he finds the disfigurement, loss of earnings, social isolation or destruction of his marriage are distinct possibilities or even probabilities. Although a frank depressive illness is rare, most patients pass through a period of dependence and depression characterized by a feeling of uselessness and inertia. This must not be allowed to culminate in withdrawal altogether from close relations and friends or from the normal environment. Too frequently, delay in settling claims for damages and compensation militate against recovery and effective return to work.

Following the period of intensive care, the whole attitude of those in contact with the burned patient must be directed towards restoring his morale and self-confidence, once again enabling him to take his place in society. This has never been more clearly demonstrated than by the success which the late Sir Archibald McIndoe, and his team of surgeons, had in treating and rehabilitating burned aircrew at East Grinstead during the Second World War.[30] His precepts should continue to guide burn surgeons today.

Nevertheless, burn scars are still too frequently permanently disfiguring. Research must be directed not only to improving the survival of patients but also to improving the quality of the healed burn scar and reducing the aesthetic problems which invariably complicate severe burns—however much we may try to ignore them.

References

1. Allison, S. P., Hinton, P. and Chamberlain, M. J. (1968). Intravenous glucose tolerance, insulin and free fatty acid levels in burned patients. *Lancet* **ii**, 1113.
2. Antia, N. H. and Somaya, P. H. (1966). An interim report on burns accidents in the city of Bombay. In: *Research in Burns*, p. 193. Eds. A. B. Wallace and A. W. Wilkinson. Edinburgh and London: Churchill Livingstone.
3. Artz, C. P. and Moncrief, J. A. (1969). *The Treatment of Burns*, p. 225. Philadelphia, Pa., and Eastbourne: W. B. Saunders.

4. Barnes, B. A. (1957). Mortality of burns at the Massachusetts General Hospital 1939–1954. *Ann. Surg.* **145**, 210.
5. Ben-Hur, N. and Soroff, H. (1975). Combat burns in the 1973 October War and the anti-tank missile burn syndrome. *Burns* **1**,217.
6. Bull, J. P. (1963). Burns. *Postgrad. med. J.* **39**, 717.
7. Bull, J. P. (1971). Revised analysis of mortality due to burns. *Lancet* **ii**, 133.
8. Bull, J. P. and Fisher, A. J. (1954). A study of mortality in burns: a revised estimate. *Ann. Surg.* **139**, 269.
9. Curling, T. B. (1842). On the acute ulceration of the duodenum in cases of burns. *Med. Clin. Trans. London* **25**, 260.
10. Denison, D. M. (1966). The fire hazards to man in oxygen-rich environments. In: *Research in Burns*, p. 41. Eds. A. B. Wallace and A. W. Wilkinson. Edinburgh and London: Churchill Livingstone.
11. Dotin, L. N. and Ritchey, C. R. (1968). White phosphorus burn, hemolysis and copper sulfate therapy—a clinical and laboratory study. *Brooke Army Medical Center Annual Research Progress Report*, sect. 39, June 30.
12. Gil, D. G. (1970). *Violence Against Children*, p. 35. Cambridge, Mass: Harvard University Press.
13. Goldstein, D. H. (1971). Electric shock. In: *Cecil-Loeb Textbook of Medicine*, 13th edn. p. 43. Eds. P. B. Beeson and W. McDermott. Philadelphia, Pa., and Eastbourne: W. B. Saunders.
14. Gabianni, G., Ryan, G. B. and Majno, G. (1971). Presence of modified fibroblasts in granulation tissue and their possible role in wound contraction. *Experientia* **27**, 549.
15. Jackson, D. McG. (1953). The diagnosis of the depth of burning. *Brit. J. Surg.* **40**, 588.
16. Jackson, D. McG. (1969). Second thoughts on the burn wound. *J. Trauma* **9**, 839.
17. Janžekovič, R. (1970). A new concept in the early excision and immediate grafting of burns. *J. Trauma* **10**, 1103.
18. Keen, J. H., Lendrum, J. and Wolman, B. (1975). Inflicted burns and scalds in children. *Brit. med. J.* **4**, 268.
19. Larson, D. L., Abston, S., Evans, E. B., Dobrokovsky, M., Willis, B. and Linares, H. A. (1971). Development and correction of burns scar contracture. In: *Research in Burns*, p. 403. Eds. Matter, P., Barclay, T. L. and Koničková, Z. Bern, Stuttgart and Vienna: Hans Huber.
20. Larson, D. L., Baur, P., Linares, H. A., Willis, B., Abston, S. and Lewis, S. R. (1975). Mechanisms of hypertrophic scar and contracture formation in burns. *Burns* **1**, 119.
21. Lowbury, E. J. L. (1975). Recent studies in the control of burn infection. *Burns* **2**, 26.
22. Lumsden, M. (1975). *Incendiary Weapons*, Chap. 3, p. 163. A Stockholm International Peace Research Institute Monograph. Cambridge, Mass: MIT Press.
23. *Ibid.*, Chap. 4, p. 199.

24. MacMillan, B. G. (1975). Burn wound sepsis—a 10 year experience. *Burns* **2**, 1.
25. McNeill, D. C. (1976). A survey of 1600 admissions to a regional burns unit. In: *Recent Advances in Plastic Surgery—1*, Chap. 7. Ed. J. Calnan. Edinburgh and London: Churchill Livingstone.
26. Mabrouk, A. W. R. (1966). Burns in the UAR. In: *Research in Burns*, p. 191. Eds. A. B. Wallace and A. W. Wilkinson. Edinburgh and London: Churchill Livingstone.
27. Milward, T. M. (1975). Prolonged gastric dilatation as a complication of lightning injury. *Burns* **1**, 175.
28. Monafo, W. W. and Bohling, C. (1975). Keratoacanthoma arising in newly healed burn scars. *Burns* **1**, 172.
29. Moores, B., Rahman, M. M., Browning, F. S. C. and Settle, J. A. D. (1975). Discriminant function analysis of 570 consecutive burns patients admitted to the Yorkshire Regional Burns Centre between 1966 and 1973. *Burns* **1**, 135.
30. Mosley, L. (1962). *Faces from the Fire*, the biography of Sir Archibald McIndoe. London: Weidenfeld & Nicolson.
31. Muir, I. F. K. (1971). Red cell destruction in burns. *Brit. J. plast. Surg.* **14**, 273.
32. Muir, I. F. K. and Barclay, T. L. (1974). *Burns and Their Treatment*, 2nd edn., p. 2. London: Lloyd-Luke.
33. *Ibid.*, p. 7; 34. *Ibid.*, p. 53.
35. Pruitt, B. A. (1974). Infections caused by *Pseudomonas* species in patients with burns and in other surgical patients. *J. infect. Dis.* **130**, S8.
36. Pruitt, B. A. and Curreri, P. W. (1971). The burn wound and its care. *Arch. Surg.* **103**, 461.
37. Pruitt, B. A., Erickson, T. R. and Morris, A. (1975). Progressive pulmonary insufficiency and other complications of thermal injury. *J. Trauma* **15**, 369.
38. Sevitt, S. (1956). Distal tubular necrosis with little or no oliguria. *J. clin. Path.* **9**, 12.
39. Sevitt, S. (1974). *Reactions to Injury and Burns*, Chap. 7. London: Heinemann Medical.
40. Summerlin, W. T., Walder, A. I. and Moncrief, J. A. (1967). White phosphorus burns and massive haemolysis. *J. Trauma* **7**, 476.
41. Teplitz, C. (1969). Pathology of burns. In: *The Treatment of Burns*, Chap. 2. Eds. C. P. Artz and J. A. Moncrief. Philadelphia, Pa., and Eastbourne: W. B. Saunders.
42. *Ibid.*, p. 27.
43. Tempest, M. N. (1966). Burns in a tropical climate. In: *Research in Burns*, p. 184. Eds. A. B. Wallace and A. W. Wilkinson. Edinburgh and London: Churchill Livingstone.
44. Wallace, A. B. (1951). The exposure treatment of burns. *Lancet* **i**, 501.

8

Injuries sustained in mining and quarrying

Mining and quarrying are high-risk occupations from the point of view of injury and death. The only more hazardous occupation in Britain is deep-sea fishing;* in the United States, the four most injury-producing occupations are all associated with mineral exploitation.

In Britain, the number of accidents and fatalities has reduced progressively over the past few decades, but much of this reduction has been due to the contraction of the industry and the *rate* of injuries and deaths has declined much less markedly.

Although a major mining disaster which involves the deaths or incarceration of a number of men immediately becomes world-wide news, there is a much greater number of fatalities and serious injuries occurring on a day-to-day basis which receives virtually no publicity at all except in the Annual Reports of various bodies responsible for mining safety. When coupled with the high risk of occupational disease, the accidents in such industries add up to a formidable technological and even sociological problem.

Confining the discussion solely to traumatic events, the most recent year for which statistics are presently available in Britain is 1973. During that year, 102 workmen were killed and 647 seriously injured in mines and quarries. Of these, coal-mines accounted for 80 deaths and 533 injuries; other mines were the site of 8 deaths and 26 serious injuries. A comparison with the 1971 figures shows that, in spite of the rapid run-down in the size of the industry, no great improvement is occurring; in that year there were 72 deaths among coal-miners, 641 serious injuries and 76 463 other injuries causing more than three days' disablement. However, recognition must be given to the fact that energetic measures in mine safety have brought about a remarkable reduction in the hazards of the occupation over the past century. For instance, in 1861 there were 230 000 miners in Britain and 1061 fatal accidents. In that year, the death rate from coal-mining accidents was eight times that in all other occupations, which themselves were relatively hazardous under Victorian conditions. The expectation of working life in coal-miners in the latter half of the nineteenth century was only 27 years, compared with 33 years in the working population at large and 42 years among farm workers.

It has been mentioned that the rate of disabling injuries in coal-mines

* This has been overtaken by oil exploration (Chapter 17)—*Ed.*

easily heads the list of all occupations in the United States; in 1971 there were over 37 disabling injuries per million man hours. This must be measured against a mean rate for all US industries of only 9 disabling injuries per million man hours. These figures refer to the *number* of injuries, but the *severity* of pit injuries was also the greatest among American industries: no less than 4232 days were lost per million man hours from injuries in 1971. compared with only 611 as the average of all industries in general. The average number of days lost from work due to injury was 113 in coal-miners and 65 in American industry generally.

A number of aspects need to be discussed in relation to this very appreciable amount of mortality and morbidity. There is, first, the traumatic pathology of the actual lesions. Apart from some broad groups, there is little in the actual surgical pathology of injuries that is specific to mining conditions. But, from the point of view of legal responsibility and the understanding of the causes and possibilities of prevention of such injuries, a breakdown of the circumstances surrounding this type of trauma is useful.

Types of injury

Injuries sustained in mines and quarries are classified into three categories:

1. Minor injuries requiring first-aid treatment only, with a loss of working time of less than one shift.
2. Injuries necessitating hospital treatment and consequent loss of working time of at least one shift.
3. Fatal injuries.

In general terms, it has been found that the minor injuries much more often affect the upper limb, especially the hands and fingers, whereas more serious injuries tend to involve the lower limbs. Bettencourt and Jensen[3] point out that this phenomenon might well be explained by the fact that a worker with a hand injury may be placed on light duty and not classed as an admission to hospital, whereas a miner with a leg injury of equal severity may have to be confined to bed and thus lose shifts. In other words, the consequence of the injury is related as much to the anatomical situation as to the traumatic severity. The same authors have presented evidence to confirm that leg injuries result in the loss of more shifts per casualty than do other injuries, especially those of the hand.

The range of really serious injuries and fatalities is limitless and extends from massive crushing under rock falls to the noxious effects of gases. The changing pattern of mining technology in recent years has also altered the type of injuries—machinery and haulage mechanisms now account for a large proportion of injuries. Falls of roof, although still a serious hazard, are not as common as they were when the bulk of the work force was exposed to direct trauma from rock falls while engaged on manual coal-getting at the face.

Even so, one of the most typical injuries a miner can sustain is the hyperflexion injury to the spine, with all the possible consequences of paraplegia, which may follow a fall of rock on to the unprotected back or head. Death may occur rapidly from multiple injuries if the rock fall is massive but the classical 'traumatic asphyxia', due to fixation of the thorax by mineral rubble or pinioning by larger masses of rock, may also occur.

Traumatic asphyxia—a particularly inappropriate name, but one which is too well established to change—is seen almost exclusively in occupational situations. Burial in iron-ore bunkers, sand-pits, grain silos, collapsed trenches and mines and quarries provide most cases, together with the overturned vehicle, especially the agricultural tractor; the remainder of cases of traumatic asphyxia are seen in crush situations such as football crowds (Chapter 15). In the mining context, burial of the thorax so that the external respiratory passages are still clear produces a characteristic syndrome. The most florid asphyxial changes are seen, with gross congestion usually confined to the area above the thoracic inlet. The other characteristic feature is the production of punctate haemorrhages of the head and neck in such profusion and severity as is seen in no other condition. Petechiae and ecchymoses in the skin, lips, eyelids and scalp are very prominent and bleeding into the eyes is frequently so gross as to produce bulging conjunctival haemorrhages. All these signs are due to inhibition of the respiratory excursions of the chest, with consequent obstruction of the venous return and anoxia (Fig. 8.1).

Accidents due to machinery and haulage equipment produce the crushed and mangled limb as well as the whole spectrum of other multiple injuries from skull fractures to abdominal visceral lacerations. The limbs are particularly vulnerable due to the possibility of their being drawn into moving conveyor-belts and coal-cutting machinery: this sometimes necessitates emergency amputation to free the victim from total entrapment.

Underground or surface transport accidents may involve crushing between rail conveyances, between a vehicle and a wall, by free-moving machinery such as track loaders or between conventional surface vehicles. All these may show any of the features of rail or road accidents in other circumstances but crushing of the head, thorax and abdomen appears to be a particularly common lesion.

Head injuries are relatively common in spite of the safety helmet worn and range from massive damage due to falls of roof, through the transport-vehicle accident to examples such as the more bizarre type of injury described by Usher[7] where a steel wedge from a roof support was squeezed out under the ground pressure and acted as high-velocity projectile.

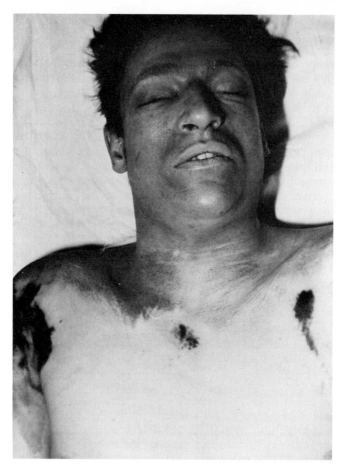

Fig. 8.1   'Traumatic' asphyxia due to fixation of chest by heavy object which has caused abrasions. The skin congestion and petechial haemorrahges are confined to the area above the thoracic inlet.

Spinal fractures

As to the actual surgical pathology of injuries, there is only one really typical lesion associated with coal-mining. This is the hyperflexion spinal fracture or fracture-dislocation, caused by a fall of roof—either of rock or of coal—upon a miner. Hyperextension injuries in this situation are very much less common. The hyperflexion lesion is due to the coal falling upon the head or shoulders of the miner, who may already be in a protective crouching position. The rock-fall impact is upon either the head—causing further flexion of the dorsal and lumbar spine —or, more commonly, asymmetrically upon one or other shoulder, thus imparting a rotational element to the hyperflexion. As the dorsal spine tends to be protected by the rigidity of the thoracic cage, most of the strain falls upon the lumbar spine and it is in this position that fractures or fracture-dislocations are common.

In a classic paper in 1949, Nicoll[4] described 166 spinal fractures or fracture-dislocations of the dorsolumbar spine, which occurred in 152 miners from the Yorkshire coalfields. According to Nicoll, the mechanism is triggered by a fall of coal on to the miner who is usually placed with his head between his knees. The dorsolumbar region is likely to be injured when the main impact is upon the shoulders; the lumbar or lumbosacral region is more vulnerable if the impact is lower down. Nicoll noted that the pelvis tended to be fixed by the tight hamstring muscles if the knees were extended at the same time—this caused greater stress in the lumbosacral region. There were no examples of hyperextension fractures in this study; such fractures are rare in the dorsolumbar region though they are occasionally seen in the cervical spine.

Nicoll's paper is especially valuable, being one of the few comprehensive analyses of such typical mining lesions. His work showed that two-thirds of the bony injuries were confined to three vertebrae—

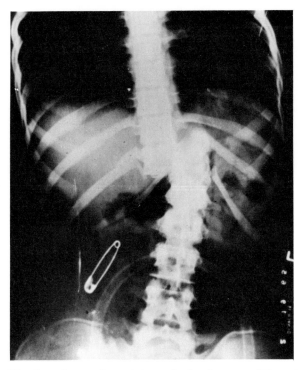

Fig. 8.2 Lower thoracic hyperflexion fracture of the spine, with marked displacement and paraplegia from cord damage. (Photograph by courtesy of Professor B. McKibbin.)

the twelfth thoracic and first and second lumbar. Twenty per cent of the 166 fractures involved the lowest thoracic vertebra, 30 per cent the first lumbar and 16 per cent the second lumbar vertebra. The incidence dropped off rapidly above and below these lesions except that the third lumbar vertebra was frequently involved.

The precise lesion was most commonly an anterior wedge fracture of a vertebral body, this occurring in almost 60 per cent of cases. The fall of coal or rock upon the upper part of the body causes great flexion strains in the lower spine; the nucleus pulposus acts as a fulcrum and the anterior margins of the vertebral bodies are compressed. In most of the cases described by Nicoll, this wedging was not extreme but, when there was extensive damage, the posterior longitudinal ligament was ruptured due to the rotational effect about the nucleus.

A lateral wedge fracture occurred in 14 per cent of cases and there was a fracture dislocation, with rupture of the posterior interspinous ligament, in almost 20 per cent of cases. This leads to displacement and is more dangerous as far as involvement of the spinal cord is concerned. Damage to the cord or cauda equina is very frequent in fracture-dislocation, occurring in over 60 per cent of Nicoll's series. There were

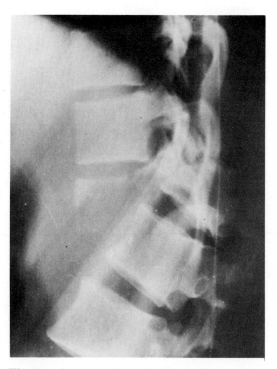

Fig. 8.3 Lateral radiograph of hyperflexion fracture of dorsolumbar spine, with gross displacement and cord damage. (Photograph by courtesy of Professor B. McKibbin.)

20 cases of paraplegia in the whole group of 152 miners; 18 of these were associated with fracture-dislocations and 2 with lateral wedge fractures (Figs. 8.2 and 8.3).

A less common bony lesion in this hyperflexion injury was isolated fracture of the neural arch, which occurred in less than 10 per cent of cases.

It can be reiterated that this type of injury appears to be the only characteristic lesion sustained in the mining profession, all other types of trauma being as are seen elsewhere in industrial, traffic and transportation accidents.

Falls of roof

The physical cause of the typical injury described above is still one of the most common and most serious of mining accidents (Fig. 8.4). Collapse of workings from the failure of roof supports is one of the specific hazards of mining and, although deaths and serious injuries due

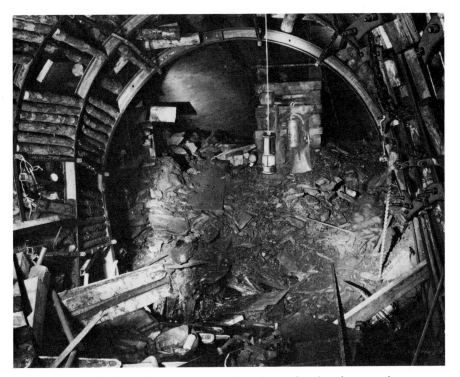

Fig. 8.4 A fall of roof in an underground roadway, showing the extensive damage and disorganization which adds to the difficulties of rescue and the identification of victims. (By courtesy of HM Chief Inspector of Mines and Quarries—Crown copyright.)

to falls of coal and rock have declined steadily in recent years, there were still 24 deaths and 148 serious injuries in 1971. By 1973 these had been reduced to 18 fatalities and 122 serious injuries, even though the latter year incorporated casualties from one major disaster involving an extensive fall of roof. The marked and progressive reduction of accidents from this cause correlates with the improvement of the older methods of working. Formerly, miners had to insert individual supports as they removed the coal and were, therefore, very exposed to falls; modern practice employs powered hydraulic supports.

The various parts of the mine workings have a markedly different potential for accidents and deaths due to falls of ground. Men in 'stables' and road-head areas of power-loaded faces are particularly vulnerable in long-wall workings. Areas ahead of the front row of props, where powered supports are used in power-loaded faces, are also markedly at risk from falls of coal, these areas accounting for over 60 per cent of all accidents associated with falls of ground. One of the most dangerous situations in this respect involves the miner who crosses the face-side of the armoured conveyor where there is a deficiency of roof support in the narrow strip between the ends of the roof beams and the coal-face. Falls of ground may also occur in the 'waste'—the area behind the coal-face where the mineral has already been removed and where the roof is allowed to fall in as the face advances. Road-heads and new headings driven through rock to reach new workings may also be sites where unexpected roof falls may cause individual or group injuries which often have the hyperflexion characteristics described above.

Accidents from haulage and transport systems

The underground haulage and transport systems provide another serious source of death and injury. More deaths occur during the movement of men and materials underground than from roof falls. Although the accident rate has been declining in recent years, 63 men were killed and 547 seriously injured in haulage accidents between 1971 and 1973. The movement of supplies along roadways causes the largest single number of such incidents and the Annual Reports of HM Chief Inspector of Mines detail numerous other dangerous situations which cause fatal and serious injuries.[5] These include the illegal riding of conveyors by workmen, accidents on man-riding systems, the transport of material on chain conveyors and numerous mishaps from moving mining cars and locomotives. Here the province of mining medicine merges into engineering, safety provisioning and colliery administration.

Conveyors, that is chain or belt systems for the moving of mineral from the face to the pit bottom, are frequent sources of injury. The chains from power-loaded haulage systems are also often responsible for accidents. In British pits, 150 accidents have been caused by these chains since 1967, frequently due to breakage of the chain or chain oscillation caused by misalignment of the face conveyor; in 1973, 4 men were killed and 51 seriously injured by machinery underground, almost half of them from haulage chains. Other accidents occur when conveyors are being advanced towards the coal-face or when they are being repaired. False starts and other defects of safety procedures are frequent causes. Men cross conveyors illegally and transport material other than coal upon belt conveyors with consequent damage. Materials falling off conveyors or sliding out of control on steep gradients may cause injuries and deaths.

Haulage of trucks along tracked systems in underground roadways is another hazard, injuries being due to actual running down, crushing between separate cars or between cars and the roadway wall; defects in the track itself are relatively frequent and include lack of fish-plates, poor track alignment and badly spaced sleepers. As with conveyors, steep gradients may lead to accidents from derailment or from cars running out of control. The period during the manual coupling or uncoupling of a sequence of mine-cars is particularly dangerous; crushing of the head, thorax or pelvis between two moving cars is relatively common. All types of accidents seen in similar surface conditions may occur with free-running trains hauled by locomotives. Misunderstanding of signals and instructions, especially during shunting operations, leads to a number of injuries and deaths, as does derailment; men may be crushed on curves where there is inadequate clearance between the rail-cars and the tunnel wall.

The author has seen a number of fatalities associated with the clearing up of spilt coal in close proximity to a moving conveyor. The moving-up of conveyors and coal-cutters appears to carry relatively high risks, especially from false starting of the electric power when workmen are not expecting this to happen. In heavy-duty coal-cutting machinery, the residual energy in a tensed but static chain may have disastrous effects if the tension is suddenly released by a workman. The cramped conditions and poor lighting at the coal-face contribute to accidents in these situations. Much trouble is admittedly due to contravention or short-cutting of established safety procedures.

Explosives and blasting

The number of deaths and injuries from explosives and blasting devices has dropped markedly in recent years; there were 2 such fatalities in 1972 and none in 1973. Similarly, the number of explosions of firedamp (methane) underground has been greatly reduced. Those which still occur are now caused by ignition from frictional sparking, by cutting or power-loading machines or from electricity rather than from the older causes of lamps and contraband; 18 out of the 20 explosions occurring in 1973 were caused in this way. In spite of the very strict regulations about shot-firing, accidents still occur from confusion over the number of charges exerted and from premature or unexpected detonation. Men may remain too near the scene of the firing and, in spite of protective screens, may be struck by material projected from the explosion.

Fire and explosions

The number of fires is relatively small, though they have not decreased in recent years—in fact, the 1973 figures for Britain showed a marked increase. The majority of fires were caused by mechanical friction from belt conveyors or by electrical faults.

Together with falls of roof, the underground explosion and fire is the classical and most feared incident associated with coal-mining. Major accidents are, thankfully, very few but it is these rare mass-casualty situations which arouse immediate interest in the news media, sometimes on a world-wide scale. The worst mining disaster in history was that due to ignition of finely divided coal-dust at the Honkeiko Colliery in China on 26 April 1942 when 1572 men were killed. The worst disaster in the United Kingdom occurred at the Universal Colliery, Senghenydd, Wales, on 14 October 1913; 439 men were killed due to ignition of firedamp, possibly by an electrical signalling device.

Deaths and injuries in mines from fires and explosions follow the same pathological pattern as do burning or blast injuries in other situations; most of the difficulties are associated with reaching victims, rescuing trapped men, performing emergency medical service in difficult situations and eventually in retrieving and identifying the victims. There have been very few deaths from fires and explosions in British mines in recent years but the danger is always present, being kept at bay only by continuous and rigorous preventive measures and maintenance of supervision. The two principal sources of widespread fire and explosion in mines are firedamp (methane) and coal-dust in finely divided form.

All coal contains methane which in itself may cause trouble even without ignition. In anthracite mines, 'outbursts' of gas and finely divided dust are common and in 1971 caused 6 deaths and 69 disablements from pure asphyxia in a single incident at Cynheidre Colliery (Fig. 8.5). A mixture of 5–15 per cent methane with air is potentially a most violent explosive.

Finely divided coal-dust is also explosive but it is less so than is the methane mixture and it requires a more vigorous ignition than does firedamp. Coal 'dust' is present even before the disturbance of mining operations; it is present in the 'cleats', the natural stratified joints in the seams. This dust is very finely divided and is liberated into the air of the workings when there is destruction of the face from any cause. It is also naturally augmented by the disruption of mined coal and by the subsequent operations of transporting it to the pit bottom.

Although a dust–air mixture is less explosive than is firedamp, a mixture of gas and dust is extremely dangerous because, if the gas is ignited, it acts as a secondary igniter to the dust cloud. This process is self-propagating; in the Universal Colliery disaster in 1913, the flame travelled along the tunnels as far as 6 km (4 miles) from its origin. A flame can move at between 20 and 2000 m s^{-1} (22–2200 yd/sec); this is in advance of the blast wave, which is considerably slower. The

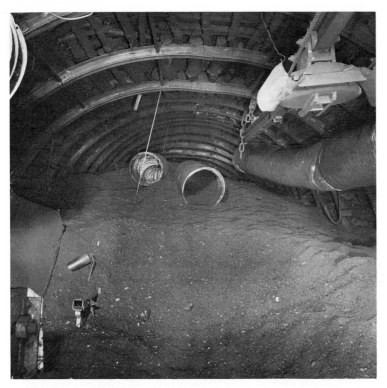

Fig. 8.5 An 'outburst' of finely divided coal in an anthracite mine in South Wales. Up to a 1000 tons of coal-dust may be released along with methane in such an occurrence. In this particular tragedy, asphyxia caused 6 deaths. (By courtesy of HM Chief Inspector of Mines and Quarries—Crown copyright.)

primary ignition of the methane–air mixture may be due to frictional causes, especially from conveyors, from electrical sparking and faults from contraband matches, etc. and from lamps; it sometimes apparently occurs spontaneously (Fig. 8.6).

One of the most important advances in the control of fires and explosions was that proposed in the early part of this century by Professor Galloway of Cardiff, who suggested that the use of an inert substance such as stone-dust could break the cycle of self-propagation of progressive flame-ignition. The aim was to form a non-combustible barrier which was automatically activated by the explosion itself. This was achieved by suspending loads of inert, non-siliceous stone-dust in the roofs of the roadways from where the explosion itself would dislodge the material into the air so as to blanket the flame effect.

As far as the traumatic pathologist is concerned, there are no particular features in colliery fires and explosions which distinguish them from non-mining accidents. Where men are exposed to flame only, they tend to show no physical trauma, but only the signs of surface burning,

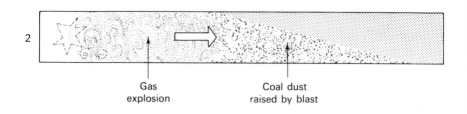

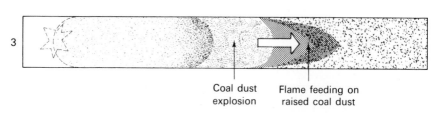

Fig. 8.6 Diagram illustrating the progression of an underground explosion. (Original drawing from Health and Safety Executive—Crown copyright.)

carbon monoxide poisoning or anoxia. On the other hand, there may be gross injuries when explosions have occurred although secondary injuries resulting from collapse of the workings may often mask those due to the original explosion. Workmen who are actually injured by the blast, or who are burnt or poisoned by carbon monoxide, may still be killed at a distance by asphyxiation from the lack of oxygen which has been used up in the fire or explosion process. Where reconstruction of the accident is attempted in retrospect, it should be remembered that men may travel long distances underground away from the origin of the explosion and also that partial carbon monoxide poisoning may make their movements and actions irrational.

The problem of identification following mining disasters rarely presents the difficulties encountered in aircraft crashes or railway accidents. It is very unusual for a large number of men to be involved in a single event and, due to the nature of the work and the very strong camaraderie, the roll-call of men underground is well known and the actual position of men in the workings is established with fair accuracy. The vast majority of mining fatalities occur in ones and twos, where identity rarely presents any problem for an appreciable length of time. Sometimes bodies are never recoverable as, for instance, when workings have collapsed or where fire and gas make it impracticable for rescue work to continue. In these cases, the workings may be closed down while still containing the bodies of the victims. It is thought that 26 bodies from the Universal Colliery disaster of 1913 still remain underground.

Causes of accidents

The causes of accidents as far as the miners themselves are concerned has been investigated extensively. Rogan[6] summarized the findings of Bettencourt and others[1, 2] which, although derived from gold-mines, probably reflects the situation in mines generally. They investigated the assumption that experienced men would be less likely to be involved in accidents than men more recently entered into the occupation. This being so, there should be an inverse relationship between the ages of the miners and the incidence of accidents due to the longer sojourn of older men in the industry. This was not, however, found to be substantiated in practice. Although the accident rate declined to the age of about 34–37 years, it subsequently began to rise again. Bettencourt and his colleagues discovered that the relevant factor was not the total experience in mining but, rather, it was the experience in a particular task. The indications were that a miner with considerable experience of one aspect of the job was little better as an accident risk than was a new man if he was transferred to another task underground. There seemed to be a minimum period of about 4 months during which accidents were more frequent.

Other workers have investigated personality traits among 'accident prone' workers and have shown that, as with vehicle drivers, a lack of inhibition and aggressive behaviour generally tended to correlate with a higher accident rate.

Quarries

Though quarrying is a surface occupation very different from deep underground coal-mining, many features are similar as far as the causation of accidents is concerned. Much depends upon contact with moving machinery and vehicles.

In 1973, 14 men were killed and 88 seriously injured in quarries in Britain (which totalled 3717). There has been a slight but progressive decline in the number of fatalities over the past few decades but the level of serious injuries has shown little decline. Incidents with vehicles—both the 'getting' vehicles such as loaders, cranes, excavators and scrapers and the more conventional trucks used for transport—formed the largest single group of accidents.

Over half the deaths in quarries involved vehicles, and haulage and transport accidents generally accounted for 40 per cent of all reportable accidents.

Falling and slipping, mainly from buildings and structures associated with the quarry rather than from rock faces, was another potent source of injuries. Falls of rock were relatively unimportant, although they caused 2 deaths and 1 serious injury in 1973. As in coal-mining, conveyor belts proved a danger, both from entrapment of limbs and from minerals falling from the conveyor on to workers.

No characteristic injuries can be attributed to quarrying; the hyperflexion injury of coal-miners is not seen in the quarrying situation due to the absence of a direct source of impact from a roof fall.

Summary

The accident medicine of mines and quarries presents little that is specific to the working conditions but the variety of mechanization now present in mines, together with the usual cramped working space and artificial lighting, adds up to a concentration of hazards which are a distillate of the dangers present in a surface environment in a more diffuse form.

An appreciation of the traumatic hazards of mines cannot be fully gained without some first-hand knowledge of the conditions underground. In attempting to reconstruct the circumstances of an accident from a retrospective study of the bodily lesions, a meaningful contribution to the investigation—which may have important medicolegal and prophylactic connotations—must take the underground environment into consideration. Because the vast majority of mining fatalities and accidents are so closely linked with the 'hardware' of intensive modern coal-getting, it is impossible to divorce the medical aspects and, indeed, the traumatic pathology from some understanding of the modern technology of mining.

References

1. Bettencourt, J. J. and Jensen, A. (1967). *An Analysis of Underground Accidents in a Gold Mine.* Unpublished Report. Chamber of Mines, South Africa, Johannesburg.
2. Bettencourt, J. J. and Jensen, A. (1967). *An Analysis of Injuries to Drilling Crews and Stope Team Labourers in a Mine.* Unpublished Report. Chamber of Mines, South Africa, Johannesburg.
3. Bettencourt, J. J. and Jensen, A. (1970). A Statistical Analysis of Accidents to Bantu Personnel in the Gold Mining Industry. *Jl. S. Afr. Inst. Min. Metall.* **71**, 105.
4. Nicoll, E. A. (1949). Fractures of the dorso-lumbar spine. *J. Bone Jt Surg. B* **31**, 376.
5. Reports of HM Chief Inspector of Mines and Quarries (Annually). London: HMSO.
6. Rogan, J. M. (1972). *Medicine in the Mining Industries.* London: Heinemann Medical.
7. Usher, A. (1964). An unusual mining fatality. *Med. Sci. Law* **4**, 42.

9

Stabbing and other knife wounds

Classification of wounds

Wounds can be divided into superficial injuries such as abrasions (grazing of the epidermis), contusions (rupture of dermal capillaries and veins with extravasation of blood) and injuries causing breaches of the intact skin. These last include lacerations, incised wounds and stab wounds.

Lacerations are splits or tears caused by blunt injury such as blows from a pickaxe handle or a bottle, or rolling or crushing injuries as sustained, for example, in road-traffic accidents; they occur particularly over bony prominences. The features of a laceration are ragged edges, crushing of the soft tissues and the driving of hair and foreign material, such as road grit, into the depths of the wound. Lacerations of the scalp following blows from a blunt weapon may sometimes superficially resemble incised wounds but more careful examination of such injuries, using a magnifying glass if necessary, usually serves to distinguish between them.

Incised wounds are caused by sharp instruments such as knives, razors or sharp-edged tools and by glass. They gape and bleed—often profusely.

Stab wounds are caused by a variety of implements. They result in penetrating injuries which may lead to rapid death from haemorrhage or air embolism or to delayed death from infection, pulmonary embolism or other complications.

Stab wounds may be due to accidents, as may occur in a butcher's shop, from suicide, although this is not common, or from an attack by an assailant. Stab wounds of the last type are usually associated with defence injuries, particularly to the hands and arms. Such injuries are incised or slashed and may be extensive and multiple. The interpretation of stab wounds is discussed later in this chapter.

In many malicious woundings the assailant and victim are under the influence of alcohol to varying degrees. It is regrettable that a large number of young men and adolescents in present-day society often carry knives or razors when they go out in the evenings—'all tooled up' in the vernacular—allegedly for self-protection but, often, to threaten or wound when arguments or fights arise; many woundings or killings are not premeditated in the true sense and the wounds are incised, as in

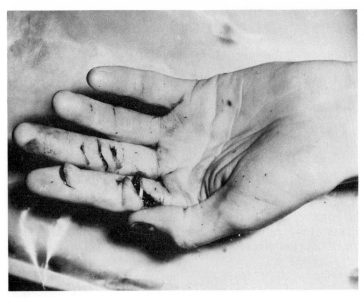

Fig. 9.1   Defence wounds of the hand caused by grasping the blade of the assailant's knife.

razor wounds of the face, or slashed, as in knife wounds of the face or arms.

Slashing injuries are, by their very nature, superficial and are fairly easy to assess, describe and interpret. Many occur on the hands and arms and are defence wounds caused by the victim attempting to ward off attacks by his assailant. He may put up his arms to protect his head and face or grasp the weapon or push it aside, sustaining cuts on the arms or palms, thenar or hypothenar eminences or on the palmar surfaces of the fingers (Fig. 9.1). Such injuries may not be obvious at autopsy when the hands and arms have been placed at the sides of the body during carriage to the mortuary and become fixed by rigor with the fingers in flexion. The pathologist should make a special point of examining the hands to the point of removing any protective plastic bags and later replacing them with fresh ones (to protect the hands from soiling during subsequent dissection).

Stab wounds

There are eleven points which must be considered in any case of stabbing:

1. The number of wounds.
2. The position of each wound.
3. The shape.
4. The length.
5. The depth of penetration.

6. The direction of thrust.
7. The force required to inflict the injuries.
8. The effects of such injuries.
9. The rapidity of such effects.
10. The ability of the.victim to carry on activity after being stabbed.
11. The interpretation of the injuries.

As to the *number* of wounds there may be one or many; the single stab wound, in many ways the easier to describe, is often the more difficult to interpret. The *position* of every stab wound must be recorded in the pathologist's notes, with photographs and drawings. The position should be related to fixed anatomical points such as the umbilicus or nipple which can be shown in photographs and which can be easily understood by a jury. The height above the heel must be recorded. The *shape* should be recorded graphically in the same way. A weapon with two cutting edges will cause a wound with sharp edges and clean-cut ends whereas a single-edged weapon will cause splitting

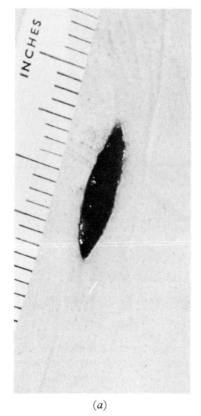 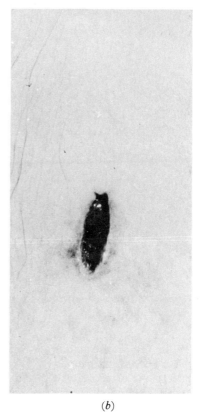

(a)   (b)

Fig. 9.2 (a) Stab wound caused by a knife with two cutting edges. (b) Stab wound caused by a knife with one cutting edge only. The blunt back of the knife has caused splitting of the upper end of the wound; so-called 'fish-tailing'.

or 'fish-tailing' at the end[3] caused by the blunt, non-cutting back of the weapon and a clean-cut end from the sharp edge (Fig. 9.2). When a double blunt-edged weapon, such as a closed pair of scissors, is used, the wound will be more rounded and will often be associated with surrounding bruising.

Whatever weapon is used, the shape of the wound will always become more rounded once the weapon is withdrawn, due to the elasticity of the skin; its slit-like character can be better seen in the deeper tissues, such as the rib cage, where a wound passing through the intercostal muscles is kept in shape by the rigidity of the ribs. The shape may be considerably distorted by the weapon being driven in one way and then pulled out at an angle, or the victim may twist or fall during the assault. The weapon may also be partially withdrawn and then driven in again. Such wounds may have a notched or scalloped appearance (Fig. 9.3).

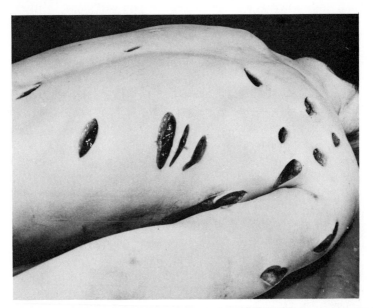

Fig. 9.3   Multiple homicidal stab wounds, many showing notching and undercutting.

The *length* of each entry wound in the skin must be measured with the sides approximated. Such a measurement can only be thereabouts due to the elasticity of the skin. It may be very misleading to photograph a rounded entry wound with a length of sticky measuring tape alongside it.

The *depth* of penetration can be difficult to assess. If there is bruising around a clean-cut wound in the skin, it suggests that the weapon has been driven in up to the hilt. Otherwise there is always the possibility that the weapon has only pierced the tissues for part of its length. The depth of penetration and *direction of thrust* are best established together by dissection. The wound in the skin may be undercut and slightly flap-like, giving a clue to the direction of thrust, be it upwards, downwards, medially or laterally.

Assessing the direction and depth of penetration has to be done on an *ad hoc* basis for each separate wound. This is rather easier in the thorax where the spine is fixed and the ribs are rigid. The chest can be opened and the site of the stab wound on the inner aspect of the rib cage inspected. The thoracic viscera can be examined in their turn, each wound being measured along the track.[4] If the track passes through the lung or heart, the viscera can then be removed and the back of the chest inspected for the final point of penetration. A probe can be passed under direct vision through the skin to the deepest point of penetration and the total length of the wound thus measured. If the wound extends only, say, into a cavity of the heart or partially into a lung, it may be possible—with the aid of a probe passed through the skin wound and chest wall into the injured viscus—to assess the depth of penetration.

When assessing the depth of penetration it is important to remember that the organs in a cadavar lying supine on a mortuary table are in different positions from those in the upright person in life where the heart is immediately behind the sternum and left ribs and the lungs fill the chest cavity.

The assessments are harder with wounds in the abdomen because the abdominal wall is soft. A thrust into the yielding abdomen may compress all the tissues; the depth of penetration, when the weapon is withdrawn and the tissues relax, may then appear to be greater than it actually is. For these reasons, it is very important to give only approximate measurements for the length of a wound track although the direction of the thrust may be reasonably easy to establish.

If necessary, for example in the neck, the track of a wound may have to be dissected by layers, this being the only way to assess the direction and depth of penetration. When a probe is used it is very easy to cause false passages or to enlarge or extend a wound track. The weapon itself should *never* be used, even if it is available, to see if it fits the wound as this will distort the wound and contaminate the weapon.

All such dissection and measuring must be performed on fresh tissue because fixation causes shrinkage and artefacts.

The correlation of the length and characteristics of the wound in the skin, the length of the wound track and its cross-section at various levels will give a profile of the weapon responsible and a minimum length for its blade. When a knife, say, is subsequently produced for the pathologist to examine, he should be able to decide whether or not such a weapon could have caused the injuries to the victim.

The *force* required to cause injury is often less than one imagines. Once the skin is penetrated the weapon slips easily through all the underlying tissues and viscera. Even the sternum and ribs do not require great force for their penetration or severance. The force required will be influenced by the victim's clothing, if he be wearing any. Multiple layers of tough cloth may render penetration much more difficult than a single layer of fabric such as a shirt. The words 'moderate force' are sufficiently non-committal and are true of the majority of cases.

The *effects* of the stabbing will vary with the direction and depth of penetration of the structures involved. Death will rapidly supervene if the aorta is severed but it is often surprising how much a victim with a potentially fatal wound can do prior to collapsing and dying. Many cases are on record where a victim with a penetrating wound of the heart or a great vessel has continued to grapple with his assailant, chased him or gone to fetch a weapon to retaliate before succumbing from fatal blood loss. It pays the pathologist to be guarded in his opinion of how long it took a victim to die.

Examination of the clothing
The pathologist should take very great note of the clothing of the deceased in all cases of wounding by a knife. The number of stab wounds in the clothing must be counted to see if they correlate with the number of wounds in the body itself. It may be that there are more wounds in the clothing than there are in the body. The usual explanation is that layers of material have been folded or superimposed before being run through with a knife. There may be a series of holes in the clothing overlying a single wound in the body if the fabric is subsequently stretched out and unfolded, perhaps during transportation of the body.[1]

It is important to see whether the positions of the holes in the clothing correspond with the wounds in the body, as this may give an indication of the position of the victim at the time of the stabbing. For example, if a hole in clothing appears not to overly a wound in the back of the body it may be that the victim's arm was raised at the time, pulling up his clothing with it. With the arm placed by the side of the body after death, the hole in the clothing will be considerably lower than the actual wound in the skin. Similarly, the skin wound may not correspond with the underlying injuries. For example, the track may appear to pass through the scapula although the bone itself is not obviously injured. This again is further evidence that the arm was raised and the shoulder-blade rotated, allowing a stab wound to penetrate the back without injuring the scapula itself.[2]

Blood stains on the clothing may appear to run down vertically over the clothing and splash on the uppers of the victim's shoes, indicating he was upright at the time of injury, or they may appear to run laterally or backwards, suggesting he was lying prone or in some other position.

Suicidal and homicidal wounds
The inexperienced pathologist may assume that multiple stab wounds in the front of the chest must be homicidal but this is not necessarily so. It is suggestive of suicide if there are one or more stab wounds in this

position and the clothing is drawn up. The surrounding circumstances, such as a room locked on the inside, a weapon in the hand of the deceased or beside him and a suicide note, may make the conclusion of suicide inescapable, particularly if the stab wounds are associated with slashing injuries elsewhere at sites of election such as the wrists or throat. Suicide by stabbing is not common but cases do occur from time to time (Fig. 9.4).

Multiple stab wounds are a feature of many homicides. The wounds vary in size, shape and depth and, the more wounds there are, the more tracks there are to dissect and measure. This may well prove tedious and time-consuming but the multiplicity of wounds does give a better

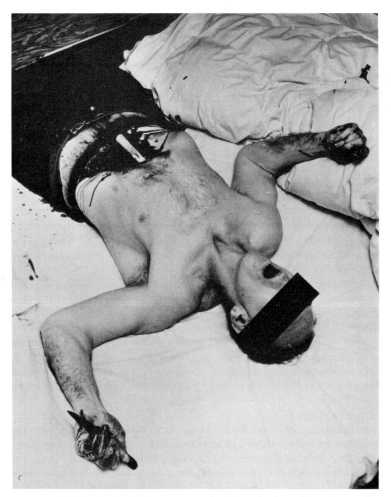

Fig. 9.4 Self-stabbing. Note the site of election in the epigastrium and a second knife fixed by rigor in the left hand.

chance of assessing the profile of the weapon responsible. One of the difficulties is that more than one knife may have been used to inflict the wounds on the deceased, as may occur in a gang fight. Here, patient dissection coupled with careful measurements should clarify the issue.

Homicidal stab wounds are frequently associated with defence wounds. Slashing wounds have already been described and some wounds may be penetrating, going, for example, through an arm—possibly severing an artery and even, on occasion, causing death. If there has been a struggle, not only will defence wounds be present but there may also be considerable variation in the stab wounds on the victim. They may be of different lengths and depths, some enlarged by rocking and twisting so that it may be difficult to assess what sort of weapon was used. However, there are nearly always one or two simple wounds where the blade appears to have gone in and come out cleanly and the pathologist should concentrate his attention on these.

He should always ask to see the alleged weapon if it is available and should have it photographed with a ruler beside it as well as describing it with measurements in his own notes. Rarely, the tip of a knife may break off during an assault. The pathologist should search for it carefully, if necessary using X-ray screening to locate and retrieve it.

Sometimes unusual weapons may be used to inflict stab wounds; such wounds may have bizarre appearances—e.g. the rectangular shape of the skin wounds caused by a chisel, or the cruciate incision caused by a drill. Really multiple wounds—40, 50 or 60—in a male victim suggest a homosexual killing, particularly if associated with sexual mutilation; the pathologist should, however, beware of reading too much into such injuries and usurping the function of the psychiatrist. It may be necessary with unusual injuries to experiment by stabbing a cadaver with possible implements to try to reproduce similar injuries to those in the victim. If such experiments are successful, the injuries produced should be photographed.

If the weapon is still lodged in the wound the pathologist must resist the temptation to pull it out himself and should agree with the police how it should be removed, bearing in mind the possibility of fingerprints being on its handle. He must also remember to collect clothing and a blood sample and hand them to the police as exhibits. He must excise the principal wounds as far as is practicable and retain them in case a pathologist acting for the defence wishes to make a further examination.

Reconstruction of events

The interpretation of some injuries is very clear—for example, the suicide scene described above, or multiple stab wounds in various parts of the body associated with defence wounds which can only be homicidal. The difficult stab wounds are those involving a single penetrating injury only. Some do happen accidentally; for example, when a boning knife slips and penetrates a slaughterman's groin or when a child at play falls on to railings which penetrate and, maybe, kill. Occasionally, a sporting event may be the scene of a tragedy such as when a javelin is thrown off target and strikes another competitor. Such incidents are unusual and others present can usually give independent accounts of what happened.

In the majority of potential homicides, an accused person will say that 'the deceased ran on the knife'. There is no doubt that the momentum of the moving body is more than sufficient to cause a fatal injury when it is impaled on a knife held rigidly. However, the knife must be held firmly and be sharply pointed; a blunt knife held limply will be turned aside by the approaching body. The combination of a victim moving forward and the stabbing thrust by the assailant is more likely to cause penetration and serious injury or death. Often the pathologist must concede in the witness box that the same injury could be caused by the victim running on a weapon held rigidly by the assailant just as by the assailant stabbing a motionless victim.

The presence of defence injuries may give the lie to the running on the knife story. The appearance and sites of wounds in the clothing may help to explain the posture of the victim as described earlier. The track of the wound may not match up with the explanation offered. Wounds that travel downwards and inwards in the body or upwards and inwards are usually caused by deliberate thrusts. A wound caused by running on a knife tends to be more horizontal in direction.

The interpretation of stab wounds is frequently made more difficult by the victim having been taken to hospital where heroic attempts at resuscitation, including major surgery, have been carried out. Wound tracks are frequently distorted or destroyed. It is imperative in such cases for the doctor who carried out such procedures to be present at the autopsy to assist the pathologist, who should not commence his autopsy on such a case until the clinician has arrived.

It is no more possible to lay down a complete set of rules which will cover every case of stabbing than it is for any other cause of violent death. The pathologist must use his common sense and alter his technique to suit each individual post mortem so that at the end of it he has all the details of each wound recorded in as many ways as possible and has retained the wounds and viscera relating to the cause of death.

Incised wounds

Apart from the stab wounds and defence injuries already described and illustrated, knives and other sharp-edged weapons, such as razor blades, may cause incised wounds. Like stab wounds, incised wounds may be caused accidentally in a great variety of ways, suicidally or homicidally.

Suicidal incised wounds are found classically in the throat, wrists, elbows or groins—the so-called sites of election (Fig. 9.5). They are nearly always multiple, they show varying depths of penetration and they are often superimposed. Some are superficial and only cut the skin—the 'tentative incisions'. Many of these self-inflicted wounds do

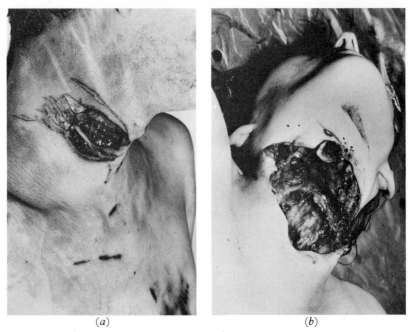

(a)   (b)

Fig. 9.5   (a) Suicidal cut throat. Note the multiple superimposed incised wounds, many of which are superficial. (b) Homicidal cut throat.

not sever major blood vessels and are not fatal. The clinician treating such cases in hospital should bear in mind the possibility of further attempts by the patient at self-destruction and guard against them; he should also consider the need for psychiatric help in treatment.

Homicidal incised wounds are often multiple; they involve the face and neck and are usually associated with defence injuries of the type already described. They lack the tentative cuts, superimposition and regular arrangement of the would-be suicidal wounds. Homicidal incised wounds may include genital mutilation.

Incised wounds of the neck may cause death either from massive haemorrhage when a carotid artery has been cut across or from air embolism, particularly where there has been partial severance of a jugular vein. In the latter case, death usually occurs within 2 or 3 minutes but some cases of delayed air embolism have been described.[5]

References

1. Cameron, J. M. (1976). Wounds and trauma. In: *Gradwohl's Legal Medicine*, 3rd edn., Chap. 15, Fig. 182. Eds. F. E. Camps, A. E. Robinson and B. G. B. Lucas. Bristol: John Wright.
2. *Ibid.*, Fig. 186.
3. Gresham, G. A. (1975). *A Colour Atlas of Forensic Pathology*, Figs. 138 and 139. London: Wolfe Medical.

4. *Ibid.*, Figs. 141–148.
5. Johnson, H. R. M. (1973). Delayed air embolism. *Forensic Sci.* **2**, 375.

Suggested further reading
6. Camps, F. E. and Cameron, J. M. (1971). Wounds. In: *Practical Forensic Medicine*, 2nd edn., Chap. 20. London: Hutchinson Medical.
7. Gee, D. J. (1975). Wounds. In: *Lecture Notes on Forensic Medicine*, 2nd edn., Chap. 15. Oxford: Blackwell Scientific.
8. Polson, C. J. and Gee, D. J. (1973). Injuries: general features. In: *The Essentials of Forensic Medicine*, 3rd edn., Chap. 3. Oxford: Pergamon Press.
9. Rentoul, E. and Smith, H. (Eds.) (1973). Medico-legal aspects of wounds. In: *Glaister's Medical Jurisprudence and Toxicology*, 13th edn., Chap. 9. Edinburgh and London: Churchill Livingstone.
10. Simpson, K. (1974). Types of injuries and wounds. In: *Forensic Medicine*, 7th edn., Chap. 5. London: Edward Arnold.

10

Sexual violence

Physical violence is not always a concomitant of sexual assault and a degree of violence may be acceptable between consenting parties. Violence may also be self-inflicted. This chapter takes little account of moral and legal questions although they are difficult to ignore in considering, for example, what constitutes rape. The law may declare carnal knowledge in some circumstances to be illegal; thus it is possible to commit an offence where there is neither violence nor lack of consent. Other texts must be consulted for details of technique in clinical examination.[15]

Considerations mainly physiological

An extended account of the physiology and psychology of sexual response has been given by Masters and Johnson.[17] Questions on such matters are frequent during cross-examination and those liable to give evidence in sexual cases should have some familiarity with them.

In sexually stimulating circumstances, the phase preparatory to coitus involves spontaneous vulval lubrication, labial engorgement and vaginal lengthening. Such changes are transient, seldom persisting beyond orgasm, although vulvar swelling is more likely to remain where such release is not obtained. The lubricant is a transudate through the vaginal walls, the production of which ceases when the stimulus is removed. Not only does production cease but the fluid quickly dries. Rugosity of the vaginal wall becomes less prominent with repeated intercourse, but not measurably so after a single act of intercourse. In summary, no invariable or reliable clinical finding is to be expected which indicates that coitus has recently taken place.

The gauge and distensibility of the introitus are frequently such that the first intercourse is accomplished without damage. Enquiry suggests that pain during defloration is common but bleeding less so. The absence of bleeding implies tearing through comparatively avascular tissue or stretching without tearing. Bleeding is occasionally so profuse as to cause death[11] or seriously to alarm the couple. In one such instance, where a bar of hymeneal tissue obstructed the vagina, its rupture caused severe bleeding and the girl's clothing became saturated. A story of rape was concocted. As she was shocked, the girl was admitted to hospital where she was examined under anaesthetic. The vagina was full of partially clotted blood and the bleeding points were ligated. Motile sperm were present and a prophylactic curettage was performed.

Positive evidence of defloration may be absent. Equivocal findings are those nicks of the free edge of the hymen which do not extend to the periphery. They may represent a small healed tear or the injury thought to be caused by repeated use of tampons. Injury to the hymen by fingers or other instruments is looked for anteriorly, whereas penile penetration causes a tear posteriorly, usually to one or other side. In the virgin, a crescentic hymen is the most common appearance, with a greater width of tissue posteriorly, so injury in this region is to be expected. Anatomical variations are legion.

Bleeding from the vagina during menstruation is a source of confusion. Menstrual blood is usually dark and characteristically does not clot. The menstrual flow is a mixture of endometrial fragments, vaginal squames and blood. As the last is derived from the dissolution of clot, its protein composition is different from shed circulating blood and it contains a much higher percentage of soluble fibrinogen. Whitehead and Divall[26] described immunoelectrophoresis of menstrual blood stains and favoured the view that its soluble fibrinogen is an early degradation product of fibrin.

When ejaculation occurs during coitus, seminal fluid is added to the vaginal pool. As the penis is withdrawn, so the pool is extended throughout the length of the vagina. Laxity of the parts or changes in the female's posture cause leakage, so allowing semen to stain the pubic hair, the perineum and the upper thighs (and, of course, bedclothes in appropriate circumstances).

Demonstration of human spermatozoa on a vaginal swab or in aspirated fluid is proof of intercourse. Can intercourse have occurred when no seminal fluid is found and clinical examination indicates virginity? Pregnancy is reported from time to time in virgins[8] but, in such cases, the definition of virginity becomes a matter of semantics. Immunological methods for identifying seminal fluid[2] cannot yet replace microscopy. Microscopic preparations are particularly well visualized by Papanicolau's cytological method, although methylene blue or haematoxylin and eosin are widely used.

The morphology of the sperm head is vital. Using Papanicolaou's technique, the head is seen as an oval body approximately 4.5 μm in length. The galea capitis covering the nucleus causes one end to be thicker and wider. The narrower cervical end takes up haematoxylin more strongly and the picture is similar to a dark-blue acorn sitting in a pale cup. Abnormal forms are frequent, increasing with the time since emission. Extruded and deformed nuclei, especially in association with thin strands of darkly stained mucus, may confuse the unwary. Wet preparations for motility are seldom of value in forensic work because live sperm are unlikely 10 hours after coitus.

Mant[16] concluded that sperm are demonstrable post mortem in the penile urethra of 75 per cent of men who have died below the age of 81 years and the percentage rises sharply when the death is anoxic. He found them less commonly in those dying of chronic infection, debilitating disease, carbon monoxide poisoning and cerebral haemorrhage. Unexpectedly, urethral sperm could be identified after prolonged immersion in water.

Failure to find sperm in material taken from the vagina soon after intercourse when there has been ejaculation may be due to poor technique by the examining doctor or in the laboratory; or sperm may be scanty, abnormal or even absent. The popularity of vasectomy has made the last more probable. Detection of seminal fluid from vasectomized males requires the demonstration of prostatic acid phosphatase, distinguishable from vaginal acid phosphatase by electrophoresis.[1] Davies and Wilson[7] found no sperm in only 1 per cent of swabs taken 36 hours after intercourse. Even after 48 hours two-thirds of the swabs were positive. Sperm complete with tails were uncommon after 16 hours.

Of the chemical tests, seminal acid phosphatase was found to be a useful factor within 24 hours of intercourse and choline (the Florence test) within 12 hours. Seminal blood group antigens were detected at useful levels only within 48 hours of intercourse. Baxter's immunological method is sensitive for 0.1 per cent dilutions of semen compared with 16 times that sensitivity using microscopy. These papers[2,7] referred to experimental results and are not likely to be reproduced in casework. Sharpe[23] indicated the perhaps more common experience in practice. He found motile sperm surviving for an average of 3 hours in the living vagina. Non-motile sperm he expected to find possibly up to 24 hours but he seldom found complete sperm after 12 hours.

Finally, in considering sexual mores from the medicolegal viewpoint, it is usual to class as abnormal various practices which are known to be widespread. These include biting (see below), fellatio and cunnilingus. Spermatozoa are occasionally found in routine throat swabs. The danger of the practice of oral intercourse lies in unintended asphyxia of the female. Several cases of sudden death from air embolism in pregnant women have been reported;[9] each involved the male in blowing into the vagina.

Bites

No classification is satisfactory which does not indicate that the teeth are not necessarily involved in causing the common 'love bite'. This lesion is an oval area of superficial punctate contusion, usually measuring at least 2.5 × 1.3 cm (1 × 0.5 in). It is seen most frequently at the side of the neck, overlying or anterior to the sternomastoid muscle. It is common also on the breast, less so on other parts of the body. The tissue 'bitten' must be loose and the mark is caused by forcible sucking applied to tissue seized by the mouth. The teeth are guarded by the lips and do not come into directed contact with the skin; indeed such an injury is easily produced by the edentulous. Within a few hours the punctate bruises coalesce and the contusion goes through the usual stages of resolution, disappearing within 5 or 6 days. Such a mark is not of odontological interest. Saliva is present and serology may assist in identification (see below).

Bites proper involve two mechanisms apart from any gripping by the teeth themselves. These are the suction already described, together with pressure by the tongue, forcing the bitten tissue against usually the palatal aspect of the teeth or the rugae of the palate. Such suckling[14] causes bruising where tissue is unsupported across any gap between teeth or at the cervical margin of the teeth. Bruises of this type may be sufficiently clear to characterize the teeth involved.

Scratches left as the teeth scrape across bitten material vary with the shape of the incisal edge and again are valuable in identification. Tooth pressure of itself, particularly if applied slowly by the incisors, leaves a crescent of pale areas caused by the incisal edges, each zone of pallor being limited by a penumbra of lividity.

The above are considered to be amorous, as distinct from aggressive, bites. Aggressive bites cause a degree of damage to the tissue. which is liable to impede identification (but see below—signs on assailant). Tissue damage, although caused by teeth, may not always be confidently so attributed and the first question for the pathologist is to ask himself if the pattern of abrasion or laceration is possibly dental. Thereafter he must seek the assistance of a dentist with appropriate experience before starting to dissect. He must also remember that biting of any description can scarcely be accomplished without the transfer of saliva, and the bite marks are swabbed with this in mind before any washing of a body.

As is the case with semen, so is ABO blood group substance present in readily detectable amounts in the saliva of the 80 per cent of the population who are secretors. To determine secretor status a sample of saliva, as the most accessible body fluid, is required. Saccharolytic enzymes in the saliva are destroyed by boiling to prevent destruction of the blood group substance.

Technicalities of the photographic and dental procedures followed in the well known murder at Biggar in 1967 have been described in detail.[12] The accused happened to have a rare degree of pitting of the teeth which added certainty to his dental identification. In that instance, the dental experts had no access to the body but worked purely from photographs.

Rape

This has been comprehensively defined as the carnal knowledge, to a lesser or greater degree, of a female not the wife of the assailant, without her consent and by compulsion, either through fear, force or fraud, singly or in combination.[22]*

It has been traditional to consider rape as requiring the victim to resist to the uttermost; no matter what degree of violence is used, she

* Rape is statutorily defined in England and Wales. A man commits rape if he has unlawful sexual intercourse with a woman who at the time of intercourse does not consent to it and at that time he knows that she does not consent to the intercourse or he is reckless as to whether she consents to it (Sexual Offences (Amendment) Act 1976, s. 1(1)).

must repel any attempt on her chastity. Successful treatment of venereal disease, ready access to therapeutic abortion and widespread use of
the contraceptive pill have tended to alter the balance. It is nowadays
asking a great deal of a girl to expect her to prefer throttling or having
her face slashed to sexual intercourse. Consent freely given has been
adduced as the significant criterion but no statute, however complicated, will relieve the Court of the duty to define consent in each
disputed case. Where the victim is alive, great assistance is given to the
Court by an experienced police surgeon but much depends on the
impression created by the complainer during her evidence.

Genital injury
There is too great a disparity between the capacity of the introitus in
the very young and the erect penis to allow sufficient vaginal dilatation.
Penetration thus causes vulvar tearing (Fig. 10.1). As seen in obstetric
injury, the tear may extend into the rectum with consequent damage to
the sphincter mechanism of the anus (Fig. 10.2). Should the posterior
vaginal wall rupture, access is gained to the peritoneal cavity. Anteriorly, the urethra is vulnerable. Tears of the vaginal wall may be in any
axis. The hymen may be impossible to identify where it splits radially

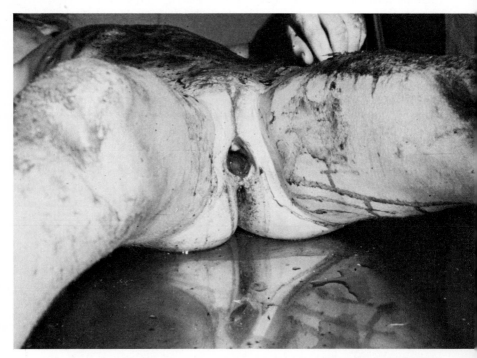

Fig. 10.1   Rape followed by throttling of a 9-year-old girl. There was wide
disruption of the rectovaginal septum. Persistent gaping of the vulva is a feature
in these cases.

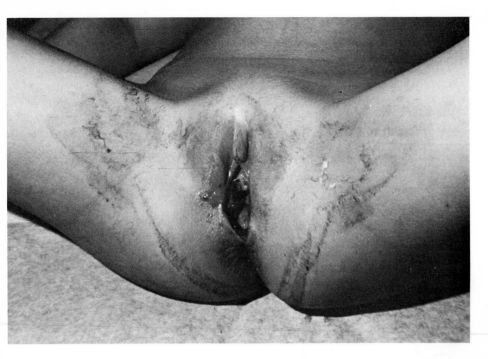

Fig. 10.2 Rape in a 7-year-old child. The perineal tear almost reaches the anus.

and at its attachment. Bleeding is often less profuse than might be expected but, where concealed, may unexpectedly very greatly increase the shock caused by the initial stretching and tearing of the vulva. Psychogenic factors initiating the state of shock should not be ignored.

The capacity of the vagina increases with puberty and injury due to simple penile penetration is probably slight. There is seldom genital injury in women accustomed to intercourse. Unwilling or insufficiently lubricated women who are otherwise accustomed to intercourse sometimes sustain small superficial stretching injuries between the labia.

Vulvar reddening and swelling are said to be clinical signs of recent intercourse. Standards of hygiene are not invariably high and reddening usually indicates no more than vulvar irritation. Some swelling after intercourse is as likely with as without consent. It has been represented during cross-examination that the absence of injury predicates consent but this is a proposition to be resisted. Conversely, relatively trivial injury, mild bruising or swelling resulting from poor technique and clumsiness have, by themselves, provoked a complaint of rape and do not really indicate force.

In uncomplicated rape, signs are most prominent in the virgin. A trivial tear of the fourchette heals within a matter of hours and leaves no sign on naked eye examination 48 hours after. A split in the hymen extends to the peripheral attachment, usually at one or other side of the mid-line posteriorly. Such ruptures are lacerations, a class of wound usually associated with extensive bruising and variable haemorrhage. Presumably because the normal tear is to the periphery, vessels are completely severed and bleeding ceases rapidly. Tiny haematomas probably represent the ends of divided vessels. The edges of the tear and other parts of the free margin of the hymen may be bruised. Within 24 hours, stretching of the introitus can be expected to cause minor fresh bleeding. Parting the posterior ends of the labia majora may again cause bleeding from an injury of the fourchette.

Small sharply defined abrasions within the vestibule or on the labia suggest finger-nail injury. More extensive abrasion is consistent with the use of other rough instruments. In one case a prostitute was subjected to a variety of practices, including being made to sit impaled upon a sports car gear lever and having stones and a hair brush put into the vagina. She was later paraded naked in the lights of the car head-lamps. Several irregular abrasions were found within the vulva. Intercourse did not take place. Clear impressions of smacks with a hand were seen on the buttocks.

The virgin introitus, unless distensible, offers resistance to penetration. The anatomical expression of resistance is felt during examination as a ring of firm tissue when the finger enters the vagina. On examination soon after defloration this resistance to penetration is still appreciable but no such resistance is felt after repeated intercourse over a period. It is a fallacy to believe that mere repetition of intercourse invariably abolishes vaginal tone. The introitus of the prostitute referred to in the last paragraph, a girl of 25 who had had one child, was still quite tight. Repeated rape by a single or several individuals may produce signs no more prominent than intercourse by a single assailant. Absence of local injury does not rule out rape, whether or not physical violence has been used against the victim.

In each instance samples of vaginal fluid and pubic hair are taken. Confirmation of intercourse apart, it may be of value to group the vaginal fluid. Combing produces relatively painless samples of pubic hair together with any loose hair from the male. Particles of vegetation and grit may be found among the hair sample or adhering to the vulva. For adequate laboratory investigation, samples of blood and saliva (for secretor status) from the complainer are also submitted. The greatest possibility of grouping the assailant's semen taken from the vagina exists when the female is a non-secretor.

Signs of restraint
Particularly in cases of multiple rape, marks of ligatures are common on wrists and ankles. These are of two types. A patterned abrasion/bruise is left when rope or similar material is used. The mark varies from mere erythema of the skin to a deep impression with distal oedema depending on the tightness and the length of time constriction is applied.

Finger-nail abrasions are common when hands are used to hold wrists or ankles. Discrete bruises may be present or widespread erythema due to 'Indian burns' are seen. In life, such marks persist for up to a few days. Many assailants may overwhelm the victim and make struggling of no avail. It may be that no sign of restraint is found in such instances.

Finger-tip bruises, seen predominantly on the inner aspects of the arms, are sustained during the preliminaries, whereas such bruises about the thighs and vulva indicate that the lower limbs have had to be forced apart.

In struggling with a girl, her assailant frequently seizes and twists clothing. The result is a patch of petechial haemorrhages or a line of punctate bruises in the skin often near the axilla or on the line of a brassiere strap. Sometimes the pattern of the material is imprinted on the skin. Haematoma of the scalp may result from violent pulling of the hair.

Signs of direct violence
Slapping, punching, kicking and beating are all employed in overcoming resistance. Evidence of such violence is frequently seen as contusions around the eyes, cheeks and lips but they are also found widely distributed elsewhere. The back of the head is often banged on the ground. If sufficiently severe, blows on such parts cause lacerations. The nose is broken; teeth are loosened; the jaw may even be fractured.

Longitudinal scratches on the trunk and lower limbs suggest dragging across a rough surface. Ingrained dirt particles may assist in identifying the locus of the attack. Other injuries typical of fights include bruising of the knuckles, of the ulnar border of forearms or of the shins. The victim's finger-nails are sometimes broken if she scratches her assailant. Material under the nails is worth collecting for scientific examination.

A quite uninjured complainer is viewed with grave suspicion but many compulsitors to sexual intercourse are used other than violence. Threats with knives, guns or other weapons are common. In one case the victim complied when her young child was threatened after several of her windows had been broken; the child was made to watch his mother's rape. Alcohol is a common adjunct to sexual intercourse. Where any moral resistance the woman has is overcome by her own acquiescent drinking, rape should not be libelled in the indictment [*or* included in the charge—*Ed.*]. Time and again one finds girls who gaily drink coma-inducing amounts of alcohol and thereby put themselves at risk. Where a man intentionally renders the female incapable of resistance by alcohol or any other drug it seems clear that intercourse in such circumstances is rape.

Asphyxia
Screaming is a useful means of raising the alarm and frightening off an assailant but is most easily stopped by clamping a hand over the mouth

or stuffing something into it. Gagging and compression of the neck both cause asphyxia; the signs are petechial haemorrhages widely scattered over the face and within the eyelids. The sexual asphyxias are discussed below.

Signs on assailant

Vaginal epithelial cells adhere to the penis during intercourse unless protected by condom. Such cells are rich in glycogen, which stains readily with iodine. A smear of the glans is stained in the vapour from 5 per cent Lugol's iodine mixed with distilled water.[24] The demonstration of sperm in the absence of exfoliated vaginal epithelium is not significant.

Penile injury is rare, although the frenum is occasionally torn in forced penetration. A similar inference is justified when a bruise of the glans if found. Blood retained under the prepuce is more likely to be derived from the female. Foreign pubic hair may be present. When apprehended shortly after the offence the suspect's hands, arms and knees may present a pattern suggestive of the surface on which the rape took place. This is especially so when open ground is involved. Foreign particles adhering to abrasions in these situations may be significant. Samples of blood and saliva are grouped for purposes of comparison.

Scratches of the face and other parts of the body are significant but it is not to be forgotten that such lesions are, at times, sustained during orgasm. Their significance is reduced if love bites caused by the complainer are also present. Bruising on the shins due to kicking, or marks caused by punching or biting elsewhere, indicate a struggle. One victim bit a piece of skin from her attacker's finger. Fortunately this lodged between her teeth and she was able to hand it to the investigating officer; dermal ridges were visible and the skin was photographed and preserved.[5] Two days passed before a suspect was arrested. This man proved to have a defect of the right index finger. Comparison photographs showed that 21 skin ridges at the margin of the suspect's wound corresponded with those of the preserved skin. He was convicted.

Murder in the course of rape

Most of the preceding sections relate to rape in which the victim survives. At death, pathological changes are, for a time, frozen. The pathologist does not have the benefit of examining a live person who is able to recount what happened or react to pain on examination. However, he does not have to contend with the difficulties and uncertainties of clinical examination nor with the over-riding duty of the clinician to treat the living when this is required. Three types of death are encountered.

Death due to the local trauma or to complications such as hypovolaemic shock or peritonitis are most often met with in the very young. Injury is gross and there is no pathological problem in directly connecting the mode of assault and the proximate cause of death.

Strangulation seems to be a common method of killing during sexual activity. The close physical relationship renders throttling easy, with the bare hands or by use of a ligature; suffocation comes into the same category. The pathological picture is that of asphyxia (see Chapter 11) with the added sexual element which is elucidated by answering the questions: was she a virgin? was penetration achieved? was there ejaculation?

Lastly, death may be accomplished by any of the other modes— kicking, stabbing and so on. Again, the pathological features are those of the principal lesions.

When death immediately follows rape, the normal forces destructive of sperm in the vagina slow down. On the other hand, bacteria multiply and putrefactive enzymes hasten proteolysis. It is to be expected that sperm survival will be prolonged by cold. Wilson[27] described the recovery of sperm from a vagina 16 days after death when the body lay in the open. Meteorological data were available from a weather station only three miles from the locus. The temperature never exceeded 15·5°C (60°F) and was warmer than 10°C (50°F) on only the last 5 days. The temperature fell to freezing point or below on 8 of the days. It must be rare to have such precise measurements of the climatic conditions. That so cold an ambient temperature is perhaps uncommon should not deter a search of the vagina in all sexual cases, however sceptical one is of the result.

It is a maxim that an assailant must take his victim as he finds him or her. Even when killing is far from his intention, death as the result of a wickedly reckless disregard for the consequences of an assault is murder, although the charge may well be reduced to culpable homicide for reasons of policy. What is the Crown to make of a death occurring at some interval after an assault where the nexus is tenuous? The question is less dramatic since capital punishment has ceased to be the penalty in most of the Western world but the pathologist's difficulties are well illustrated in the following case.

A parous woman of 74 was attacked by a young man in her own home late one evening, was forced to undress and to have intercourse. Examined some 12 hours later, she was seen to be distressed and to be orthopnoeic. She complained of generalized aching and nausea. Many bruises were present on the trunk and limbs. The vulva showed senile changes. The labia were swollen and tender, their inner aspects being bruised and abraded. There was a slight blood-stained discharge and a small tear at the back of the vestibule. She would permit no further examination. On microscopic examination of smears from the outer part of the vulva only blood was seen. The opinion was given that the findings were consistent with forcible intercourse.

Despite admission to hospital and adequate care, she died 5 days later. At post mortem mild oedema of the legs was noted. Her bruises had, of course, faded and become less well defined. The lungs were congested and oedematous and a small amount of pleural fluid was present. The pericardium contained liquid and clotted blood from a rupture in the anterior wall of the left ventricle. Ischaemic change in the myocardium was confined to the immediate area of the rupture.

The relevant coronary branch was considerably narrowed but all the vessels showed moderate atheroma.

Here, then, was an old lady in some congestive failure whose ECG showed old ischaemic changes. She had had no treatment before the assault. Did the assault hasten her demise?

Rape in the course of other crime

There have been several instances of housebreakers who, finding themselves alone in a room with a sleeping woman, have taken advantage of the situation. In Scotland, this offence is one of a group known as clandestine injury to women. Where the victim is not asleep, intercourse is simple rape. Damage to premises that have been broken into is frequently far greater than that necessary to enter the premises or to rifle potential hiding-places. It is thought that there may well be a sexual element in such disproportionate destruction.

In one case two persons, male and female, entered a house to break open the gas meter. They were interrupted by the householder, an elderly woman. She was severely beaten and dragged from the kitchen, where the meter was, into her living-room. The house was ransacked and the intruders departed. Shortly after, the male returned to the house to rape the woman who died after being trussed and thrown under a table.

Necrophilia

Sexual acts committed with the dead are of two essential types. In the more important, the death and the defilement are part of the same delict. Intercourse is not an invariable element. The pathological investigation has been discussed above. Consideration is also given to deciding which injuries, if any, have been inflicted after death. In the absence of appropriate genital injury (and histological examination of the tissue involved), it is impossible to say that intercourse took place after rather than during or immediately before death. Christie is a celebrated example of an individual whose libidinous proclivity was towards a newly killed female. He is known to have strangled at least three women for the purpose of having intercourse.[13] It seems likely that he was incompetent if not impotent in other circumstances, being afraid of rejection by a normal woman. He made a collection of pubic hair from some of his victims, perhaps for use as a fetish.

Intercourse or lesser acts with the dead by those who have access to cadavers forms the second category. Price[19] raised a number of interesting points in the course of describing such a case. An elderly woman was stabbed but the reason for her death was not appreciated until post mortem was conducted the following day. As she was being undressed by the mortuary attendant he noticed blood staining of the lower part of the vest and some blood between the legs. Not until the body was opened was the possibility of murder realized. There was a tear 2·5 cm (1 in) long, with bleeding of the posterior wall at the introitus. Spermatozoa were present in the vagina.

Enquiry among male staff who had access to the body led to a confession by a young porter. Intercourse took place about 1 hour after death. Penetration was difficult, probably due to senile change in a virgin, and tearing occurred. He was adamant that no instrument was used. He denied that there had been previous incidents of this kind. This was his first experience of intercourse. The Director of Public Prosecutions decided against proceedings.

Post-mortem dissection cannot be performed vicariously. External examination and evisceration are important steps in the autopsy and should not be lightly delegated.

Factitious injury
False allegations of sexual assault are common. In many of these no injury has been suffered but the complainer's need to embellish is demonstrated as superficial, usually incised wounds. The favourite site is the forearm. Similar lesions are occasionally seen on the trunk but are unlikely on those parts open to view when fully dressed.

Masturbation using an instrument which causes damage and bleeding may similarly be explained as resulting from sexual attack. Rape was alleged by a young woman who had some bruising of the face but also many abrasions. These were characteristic finger-nail injuries which were much more typical of a fight between females; enquiry showed this to be the case.

Assault not involving intercourse

Lewd conduct has many variations, including voyeurism, exposure of genitalia and importuning children. Such acts are not always committed by males towards females. A woman of proportions so vast that she could not leave her own home induced her mentally retarded son to procure on her behalf young boys who literally crawled all over her. In few of these cases is there likelihood of physical injury. There may well be transfer of trace evidence. For example, seminal staining or pubic hair found on the clothing of a prepubertal child have clear implications. Many of these offences are committed in public parks— vegetation or soil is to be sought adhering to the victim or retained on clothing.

Intercrural intercourse is common as a substitute for incest. The problem here is to assess the significance of any vulvar reddening or swelling and thickening of the hymen which is seen from time to time in girls subjected to vulvar intercourse and fingering.

Homosexuality

Homosexual conduct of itself seldom leads to death or even palpable physical injury. The pathologist becomes involved because the male homosexual is more prone to sudden and unexpected violent death than is the average citizen.[20] Because of the clandestine nature of homosexuality, assaults are frequently not reported by those who would have difficulty in explaining their presence in haunts frequented by male prostitutes. When desire overcomes discretion, the homosexual falls prey to those who allow themselves to be picked up for the purpose of robbing such persons. Homosexuals tend to be promiscuous and provide a major reservoir of venereal disease. Many do not confine sexual acts to other males.

Homosexual acts between males range from mutual masturbation through intercrural and intergluteal to oral and anal intercourse. The Sexual Offences Act 1967 legalized such conduct in England and Wales where the participants are adults, the acts are by mutual consent and are conducted in private. Paedophilia, where the boy is usually the passive agent, was not sanctioned. Soliciting for boys in public is still rife.

Sodomy is the typical practice. Penetration of the anus is easily accomplished only when lubricants such as petroleum jelly are employed. Repeated acts slacken the sphincter and render the anus patulous. The perianal skin becomes thickened. A funnel anus is rarely seen. The anal canal becomes excoriated, fissures develop and signs of chronic inflammation are found. The anal canal is usually empty of faeces but a bowel movement subsequent to the sodomy will take ejaculate with it. Anal tone cannot be reliably assessed at post mortem. In a case of murder by strangulation of a young girl who had gross vulvar tearing extending into the rectum a man was arrested within a few hours. What was obviously faecal material was seen under the foreskin when it was retracted.

The allegation that the victim made persistent but unwelcome homosexual advances is often adduced as an excuse for great brutality (Fig. 10.3). One middle-aged man picked up two youths in a pub. They drove him in his own car some 16 km (10 miles) into the country where the car became bogged down in a field. Such a beating was administered that much of the interior of the car was spattered with blood. The man was then taken out of the car and jumped on until his head was battered into the soft earth. The skeleton of the middle third of the face was depressed by 2·5 cm (1 in).

Most homosexual activity, whether or not it comes under the saving provisions of the 1967 Act, is with consent. The analogue of rape is uncommon. One youngster was seen who had been abducted by two men to a disused railway line where he was severely beaten about the trunk with a belt, stripped and the belt tightened round his neck before being buggered. He lost consciousness when penetrated, probably due mainly to asphyxia, and was left lying on the ground.

Homosexuals who attempt to conceal their predilections from family and employer are vulnerable to blackmail. A proportion of these opt for suicide and one authority suggested that homosexuality should be considered as the underlying cause for suicide until proved otherwise in any young man with no significant medical history.[20] Checking the trachea for seminal fluid in any suspicious death where there is possib-

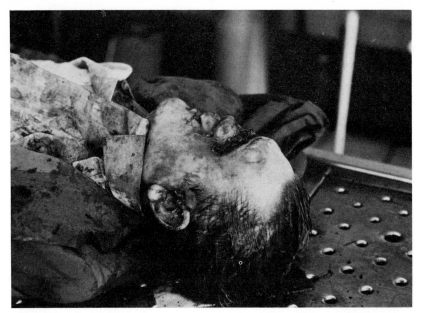

Fig. 10.3 Violence associated with the rejection of homosexual advances.

ility of accident during oral intercourse was also thought to be worthwhile.

Lesbian conduct has long been accepted legally if not socially. Physical findings as a result of mutual masturbation are nil. Love bites may be present. Murder from motives of jealousy involving lesbians is of a brutality not otherwise associated with female crime.

Bestiality

Intercourse by male humans with animals has long been associated with rural life. Hens, ducks and sheep are commonly employed, although larger animals like cows are also abused. Unless caught in the act, detection depends on the discovery of appropriate trace evidence on the accused and around the genitalia of the animal.[3] Domestic fowls frequently die following the assault and the body should be examined by a veterinary surgeon aware of the need to take the necessary specimens. It is neither necessary nor pleasant to have delivered to one a parcel containing the pelvic organs of a sheep.

Certain pornographic books carry illustrations of intercourse between male animals, usually dogs, and human females. Whether or not these practices are to be found away from such a milieu is not known. Danger to the human arises when the larger animals are provoked into retaliation. Some savage treatment of animals is bestial not only in the commonly accepted sense. Although it does not involve overt sexual contact, the infliction of pain provides sexually based pleasure to some persons. This is analogous to the pleasure derived by some fire-raisers from a conflagration.

Sado-masochism

In the archetypal sadistic murder, the killing is a substitute for coitus.[18] There is no attempt at intercourse: satisfaction is obtained from the act of throttling, biting, ripping of the vulva or multiple stabbing of the breast. Some phallus substitute may be left where it has been forced into the vagina or rectum. The key for the pathologist is in the gross mutilating nature of the injuries. Frequently the infliction of injury has continued after the victim's death. Such murders are seldom committed by females. Where the victim is male there is probably a homosexual element in the murderer.[4]

Brutal injury need not be sadistic but it falls into this category where the motive is partly sexual. Some cases of child battering, for instance, are of such a nature. Again, the man who feels called on to consort with prostitutes and then 'punish' them is a sadist. One prostitute told of a client who used her at intervals for the sole purpose of driving her into the country where he slapped her violently on the face, paid her for her trouble and took her back to her beat.

A woman reported to the police that her dog had bitten off her infant son's genitalia. The amputation wound had an appearance of incision rather than laceration and it became apparent that the mother had used a knife for the amputation and had then attempted to incriminate the dog. The clinicians concerned were left with the difficult problem of how the now neutered child should be reared.

The masochist is gratified by submitting to such practices as flagellation. Death during these acts is accidental—at least from the point of view of the participants—and likely to be asphyxial, perhaps from the incautious use of bonds. In any one individual there is frequently a mixture of sadism and masochism.

Self-inflicted sexual injury

Male and female patients presenting with foreign bodies in rectum or urethra are presumed to have been seeking sexual pleasure. The patient is seldom in great danger, although sharp objects are prone to penetrate the wall of the viscus, with the attendant danger of infection. Other masturbatory activity includes the use of electric shocks, vibrators and apparatus designed to cause mainly painful stimuli. Applying the tube of a vacuum-cleaner over the penis for pleasure has caused gross lacerations.[10] However plausible the explanation offered, it is naïve to consider such injuries as accidental.[28] Genital injury need not have a sexual basis, as in the case of a man who, because of pain and depression from a peptic ulcer, amputated the right testis with a broken glass.[6]

Although now well documented, death from sexual asphyxia is still likely to perturb an investigating officer who has not previously encountered such circumstances. Details in each instance are peculiar to the case itself. The composite picture is of a male in early adult life, of no particular social background, but an Anglo-Saxon. Typically using female clothing, he goes through a ritual of masturbation assisted by erotic pictures while trussed in bonds. These he is able to manipulate in such a way as to cause cerebral anoxia, thus heightening his fantasy. He always uses the same place where he knows he is unlikely to be disturbed (perhaps a garden shed or an attic). He protects his neck by padding ligatures and he has no thought of suicide. Usher[25] considered that the presence of four or five of these features should raise suspicion that a death is due to a fatal sexual accident.

A typical case concerned a 44-year-old man who was found locked in a small boxroom situated on a common landing (Fig. 10.4). The key was lying on the floor inside, with no room to slip it under the door. He was known to disappear for hours at a time. Being missed for a couple

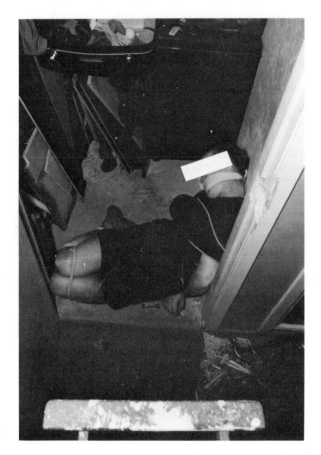

Fig. 10.4 The locus in the case of sexual asphyxia described in the text. (Photograph by courtesy of the Chief Constable, Strathclyde Police.)

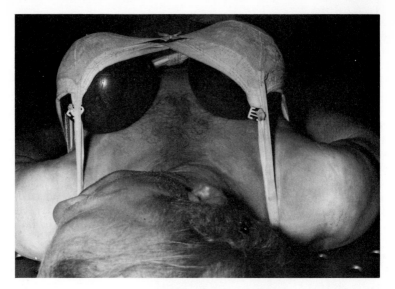

Fig. 10.5   Simulated female appearance as described in the text. (Photograph by courtesy of the Chief Constable, Strathclyde Police.)

of days, this door was forced and he was found slumped partly against the door. His clothing was female except for the underpants. There were two wooden balls in the brassiere (Fig. 10.5). A heavy metal wedge, the base of which measured 6 × 2·5 cm (2·5 in × 1 in) was held in the mouth by a gag. Rope tied the legs at the ankles and knees, the wrists and the chest. The slip was gathered between the legs by wire. The face was cyanosed but there were no petechiae about the eyes and face. Petechiae were present on the trunk and legs. A small amount of aspirated vomit was found in the trachea. A few petechial haemorrhages were seen on the heart and pericardial fluid was increased. The heart was enlarged and flabby. The cerebrospinal fluid was blood-stained both within the brain and on its surface.

It has been considered[25] that females do not indulge in such conduct, but this view is challenged by Sass[21] who described sexual asphyxia in a woman aged 35.

Conclusion

Aspects of varied sexual habits have been alluded to above. The categories used to describe departures from the norm are aetiological rather than pathological. Patterns of human behaviour are moulded by many factors. The results of sexual violence arising from these patterns are modified by the circumstances of the encounter, the resistance offered and the probability of interruption. The pathologist will do well to remember this as he attempts to reconstruct a dynamic situation from the static picture before him.

References

1. Adams, E. G. and Wraxall, B. G. (1974). Phosphatases in body fluids: the differentiation of semen and vaginal secretion. *Forensic Sci.* **3**, 57.
2. Baxter, S. J. (1973). Immunological identification of human semen. *Med. Sci. Law* **13**, 155.
3. Berg, S. (1957). Medico-biological interpretation in cases of sexual delinquency. *J. forensic Med.* **4**, 82.
4. Brittain, R. P. (1970). The sadistic murderer. *Med. Sci. Law* **10**, 198.
5. Butler, O. (1966). Unusual identification. *Police Journal* **39**, 605.
6. Chandulal, R. (1973). An unusual method of suicide. *Forensic Sci.* **2**, 379.
7. Davies, A. and Wilson, E. (1974). The persistence of seminal constituents in the human vagina. *Forensic Sci.* **3**, 45.
8. Farn, K. T. (1975). Sexual and other assaults on children. *Police Surgeon* **8**, 37.
9. Fatteh, A., Leach, W. B. and Wilkinson, C. A. (1973). Fatal air embolism in pregnancy resulting from oro-genital sex play. *Forensic Sci.* **2**, 247.
10. Fox, M. and Barrett, E. L. (1960). Vacuum cleaner injury of the penis. *Brit. med. J.* **1**, 1942.
11. Georgiades, J. and Eliakis, C. (1939). Fatal haemorrhage due to rupture of the hymen. *Med. Crim. Rev.* **7**, 89.
12. Harvey, W., Butler, O., Furness, J. and Laird, R. (1968). The Biggar murder—dental, medical, police and legal aspects. *J. forensic Sci. Soc.* **8**, 153.
13. Jesse, F. T. (Ed.) (1957). *Trials of Evans and Christie*. Edinburgh: William Hodge.
14. MacDonald, D. G. (1974). Bite mark recognition and interpretation. *J. forensic Sci. Soc.* **14**, 229.
15. McLay, W. D. S. (1975). Sexual assault—the role of the police surgeon. *Police Surgeon* **8**, 9.
16. Mant, A. K. (1962). The significance of spermatozoa in the penile urethra at post mortem. *J. forensic Sci. Soc.* **2**, 125.
17. Masters, W. H. and Johnson, V. E. (1966). *Human Sexual Response*. Boston, Mass: Little, Brown & Co.
18. Podolsky, E. (1965). The lust murderer. *Med.-leg. J.* **33**, 174.
19. Price, D. E. (1963). Necrophilia complicating a case of homicide. *Med. Sci. Law* **3**, 121.
20. Rupp, J. C. (1970). Sudden death in the gay world. *Med. Sci. Law* **10**, 189.
21. Sass, F. A. (1975). Sexual asphyxia in the female. *J. forensic Sci.* **20**, 181.
22. Schiff, A. F. (1969). Statistical features of rape. *J. forensic Sci.* **14**, 102.

23. Sharpe, N. (1963). The significance of spermatozoa in the victims of sexual offences. *Canad. med. Ass. J.* **89**, 513.
24. Thomas, F. and van Hecke, W. (1963). The demonstration of recent sexual intercourse in the male by the Lugol method. *Med. Sci. Law* **3**, 169.
25. Usher, A. (1974). The sexual asphyxias. *Police Surgeon* **5**, 76.
26. Whitehead, P. H. and Divall, G. B. (1974). The identification of menstrual blood—immunoelectrophoresis characterisation of soluble fibrinogen from menstrual blood-stained extracts. *Forensic Sci.* **4**, 53.
27. Wilson, E. F. (1974). Sperm's morphologic survival after 16 days in the vagina of a dead body. *J. forensic Sci.* **19**, 561.
28. Zufall, R. (1973). Laceration of penis from hand vacuum cleaner. *J. Amer. med. Ass.* **224**, 630.

11

Violent forms of asphyxial death

Asphyxia results from occlusion of the air passages. It is one of several causes of failure of proper oxygenation of tissues and, by contrast with other causes, it is often a violent event. The Greek origin of the word can be freely translated as 'pulseless' and it is perhaps because of its etymology that the term is often misused. It should not be confused with other anoxic states due to impaired circulation of the blood, deficiency of haemoglobin or some poisonings, such as cyanide, when the uptake of oxygen by the tissues is impaired. These forms of anoxia are called stagnant, anaemic and histotoxic respectively.

To the forensic pathologist the word 'asphyxia' means anoxic anoxia and implies some compromising of the air passages which may come about in a variety of ways. It is a common event in forensic practice and can be accidental, self-inflicted or the result of homicidal attack. Suicide by hanging is common particularly in those places where coal gas, which used to be a frequent method of self-poisoning, has been replaced by natural gas; in parts of the United Kingdom, some 90 per cent of suicides are due to hanging.

Asphyxia may be brought about in a variety of ways. Strangulation with a ligature such as a rope, electric cable, belt, scarf, tie or stocking may be self-inflicted or done by some other person. Tight clothing around the neck of an infant may cause death if the child contrives to hook the edge of the garment over a point of suspension such as a projecting bolt on the top edge of a cot. Smothering is a particularly important form of asphyxia to recognize. Essentially it is the covering of the nose and mouth by a soft object which occludes the airway. It might occur accidentally but it is not infrequently a mode of death in children who suffer non-accidental injury. Smothering can be difficult to detect because pressure marks may not be found on the face if the object used is a soft, thick pillow. It is important to pay particular attention to the sides of the head and neck in such cases as the fingers of an assailant may slip over the edge of the object used for smothering and nail marks may be found on the lateral sides of the neck.

Suffocation is another mode of asphyxia where the supply of air is restricted and in which death tends to occur gradually. It comes about accidentally if small children pull plastic bags over their heads or become shut in refrigerators, boxes and the like. Suffocation is not uncommon in mental institutions when patients may get into confined spaces and become trapped. Choking, another form of asphyxia, is also seen in mental hospitals. Schizophrenics and patients taking tranquillizing drugs are liable to choke—that is to say the larynx or trachea becomes obstructed by a bolus of food or by false teeth (Fig. 11.1). Children may accidentally inhale foreign objects such as bolts, ball-bearings and the like, which may lodge in the larynx.

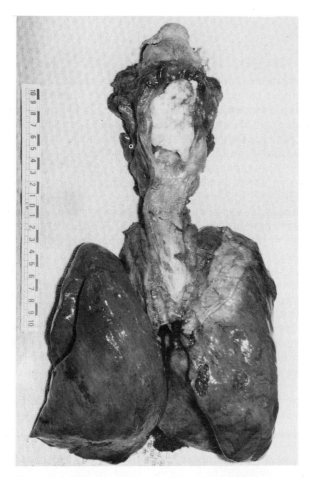

Fig. 11.1 Larynx, trachea and lungs showing a bolus of food impacted in the laryngopharynx.

Constriction of the neck can be by strangulation or by throttling with the hands. Constriction of the chest occurs by a fall of earth on those working in ill-prepared trenches or by the weight of a vehicle, as not infrequently happens when tractors overturn on agricultural workers. This latter event is one of the commonest forms of accidental death in farm workers.

Patterns of injury in asphyxia

Cardiac arrest
It is important, at the outset, to realize that there may be few or no abnormal findings in a sudden asphyxial death. The various features which we shall discuss in this chapter may be absent and death in such cases is usually attributable to cardiac inhibition caused by sudden pressure on the neck. The mechanism is probably very similar to that which occurs in carotid sinus syncope when, for example, the wearing of a tight collar can induce profound bradycardia and loss of consciousness. It is not at all uncommon that few signs are present in cases of suicidal strangulation with ligatures. The usual conclusion is that circulatory arrest is so rapid that there is not sufficient time for the appearance of petechial haemorrhages and other phenomena to occur. However, a diagnosis of cardiac arrest in cases of asphyxia should not be made readily. It is more a diagnosis by exclusion and demands rigorous enquiry and investigation before it is made.

Petechial haemorrhages
A common finding in asphyxia is the presence of petechial haemorrhages in the loose skin of the eyelids (Fig. 11.2), behind the ears and in the conjunctivae. It is by no means certain whether the haemorrhages

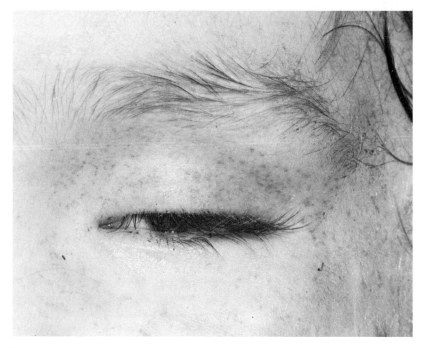

Fig. 11.2 Petechial haemorrhages in the upper eyelid.

are due to hypoxia or to increased pressure within the capillaries, as for example when mechanical constriction occurs leading to occlusion of the venous return. It is true that they are more frequent in the skin above a ligature, suggesting elevated venous pressure as a cause. Equally, they may be found in other parts of the skin unrelated to a ligature. For example, a cluster of petechiae may be found on the leg in people who hang themselves. They are probably caused by active movement of the body before death, causing the limb to bump against an adjacent object. Hypoxia and hypercapnia develop together in asphyxia; there is a rapid rise of blood pressure, an increase of cardiac output and profound secretion of catecholamines—particularly nor-epinephrine. The last has been shown to increase endothelial permeability in isolated perfused arteries in the rat. This it does by causing the endothelial cell junctions to widen.[2] A number of factors such as pressure and cell dehiscence clearly conspire to produce petechiae.

The distribution of asphyxial haemorrhages is often easy to explain and their predilection for loose soft tissues such as retroauricular skin, conjunctivae, thymus, subpleura and atrioventricular grooves is well known. Occasionally in infant sudden deaths, large numbers may be found over the entire parietal and visceral pleura, pericardium and thymus; this sort of grouping is less easy to explain.

Petechial haemorrhages occur in other cases where asphyxia is not the prime cause of death. They are commonly seen along the thoracic aorta and occasionally in the conjunctivae in deaths from acute myocardial failure due to coronary artery disease. Another problem is the occurrence of artefactual haemorrhages post mortem. They can readily be produced in the deep scalp when the skin is reflected to remove the skull; they are the result of tearing many small vessels during the manoeuvre. Artefactual haemorrhages are also seen in dependent skin, particularly over the lower posterior thorax. These are usually larger than petechiae, though petechiae themselves can enlarge post mortem if they occur in dependent parts of the body when blood can continue to ooze from damaged vessels. On the contrary, petechiae may be difficult to spot in intensely congested skin and it is a good policy to examine the skin again after the autopsy has been done. Petechiae in the skin behind the ears may then be much more readily seen after blood has drained away from the tissues. This is particularly the case in child deaths.

Cyanosis and congestion

Asphyxia is not the only fatal condition causing cyanosis and this feature is consequently an unreliable aid in the recognition of an asphyxial death. To be of any significance, it must be present when the body is examined a few hours after death. In the course of a day or so, oxygen is gradually lost from the blood and cynosis is then meaningless.

Dilatation of the great veins and of the right side of the heart is also often cited as an indication of asphyxial death. It is true that this is often the case but, like cyanosis, these changes are found in so many other causes of death that they cannot be used as reliable indications of asphyxia. Yet another feature which has been regarded as an accompaniment of asphyxial death is the finding of fluid blood in the heart and vessels at post-mortem examination. This is most probably due to liberation of antithrombins such as heparin from mast cells or to the development of profound fibrinolytic activity in the blood after death. Fluid blood is found at necropsy in many rapid deaths and is more closely related to the speed of death rather than being specifically related to asphyxia.

Findings in the air passages

The inhalation of a wide variety of materials occurs frequently. Sometimes this is clearly related to the cause of death but often it is not; the impaction of a bolus of food or some other foreign body in the larynx leaves no doubt about the cause of death but the role of inhaled fluids such as water and gastric contents is more debatable. Inhalation of stomach contents is frequently a feature of the terminal phase of asphyxia when respirations are irregular and gasping and when consciousness is lost.

Stomach contents can be found by both macroscopic and microscopic examinations in the lungs of children who die suddenly and unexpectedly in their cots. Until comparatively recently, it was widely held that these infants died as a result of asphyxia. Knight[5] has shown that vomit is found in the lungs with a similar frequency in an unselected series of adult deaths investigated by the coroner; it does therefore seem unlikely that direct airways obstruction is the prime cause of death in these infants. However, it does not rule out the possibility; Parish et al.[8] have suggested that death results from a hypersensitivity to artificial foods which have been inhaled into the bronchial tree.

Petechial haemorrhages are not infrequently found in and on the surface of the thymus in cot deaths. Sometimes they are more extensive within the thoracic cavity but frequently they are difficult to find at all. It is therefore most unlikely that asphyxia is a factor in cot death. Indeed, Woolley[12] has shown that active infants roll over and avoid experimentally contrived smothering and that they do not readily allow their airways to become obstructed. Over-lying of infants is occasionally said to be a cause of asphyxial death. It is possible, although uncommon, for the parents of a child found dead in suspicious circumstances to assert that death was due to an accident of this type; such an assertion is difficult to disprove if it is stoutly maintained. Death is due to pressure on the chest by a larger person, which prevents breathing, and signs of asphyxia can be scanty. The critical age beyond which over-lying is deemed to be physically impossible is not clearly defined although, legally, the Children and Young Persons Act 1933 (S. 2(b)) makes it neglect of an infant in a manner likely to cause injury to its health if a child under 3 years of age occupies the same bed as a person over the age of 16 years. The frequency with which this type of association must occur emphasizes the rarity of over-lying as a cause of asphyxial death.

The finding of stomach contents in the air passages in any of the preceding types of cases must therefore be regarded critically. It is particularly liable to occur in infants as a result of post-mortem manipulation of the body. True ante-mortem regurgitation can be recognized only when acid digestion and necrosis of lung tissue have taken place, as in Mendelson's syndrome.[6] Of autopsies on medical patients, 5·7 per cent revealed this state of affairs,[3] which is considerably less than 25 per cent of cases where food was found in the lungs.[5] This, again, suggests that the finding of stomach contents in the air passages is, in many cases, an artefact.

A variety of other liquids may be inhaled into the lungs but they cause death by poisoning or induced biochemical changes rather than by asphyxia. Water may enter the lungs in drowning but it is now well recognized, and has also been established experimentally,[10] that it is rapidly absorbed from the bronchial tree. This is particularly so with fresh rather than salt water. Death results from haemodilution with lysis of erythrocytes and the release of potassium in quantity from the cells. The subsequent hyperkalaemia causes altered repolarization in cardiac muscle with atrial paralysis; finally, all cardiac fibres become unexcitable and the heart stops in diastole. It is not surprising that, although pulmonary oedema is not infrequent, excess water is rarely found in the bronchi of drowned persons. A much more reliable macroscopic indication of drowning is the presence of abundant water in the stomach that has been gulped in the terminal phases.

The inhalation of liquid petrol, which occasionally occurs in passengers in rear seats of cars involved in a collision, is worthy of special mention. The concussed individual is found on the floor of the vehicle with the head bathed in petrol derived from a leaking fuel pipe. Quite often the vehicle bursts into flames and evidence of petrol poisoning is then destroyed.

Laryngeal injury

Investigation of the state of the larynx is of paramount importance in the study of violent asphyxial death. It is particularly liable to be damaged in throttling, mugging, homicidal strangulation and even accidentally during violent sexual activities. By contrast, it is rarely found to be damaged in suicidal strangulation.

Laryngeal injury in violent asphyxial deaths is rare in children; the hyoid is still pliable because there is a cartilaginous union between the body of the bone and its greater cornua. The thyroid cartilage and its cornua are also unlikely to be damaged in children because ossification or calcification has not yet occurred. Calcific rigidity of the thyroid cartilage occurs earlier in men than in women and can be seen as soon as the third decade. The superior cornua are most liable to be injured in asphyxia and the degree of force needed to do this can be slight (Fig. 11.3). It is consequently particularly important to avoid producing artefactual fractures when the thoracic organs are 'plucked' out of the

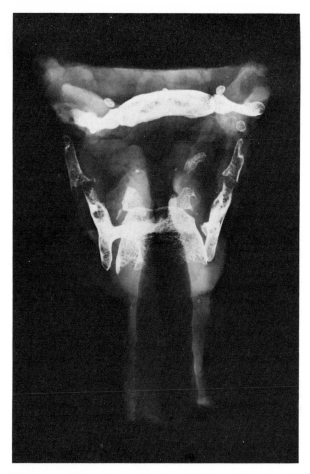

Fig. 11.3 Bilateral superior thyroid cornual fractures. From an elderly woman assaulted by a young man.

thorax at autopsy. The trachea and lungs should be freed by incising the posterior parietal pleura along the line of the vertebral bodies and then lifting the thoracic organs out of the chest by placing the hand around the middle of the trachea.

Fractures of the body of the thyroid cartilage are rare and are usually caused by a direct blow to the front of the neck. They can also occur in mugging where the neck is constricted by applying a strangle hold with the forearm across the front of the neck. In such circumstances, the rare event of a fracture of the cricoid cartilage may be found as well. Bruising of the deep tissues surrounding the larynx is often extensive in these cases. It is readily seen when the organs are still in situ and indicates the need not only for careful handling of the neck organs but also for a radiological examination of the larynx to determine the exact injuries. Mere palpation of the larynx is an unreliable way of examining the organ, and dissection is also not entirely satisfactory in that artefactual fractures may be created; furthermore, the undue mobility of the young larynx and hyoid might suggest fracture when none is present. Fractures which are unaccompanied by any extravasations of blood in their vicinity should be regarded with caution as they are most often the result of post-mortem damage from handling the larynx. It is also true that haemorrhages in the laryngeal mucosa do not always indicate the presence of fractures. Voigt[11] has shown that they may occur not only in strangulation or other trauma to the neck but also in fatal poisonings by sedatives, after intubation of the larynx, in drowning, in traumatic asphyxia caused by pressure on the chest and also in deaths from natural causes such as ischaemic heart disease (Fig. 11.4). Paparo and Siegel[7] also emphasize the importance of not always considering posterior cricoarytenoid haemorrhages to be the result of trauma. These mucosal haemorrhages are not infrequently found in deaths from a variety of causes including natural disease, drugs and physical agents. They lie on the posterior larynx in the upper pharyngeal mucosa and have, in the past, been considered to result from pressure of the larynx against the cervical spine which lies posteriorly. It is more likely that they are due to the rupture of veins which form the laryngopharyngeal plexus and that the veins burst because of increased pressure within them rather than from trauma to them from without.

Fractures of the hyoid bone are seen less commonly than are those of the thyroid cornua. Two mechanisms have been postulated to explain them. The greater cornua may be fractured from lateral pressure high in the neck, as for example in manual strangulation when the hands are applied on either side of the neck below the angles of the jaw. The other possibility arises as a result of downward pressure on the larynx. Traction on the stylohyoid or the thyrohyoid ligaments will prevent movement of the hyoid bone inferiorly and cause it to break anteriorly.

In addition to the possible production of artefactual fractures, there is also a risk of post mortem oozing of blood into the tissues of the neck and of thus creating a false impression of bruising. It is wise to allow blood to drain from the neck structures before they are dissected—preferably in situ rather than after removal from the body. This can be done by removing the heart and brain before making an incision in the neck. Probably the best neck incision is that which runs transversely across the clavicles and then proceeds vertically along the posterior borders of the sternomastoids to join with the scalp incision made for the removal of the brain. A large skin flap can then be reflected over the face and further reflection upwards of the skin of the chin and lower lip gives a clear view of the lip mucosa (Fig. 11.5). Bruises and laceration of the lips can be readily seen in this way. Injuries of this sort are not infrequent in cases of violent asphyxia.

Pulmonary appearances
Pulmonary oedema is one of the most frequent of the other changes in

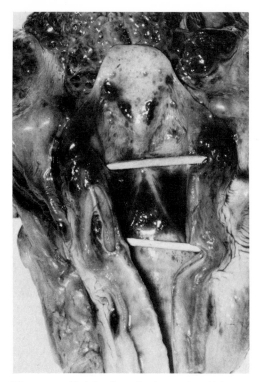

Fig. 11.4 Epiglottic and cricoarytenoid haemorrhages in sudden death from ischaemic heart disease.

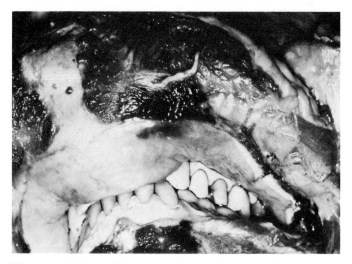

Fig. 11.5 Reflected lip mucosa showing bruising of the lip, from a case of suffocation.

the air passages which are found in asphyxia. This results partly from the effects of hypoxia on the vasomotor centre and is of variable degree. It may be so severe that abundant, pink froth exudes from the nose and mouth or it may be so slight as to be detectable only by histological examination of the lungs. Blood is seen in the bronchi and trachea in traumatic asphyxia when the chest has been compressed, usually in road traffic victims. The condition is more frequent in the pliable chest of young people which can be squashed without rib fracture and then returns to its usual shape. In these circumstances, haemorrhage occurs as a result of contusion and internal laceration of the lung substance and frequently develops without any tearing of the pleural surfaces; it is this blood which is the cause of the asphyxia so often seen in road traffic deaths. More important is the asphyxial bleeding in concussed victims of road traffic accidents; the blood is inhaled from injured nose, lips or jaws. Life may be saved if the condition is recognized at the time and the air passages are cleared by suction.

Marks and other injuries in asphyxial deaths

Marks about the head and neck are frequently present in cases of accidental, suicidal and homicidal asphyxia. Most often, death is caused by strangulation and the degree of damage to the external tissues and internal organs is more closely related to the position and force of the constriction than to its nature. For example, the view that broad ligatures, such as stockings, cause less damage to neck structures than, say, a thin rope cannot easily be sustained.[4]

A wide range of objects have been the cause of strangulation and they vary according to the circumstances. Accidental strangulation is most often seen in infants and young children and is usually caused by clothing becoming tight about the neck, as for example when the neck of a garment becomes hooked over a projecting part of a cot. Occasionally, clothing entangled in machinery can cause asphyxia in adults. The author has found suicidal strangulation to be common in East Anglia— all sorts of ligatures have been used including ropes, stockings, wires, straps and belts. Homicidal strangulation is most often manual though, occasionally, a ligature may be used either alone or in combination with manual strangulation (Fig. 11.6). Green[4] emphasized that there are marks on the neck in most cases of strangulation and the only occasion when they are not found is when asphyxia has been produced by mugging with the forearm. While he frequently found bruising of the sternomastoid and of the strap muscles in cases of strangulation, injury to the hyoid or larynx was rare. He also found injuries to the carotid arteries in his series. These take the form of subintimal haemorrhages or splits in the intima of the upper parts of the common carotid arteries. There may also be fracture of atheromatous plaques in the carotids. Carotid artery damage must be sought with care because the process of opening the vessel may destroy the torn area.

Perhaps the most important evidence in a case of strangulation is

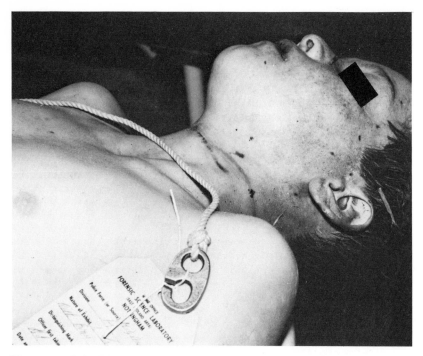

Fig. 11.6 A double ligature mark due to homicidal strangulation with a lanyard. Note finger-nail abrasions near to the ligature mark.

afforded by the nature and position of the mark caused by the ligature. Not only does it indicate the possibilities of accident, suicide or murder but it also provides evidence as to the type of ligature which had been used. In addition, the position of the ligature mark can help in deciding the length of time which may have elapsed between the application of the constriction and death. This period of time depends upon the intensity of constriction and also upon the position of the noose. Hanging or suspension of the body is usually done by means of a running noose. The body may be completely suspended above the ground or sag with the feet touching the surface. It is possible to achieve suicidal strangulation in a variety of positions such as sitting, kneeling and lying prone; asphyxia occurs as long as the weight of the body tightens the noose. Constriction is intense when the body hangs above the ground and death occurs rapidly in such circumstances; when the ligature is not so tight, death may occur slowly with a period of coma developing beforehand.

Rentoul and Smith[9] describe experiments which have been done in order to determine the effect of the position of the noose upon the speed of death. If the ligature is placed between the jaw and the hyoid bone and tightened moderately, breathing is affected but nevertheless continues. It is necessary to release the constriction after about 2 minutes. If, however, the ligature is placed over the larynx itself, the subject requires to be released within 1·5 minutes. If placed lower still, over the cricoid cartilage, a ligature causes such respiratory embarrassment that the experiment cannot be allowed to go on for more than a few seconds.

The effect of constricting the neck structures is due to a variety of factors such as occlusion of the cerebral circulation, pressure on the vagal and phrenic nerves, and obstruction of the airway. The last occurs in suicidal hanging, when the ligature usually lies between the larynx and the hyoid or between the hyoid and the lower jaw. This causes the tongue to be forced upwards and forwards and, in the process, it is clenched between the teeth. Marks of teeth can often be found on the tongue in such cases (Fig. 11.7). These give a useful indication of suspension while the person was alive and provide one of

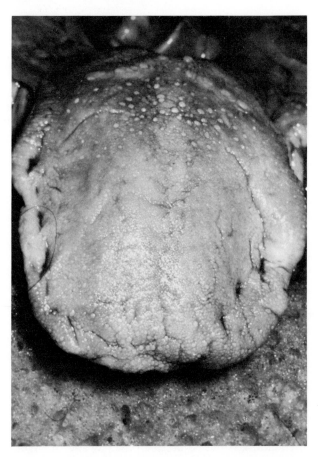

Fig. 11.7 Teeth marks at the edge of the tongue in suicidal strangulation. (The hair-like mark is an artefact.)

the adjuncts in excluding the possibility of post-mortem suspension of a body. A curious oral feature of violent death from asphyxia is the occasional finding of pink teeth.[1] A likely factor in producing the appearance is the presence of blood saturated with carbon dioxide, probably because of the lack of oxygen in the tissues post mortem. It is another helpful indication of the mechanism of death but is by no means specific for asphyxia. Turgescence of the penis and the presence of semen at the urethral meatus have been regarded as other features of death from strangulation. However, they occur in many types of death and are probably explained by hypostasis and the effects of rigor mortis.

Ligature marks on the neck require careful study; a detailed photographic record, including a scale of measurement, is essential. They may be single or multiple. Attempts at suicidal hanging may be unsuccessful at first because the rope breaks. A second attempt may succeed and the final result will leave several marks on the neck. There may, in addition, be evidence of suicidal attempts in other ways such as by wrist cutting or self-stabbing and, if the individual has wandered around in a confused state before hanging himself, the appearances at the scene might be interpreted as those of a struggle. In cases like this the ligature mark will provide useful evidence of the way in which death was effected.

The hanging groove on the neck varies in intensity. In general, the broader and softer the object, the less distinct the mark is likely to be. In most cases, however, there is a wealth of detail to be seen. Marks of knots, irregular thickening and twisting of the ligature and the like can be easily detected and the width of the ligature can be measured readily. In self-strangulation, the mark around the neck is usually single unless a double ligature is used or the cord slips up the neck after the first application. The groove has a yellow parchment-like appearance and is deepest at the point where the weight of the body is taken up by the ligature. At this point, the superior edge of the mark usually shows some creasing of the skin when the body is suspended vertically. Away from the area of maximum weight bearing the ligature mark becomes less distinct as it rises to a suspension point behind an ear or to the nape of the neck. Homicide should be suspected if the mark runs horizontally around the neck and if there are more than one. Usually, however, there are finger marks from the assailant at the sides or back of the neck. Horizontal marks fading posteriorly can be found in suicidal hanging when the body lies in a semi-prone position. The position of a knot on the ligature is important; right-handed persons usually place the knot on the right side, and vice versa for the left-handed.

Artefactual marks on the neck may be produced by tight clothing in young children and in obese or oedematous adults. Similar marks may also be produced after death by the application of a tight-fitting shroud or bandages placed around the jaws in order to keep the mouth shut. These marks are usually of slight degree and are not accompanied by damage to neck structures; it is seldom difficult to recognize their cause

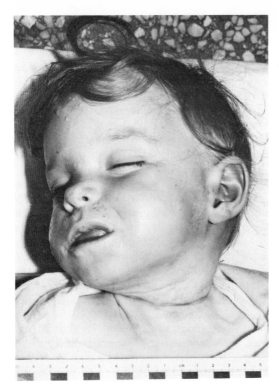

Fig. 11.8   Artefact mark due to a tight nightie.

(Fig. 11.8). On the other hand, ligature marks may disappear in severely decomposed bodies or in corpses immersed in water for a period. Careful macroscopic and microscopic examination of skin and neck structures will be needed to discover evidence of bruising in decomposed bodies.

In cases of strangulation, the ligature has often been cut or removed before the pathologist has arrived. There is clearly no justification for doing this if a body is decomposed but the ligature must be removed if life might be saved. Ideally, it should be gently slipped over the head of the victim; if not, it should be cut. In no circumstances should any knot be undone. The position and type of knot provide valuable evidence as to whether the individual could have tied it. It is also important when removing or handling ligatures removed from corpses that they should not be stretched. This is particularly so in the case of articles of cloth-ing which have been used to constrict the neck. The degree of defor-mity of synthetic fibres in a stocking, tie or pair of tights might indicate the tightness of the ligature when the neck was constricted; such evidence can make a great deal of difference in deciding whether death was caused accidentally or deliberately. A husband claimed that he was attempting to restrain his infuriated wife with a pair of tights put around her neck. The degree of deformation of the fibres strongly suggested that far greater force had been applied than that which might reasonably be used in restraint.

Additional injuries to the neck are often seen in cases of throttling—which is strangulation with the hands. They are usually abrasions caused by finger-nails digging into the neck skin and bruises caused by finger-ends or knuckles. In general, bruising is more conspicuous on the thin skin over the front of the neck rather than on the thicker skin of the neck posteriorly. Abrasions are usually curved when produced by finger-nails, though it is often difficult to say which digit was responsible for a particular injury. Abrasions and bruises are often grouped together and the conformation of the group may indicate the way in which the hands have been applied to the neck. The size, shape and distribution of such injuries must be carefully recorded by measurement and photography. Considerable ingenuity in the use of ordinary or ultraviolet light is often needed to produce adequate photographs.

When ligature marks, abrasions and bruises occur together, the likely possibility of homicide should be carefully considered. However, nail marks might be found in suicidal strangulation if the victim's fingers become trapped between the noose and the skin of the neck. Such abrasions may cause confusion if the ligature has been removed from the neck and careful records have not been preserved. Clusters of numerous abrasions on the neck are not infrequently the result of heterosexual and homosexual activity. Usually they have little to do with the cause of death and similar marks will be found elsewhere on the thighs, genitals and abdominal wall when a detailed examination is made.

Traumatic or crush asphyxia

This is the result of intense compression of the chest and abdomen by a fall of earth in a trench, a heavy vehicle, the pressure of an unruly crowd and so on. The post-mortem appearances are often dramatic. There is intense congestion of the tissues above the compressed area and petechial haemorrhages are abundant in the skin and conjunctivae, which are also oedematous and suffused with blood. Despite the dramatic signs that are seen in traumatic asphyxia, it is remarkable that recovery can nevertheless take place. The subject is considered in greater detail in Chapters 8 and 15.

Conclusion

Most cases of violent asphyxia yield features which lead to a prompt solution. Several problems do, however, remain. For example, the degree of pressure on the neck which might prove fatal is not clearly defined; it may be remarkably slight. This sort of situation may arise during vigorous sexual activity when death may ensue from relatively slight compression of the neck. Another difficulty arises from smothering with soft objects. Very little evidence to prove asphyxia or injury may be present if a pillow is used. The only indication leading to suspicion of foul play may be ill-defined pressure marks from teeth on the inner lips and a few petechial haemorrhages in the conjunctivae.

As in all types of forensic work, the pathology is but one facet which cannot always provide a solution of itself. The answers are generally more forthcoming when the pathological features are considered in association with the circumstantial evidence and the results obtained by other forensic scientists.

References

1. Beeley, J. A. and Harvey, W. (1976). Pink teeth seen post mortem. In: *Dental Identification and Forensic Odontology*, Chap. 8. Ed. W. Harvey. London: Henry Kimpton.
2. Constantinides, P. and Robinson, M. (1969). Ultrastructural injury of arterial endothelium. II. Effects of vasoactive amines. *Arch. Path.* **88**, 106.
3. Fetterman, G. H. and Moran, T. J. (1942). Food aspiration pneumonia. *Penn. med. J.* **45**, 810.
4. Green, M. A. (1973). Morbid anatomical findings in strangulation. *Forensic Sci.* **2**, 317.
5. Knight, B. H. (1975). The significance of the post-mortem discovery of gastric contents in the air passages. *Forensic Sci.* **6**, 229.
6. Mendelson, C. L. (1946). Aspiration of stomach contents into the lungs during obstetric anesthesia. *Amer. J. Obstet. Gynec.* **52**, 191.
7. Paparo, G. P. and Siegel, H. (1976). On the significance of posterior crico-arytenoid muscle haemorrhage. *Forensic Sci.* **7**, 61.
8. Parish, W. E., Barrett, A. M., Coombs, R. R. A., Gunter, M. and Camps, F. E. (1960). Hypersensitivity to milk and sudden death in infancy. *Lancet* **ii**, 1106.
9. Rentoul, E. and Smith, H. (Eds.) (1973). Asphyxia. In: *Glaister's Medical Jurisprudence and Toxicology*, 13th edn., Chap. 6, pp. 171–172. Edinburgh and London: Churchill Livingstone.
10. Segarra, F. and Redding, R. A. (1974). Modern concepts about drowning. *Canad. med. Ass. J.* **110**, 1057.
11. Voigt, G. E. (1974). Petechial bleedings in the larynx. *Forensic Sci.* **3**, 256.
12. Woolley, P. V. (1945). Mechanical suffocation during infancy. *J. Pediat.* **26**, 572.

12

Blunt head injury

The effects of head injury are complex[1,4,7,8,23] and depend not only
on the mechanism of injury and on the severity of the applied force but
also on the site of its application to the skull and on the presence or
absence of injury to other parts of the body.

The scalp, skull and meninges, superficial vessels and the brain may
be damaged singly or in varying combinations at the moment of impact.
While the immediate injury to the brain may be so severe as to preclude
survival, many individuals who sustain less severe initial injury die,
often needlessly, from the secondary effects—haemorrhage, oedema,
cerebral displacement and stem haemorrhages and, less commonly,
infection and hydrocephalus. The disparity between the gross appearance of the brain and the eventual outcome is a puzzling feature of some
cases. Whereas there is obvious structural damage to the brain and/or
an intracranial haematoma in most fatal cases, in a few instances, particularly in children, brain swelling and 'oedema' may be the main
finding and careful scrutiny reveals only minor cerebral contusions.
Nevertheless, detailed histological study of such cases may show
numerous widespread foci of injury.

Injury to the head may be direct or indirect. Indirect injuries may
result from a heavy fall on to the feet or buttocks, the force of the
impact being transmitted via the vertebral column to the base of the
skull; this type of injury, although well documented, is, in fact,
relatively rare in practice except in unusual situations such as parachuting.

Direct injuries, which are much commoner, may be caused by the
following mechanisms:

1. Compression of the stationary head.
2. A blow to the stationary head from any type of moving object,
ranging from a large, relatively slow-moving object such as a club or
stone to a small, high-velocity bullet. Impact by large objects is complicated by the development of acceleration effects in skull and brain
even at relatively low velocities if the head is unsupported. The so-
called 'punch-drunk' syndrome (see Chapter 15) is a unique example of
the cumulative effects of repeated heavy blows to the face and head.
3. The majority of head injuries encountered in civilian practice are
deceleration—or negative acceleration—impact injuries of the type

which occur in road traffic accidents and falls and are due to the moving head being more or less suddenly brought to a stop against a large, unyielding, usually stationary object. Most blunt head injuries come into this category and it is with these that the present account is concerned.

Blunt injuries are liable to be associated with a variable degree of transient deformation of the skull. When the head is accelerated or decelerated as the result of impact with a blunt object, movement of the

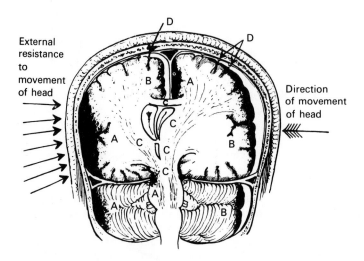

Fig. 12.1 The mechanism of cerebral injury by linear deceleration.[23] A: Injury by impact; B: injury by suction; C: injury by distortion; D: rupture of vessels by stretching. (Reproduced by kind permission of the author, Dr. G. F. Rowbotham, and the publishers, Churchill Livingstone.)

brain in relation to the skull may be either linear or angular (Figs. 12.1 and 12.2) to the direction of the applied force or a combination of these types of movement may result. According to Gurdjian,[9] injury to the brain results from:

1. Compression or pushing of the tissues together.
2. Tension or pulling of the tissues apart from one another.
3. Shear or sliding of one portion of tissue over another.

The lesions observed within the skull are therefore frequently complex and since any of these mechanisms can operate individually or collectively in a given case, their interpretation may be difficult.

Apart from any obvious immediate effects of head injury such as cerebral contusions, lacerations and haemorrhages for which a clear-cut mechanical explanation may be established by correlating the position of scalp or facial injuries and skull fractures with the circumstances of

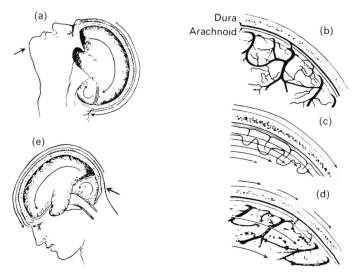

Fig. 12.2 Injury of the brain by rotation.[23] Whenever the head is struck by a force not directed along that line which passes through the centre of gravity of the head and the occipitoatlantal joint (the fulcrum), it is set into rotation. The skull necessarily takes the first impact of the blow and moves before the brain. Then the brain is secondarily set into motion by the skull and, particularly, by projecting bony prominences and dural septa. Since the brain is soft and not rigid, it rapidly becomes deformed. In closed injuries it is the shearing forces associated with deformity which cause the maximum damage to the cerebral tissues and tear the cerebral arteries and veins.

(*a*) When a patient is struck on the chin the head is thrown backwards. (*b*)–(*d*) The resulting deformity of the brain in relation to the vault of the skull. (*e*) If a patient falls backwards and strikes his head on the ground, the head will be knocked forwards into an anterior rotation, the shearing forces in this case being the opposite direction. Probably in most accidents, the head is set into violent rotation about different axes at different phases of the infliction of the violence. (Reproduced by kind permission of the author, Dr. G. F. Rowbotham, and the publishers, Churchill Livingstone.)

the accident, consideration must also be given to the possible effects of mechanical injury, short of actual rupture, on the vasomotor activity of the smaller blood vessels of the brain. As Langfitt[16] has shown experimentally, vasomotor changes do occur following injury and may be responsible for the development of brain swelling (oedema). It is the amount of brain damage inflicted at the moment of impact which is the major determinant of the outcome and this does not necessarily bear any relationship to the severity of any scalp lesion present or to the presence or absence of skull fractures. Nevertheless, a careful study of scalp lesions and skull fractures is essential not only with a view to their treatment but also as evidence of the cause of injury, the direction of forces applied to the brain and the location of the brain injuries which may be expected to have occurred, all of which are matters of importance to clinician and forensic pathologist alike.

It is unnecessary here to dwell on facial and scalp injuries. They range from simple bruising through abrasions to extensive lacerations. The last, even when they follow blunt head injury, may superficially resemble incised wounds and be responsible for excessive blood loss or provide a portal for the entry of organisms. Bleeding from the ears or nose is common in basal fractures.

The importance of skull fractures has, perhaps, been somewhat exaggerated in the past. Their intrinsic importance is that they confirm beyond doubt that a significant amount of violence has been applied to the head and, if depressed or comminuted, they indicate not only the site of impact but also give a clue as to the likely position of contre coup brain lesions. Fractures, particularly those involving the squamous temporal bone, may be responsible for extradural bleeding. Depressed fractures may be associated with tearing of major dural venous sinuses and/or cause severe focal damage to the cerebral cortex and increase the risks of sepsis and post-traumatic epilepsy. Fractures which involve the paranasal air sinuses, cribriform plate or middle ear are all compound fractures which may subsequently be associated with infection and, in the case of the cribriform plate, cerebrospinal fluid rhinorrhoea or aerocele.

Concussion

The immediate effect of a significant degree of injury to the head is loss of consciousness. The term 'simple concussion' is usually applied to those cases in which the conscious level returns to normal within a few moments, hours or, perhaps, 2–3 days without any permanent neurological sequelae. Concussion therefore refers to a clinical state of depressed or absent cerebral function which may be accompanied by evidence of depressed medullary function. As recovery is the rule in uncomplicated cases, little is known about either its pathogenesis or its pathology. It has been variously ascribed to:

1. A generalized shake-up of neurones by widespread vibrations set up within the brain at the moment of impact or by pressure waves transmitted by the cerebrospinal fluid.

2. Acute momentary brain shifts through either the incisura of the tentorium or the foramen magnum.

3. Sudden anoxaemia caused by traumatic vasomotor paralysis.

Concussion is always more severe in acceleration or deceleration injuries than in crushing injuries. Examination of the brain of an individual who has recently recovered from an episode of concussion and died from some other cause may reveal either no intracranial abnormality or only slight swelling, scattered petechial haemorrhages or minor contusions or lacerations. It is hardly surprising that there are no constant pathological findings in such cases, as the reversible nature of the condition must presumably indicate that the disturbance giving rise to the loss of consciousness is physiological and therefore need not be accompanied by structural changes demonstrable by any of the methods presently available to us.

Brain swelling

One of the basic reactions to injury anywhere in the body is development of a greater or lesser degree of swelling of the part affected. This is due to the accumulation of extracellular fluid as a result of an alteration in the vascular permeability. Swelling occurs in the traumatized brain and sometimes, especially in the young, is so severe as to be the most important single factor leading to the patient's death.

The presence of brain swelling is to be suspected when the unopened dura is found to be tightly stretched, difficulty is encountered in dividing it without damage to the brain and the cerebral gyri are wide, pale and flattened while the intervening sulci are narrowed. Bilateral uncal herniation is present and the cerebellar tonsils may be impacted in the foramen magnum. Section of the brain reveals compression of the subarachnoid space and of the ventricles. Much of the increase in cerebral volume is due to expansion of white rather than grey matter and the cut surface may be wet or dry. These features are asymmetric when associated with focal injury to the brain, being usually most marked in relation to the traumatic lesions.

The increase in cerebral volume is due to accumulation of fluid but, whereas it has long been accepted that elsewhere in the body this fluid is located in the intercellular spaces, the term 'oedema' being appropriate, the situation has been far less clear in the brain. It is well recognized that, even in the presence of severe swelling, the cut surface of the brain does not always weep fluid as do oedematous tissues elsewhere, and the early electron microscopic studies, by their denial of the existence of extracellular space in the brain, encouraged the view that brain swelling differed from oedema in that the fluid accumulation was intracellular. More recent studies reviewed by Klatzo,[14] however, have indicated that an extracellular space does exist and that its dimensions in the white matter differ from those in the grey. In the white matter the spaces are irregular, and may attain a width of 80 nm (800 Å); in the grey matter adjacent cell membranes are separated by no more than 10–20 nm (100–200 Å). Subsequent investigators have concluded that a degree of intracellular swelling does occur and that in any one case fluid accumulates both in the extracellular space and in the cytoplasm of the glia, most notably of the astrocytes.

Intracranial haemorrhage

A variety of lesions may be found within the skull as a result of a blunt head injury and these may occur singly or in combination. These are considered most simply in the anatomical sequence in which they are encountered at necropsy and are as follows:

Extradural haemorrhage
Subdural haemorrhage
Subarachnoid haemorrhage
Brain injury.

Extradural haematoma

Fracture of the skull, most commonly one which involves the temporal bone, may be complicated by the accumulation of a lenticular mass of clotted blood between the bone and the dura. Very rarely, no fracture is demonstrable at necropsy. As an isolated lesion, such a haematoma is rare at any age and is almost unknown in infancy. It acts as a space-occupying lesion and where there is little room for its expansion, as in the posterior fossa, a small haematoma may assume major significance—the possibility of its occurrence at this site also tends to be forgotten by the clinician.

The source of bleeding is usually one of the middle meningeal vessels but it may be from a venous sinus or an un-named diploic vessel. The haemorrhage is usually thought of as being arterial but there is no doubt as to its venous origin on occasion. There is good evidence that separation of the dura from bone occurs at the moment of impact and it is into this preformed space that bleeding takes place.[5] Although, initially, both separation of dura and the extent of haematoma tend to be limited by the dense adhesion of the dura to the suture lines, this boundary may be transgressed by a haematoma which may come to cover much of one cerebral convexity.

Characteristically, after a period of several hours, or even days, of apparently total recovery from a concussive head injury (the so-called 'lucid interval') cerebral function deteriorates over a few hours, unconsciousness recurs and symptoms of progressive cerebral compression appear.[11] The delay in the onset of these symptoms relates either to systemic hypotension (shock), to slow oozing from a lacerated vessel in which spasm and partial plugging of the leak by thrombus has occurred or to the time necessary for the haematoma to attain a critical volume.

Removal of the calvarium at necropsy necessitates opening into the haematoma cavity and this may lead to loss of blood. The volume of the haematoma may thus be difficult to estimate; it is best recorded by direct measurement in a graduated vessel or in terms of its area and maximum thickness. An average volume in fatal cases is between 100 and 150 ml.

The situation is complicated, both clinically and pathologically, by the presence, in about half of the cases, of cerebral contusions and lacerations which are usually contralateral. In a number of cases, a subdural haematoma occurs either on the same or the opposite side; when it is on the same side and in direct relationship to the extradural haematoma, the subdural haemorrhage may be a simple extension of the extradural bleeding through a dural tear rather than a separate lesion.

Subdural haemorrhage

Subdural haemorrhage may be either acute, subacute or chronic; in its acute variety it is a common post-traumatic lesion which is present in most patients dying within a few days of their head injury.

Acute subdural haematoma

Acute subdural haemorrhages are considerably more common than are extradural haemorrhages and neither a fracture of the skull nor a contusion of the brain is present in at least half of the cases.

Minor degrees of acute subdural haemorrhage take the form of a thin film of clotted or unclotted blood which diffusely overlies the cerebrum or cerebellum, possibly related to a trivial surface contusion or laceration. It may occur either at the site of injury, on the opposite side or, as is frequently the case, bilaterally. The bleeding probably results from the laceration of a cortical vein as it traverses the subdural space en route to one of the venous sinuses; this origin is not by any means invariable and the haemorrhage may result from laceration of the superficial brain substance. The haemorrhage presents as a poorly defined lenticular mass of partially clotted blood which usually overlies the convexity of the cerebral hemisphere; a tapering sheet of blood extends peripherally into the cranial fossae. The major mass of a subdural haemorrhage may occur at other sites, such as alongside the falx or in the posterior fossa.

The size of the haemorrhage may be considerable and should be recorded at operation or necropsy; as with the extradural haematoma, it is possible that loss of blood during removal of the brain may lead to an underestimate of its original volume and a corresponding failure to appreciate its significance as a major space-occupying lesion.

Very occasionally, but often enough to be worth stressing, an acute subdural haematoma results from rupture of a congenital aneurysm; this is usually on the posterior communicating artery which, because of a previous leak, has become fused to the overlying arachnoid so that subsequent haemorrhage occurs directly into the subdural space.

Subacute subdural haematoma

These lesions are clinically directly related to a traumatic incident but the onset of symptoms is delayed for a few days or even a week or two. They are usually accompanied by a fracture of the skull or cerebral laceration. The occurrence of a subacute lesion is to be suspected when a patient who has been maintaining a steady improvement levels off or deteriorates.

The distinction between acute and subacute post-traumatic subdural haematoma is largely clinical; pathologically they may be indistinguishable, but commencing organization of the haematoma from the dura may be seen.

Chronic subdural haematoma

It might be supposed that a chronic subdural haematoma is simply an acute one which has been present for a long time. This, however, does not appear to be the case. Frequently, no reliable history of head injury is available and it is exceptional to find evidence of one at necropsy. They tend to occur at the extremes of life and, being commonly bilateral, they give rise to symmetric brain compression; the slowly evolving and subtle mental and physical changes so produced in children and the elderly tend to be unnoticed until the volume of the clot and granulation tissue has reached considerable proportions.

The haemorrhage most commonly occurs from a ruptured bridging vein, i.e. one which traverses the subdural space en route from subarachnoid space to dural venous sinus. Rupture of such a vein occurs most readily when relative movement of brain and skull is easiest—when the skull is most pliable as in childhood and the brain is atrophic as in the aged.

A chronic subdural haematoma is essentially a mass of subdural clot which has been partly organized by the growth of granulation tissue from the dura (Fig. 12.3). This growth occurs not only into the dural

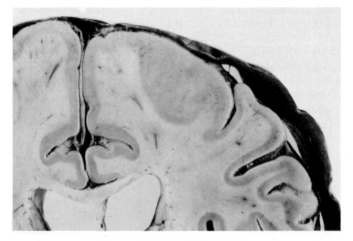

Fig. 12.3 Chronic subdural haematoma over cerebral convexity. Elderly patient, no history of injury; note compensatory ventricular dilatation due to brain atrophy.

aspect of the clot but also along its interface with the outer surface of the arachnoid, which rarely becomes involved in the reparative process. The appearance is thus of a brownish mass of spongy, partly cystic, granulation tissue which is adherent to the dura and is bounded on its deep (i.e. arachnoidal) surface by a smooth 'false' membrane. It is clear from microscopic examination of any chronic subdural haematoma that repetitive haemorrhage occurs into the granulation tissue and leads to 'growth' of the haematoma in a way which makes attempts at ageing it abortive.

A small haematoma may become completely organized and is seen as a more or less thin brown membrane adherent to the deep surface of the dura, whereas a larger one becomes extensively cystic and is essentially a fibrous-walled sac of yellowish fluid attached to the dura.

The effects of chronic subdural haemorrhage are those of cortical compression and chronic cerebral displacement. The cortex immediately related to the haemorrhage shows neuronal depletion and astrocytic gliosis which is most readily detected in the marginal layer (Fig. 12.4). The leptomeninges show mild fibrosis, chronic inflam-

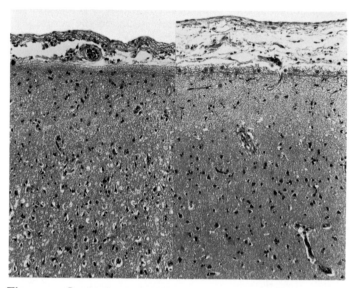

Fig. 12.4 Cerebral cortex and leptomeninges: (*right*) from normal hemisphere; (*left*) beneath chronic subdural haematoma (not seen), displaying leptomeningeal fibrosis and gliosis of subpial layer of cortex. (H & E, × 110)

matory cell infiltration and haemosiderin pigmentation which may also extend for some way into the cortex.

A careful examination of the brain should be made for the presence of cerebrovascular disease or other type of organic dementia in all cases of chronic subdural haemorrhage in the aged. The effects of these, separately or together, may be added to those of the subdural haemorrhage, a situation which is of obvious forensic significance.

Subarachnoid haemorrhage
Subarachnoid haemorrhage, either focal or diffuse, is probably the commonest post-traumatic intracranial lesion. It varies greatly in amount and may or may not complicate the presence of an overt cor-

tical contusion or laceration. It naturally tends to be greatest in amount along the sulci and, occasionally, a focal subarachnoid haemorrhage attains such a size as to constitute a space-occupying lesion; this feature is commonly seen over the insular cortex.

Subarachnoid haemorrhage elicits a variable degree of sterile leptomeningitis; the resultant fibrosis (which may occur at any site from the exit foramina of the fourth ventricle to the superomedial border of the cerebral hemispheres) is usually accepted as an explanation of the transient or permanent hydrocephalus which develops following some head injuries.

Cerebral contusions and lacerations
Contusions are traumatic lesions of brain tissue which stop just short of macroscopic tearing or laceration. They may occur on the cerebral or cerebellar cortex or deep within the brain and are essentially coalescent punctate haemorrhages around which focal swelling has occurred. When superficial, they appear as mottled purplish areas on which are superimposed variable numbers of small subpial haemorrhages. The lesion is often wedge-shaped on section, with its base on the surface of the brain.

Lacerations are macroscopically visible tears of the brain and may be considered as contusions in which traumatic disruption of brain tissue has occurred. They are often located on the orbital surfaces and supraciliary borders of the frontal lobes and on the temporal poles. They are usually superficial but are occasionally deep enough to open into a ventricle; the deeper lacerations are commonly associated with comminuted, depressed fractures. The pia is always torn and ruptured cortical vessels may bleed into the subarachnoid space. Tearing of the arachnoid is also usual and this permits blood and cerebrospinal fluid to escape into the subdural space, thus giving rise to an acute or subacute subdural haemorrhage. Dural tears are less common and, when they occur, are usually directly related to a fracture. Irregular blood-filled cavities may be found within the brain in severe injuries and, occasionally, there may be total disintegration of one or more lobes—the so-called 'burst lobe' effect.

Vertical lacerations through part of, or the whole thickness of, the corpus callosum are common even when superficial contusions and lacerations are inconspicuous elsewhere. They are still considered by some to be due to a slicing action of the falx cerebri caused by vertical compression of the cranial vault but they are, in fact, almost certainly due to mass disparate movement of the two cerebral hemispheres, one of which is prevented from moving laterally at the same rate as its fellow because of the intervening falx.[18]

Microscopic examination of recent contusions and lacerations shows interruption of cytoarchitecture by haemorrhages of varying size, the smaller of which are of 'ball' or 'ring' shape. The nerve cells, their processes and the neuroglia at the site are destroyed. Cellular alterations seen at the margins of the haemorrhage depend upon the time interval between injury and death and, in general terms, resemble those following infarction—interstitial oedema, chromatolysis, ischaemic nerve cell change and swelling with eventual disintegration of both myelin and axis cylinders. Polymorphonuclear leucocyte diapedesis occurs after a few hours and is followed by proliferation of microglial cells and their transformation into compound granular corpuscles which remove the dead tissue and, later, by proliferation of capillaries and surviving astrocytes. After 7–10 days, the area of injury is fairly well demarcated from the surviving brain by cerebral granulation tissue which grows into and replaces the necrotic debris. Eventually, all that remains is a loose, sparsely cellular and relatively avascular glial scar which may be cystic and is usually stained by haemosiderin. Fibroblastic proliferation accompanies the healing process in superficial lesions associated with injury to the meninges; the resultant scar contains both collagen and glial fibres and there may be adhesion to the dura. It is usually fairly easy to distinguish old areas of traumatic cortical scarring from healed infarcts as the former characteristically involve the summits of gyri and the latter the cortex in the depth of sulci. Contraction of the scarred regions of brain may lead to deformity of the affected lobe, with distortion and compensatory dilatation of the ipsilateral ventricle. Large post-traumatic cysts may communicate with the ventricular system.

Localization of contusions and lacerations

The anatomical location of contusions and lacerations is of particular importance in the elucidation of the mechanism of injury in a given case. In the more common type of injury, which results from deceleration of the moving head against a stationary or relatively stationary object, lesions are seen at two sites:

1. direct (coup) injuries occur at the site of impact; and
2. subdural and subarachnoid haemorrhages, cerebral contusions or lacerations which may be found, singly or in combination, more or less diametrically opposite the site of direct injury (*contre coup*).

The latter, indirect, injuries are frequently of much greater severity than are the direct injuries and their occurrence is of considerable importance (Fig. 12.5).

In the case, for example, of an individual who falls to the ground and strikes the back of his head, examination of the brain will reveal not only injury in the occipital region but also severe contre coup contusions and lacerations which are almost invariably found in the subfrontal and anterior temporal regions; the nearer the mid-line the impact occurs, the greater the liability for the contre coup lesions to be bilateral, and the further laterally the point of impact moves from the occiput, the more involved is the opposite frontotemporal region. In most striking exception to these general observations, contre coup

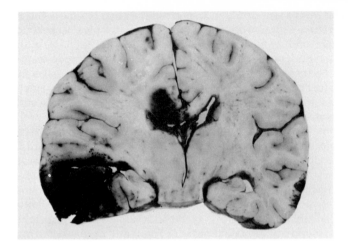

Fig. 12.5 Coronal slice of cerebrum showing trivial coup contusions (right temporal) and severe contre coup lacerations (left temporal). There is also laceration of the corpus callosum.

lesions are virtually never seen in the occipital lobes. They may be observed on the inferior surface of the cerebellum.

Numerous theories have been propounded to explain the occurrence of contre coup lesions.[2]

1. *The struck hoop theory.* Indentation or flattening of the skull at the site of impact causes deformation of the skull as a whole; the skull momentarily tends to assume a more ovoid shape and that portion diametrically opposite suddenly impinges on the underlying brain.

2. *Russel's theory of brain displacement.* The skull is immediately arrested at the moment of impact, but the brain, being of greater mass and having a jelly-like consistence, continues in motion for a fraction of time and deforms in such a manner that there is a potential space between brain and skull at the pole opposite the site of impact. The sudden separation of brain and leptomeninges from the dura is liable to cause rupture of vessels traversing the subdural space and result in cortical lesions.

3. *Goggio's pressure gradient theory.* At the moment of injury there is a high positive pressure at the site of impact and a corresponding negative pressure diametrically opposite. This negative pressure causes a bursting or explosive effect, with disruption of vessels and nervous tissue.

4. *Rotational forces* set up at the time of impact in either acceleration or deceleration injuries may also account for the production of contre coup lesions.[10, 22]

None of these satisfactorily explains the rarity of contre coup lesions on the occipital lobes. The floor of the anterior, middle and, to a lesser extent, the posterior fossae is markedly irregular and the sharp cutting edge of the lesser wing of the sphenoid bone is situated between the anterior and middle cranial fossae; localization of contre coup lesions to the frontotemporal regions, particularly following deceleration injury, does suggest that sudden differential movement of the base of the brain over the irregular floor of the skull after impact probably plays a prominent part in their pathogenesis. The occipital lobes relate to the much smoother contours of vault of skull and tentorium. Clearly, no simple explanation is likely to be adequate for all circumstances.

Brain stem lesions

Lesions found in the brain stem in fatal head injury cases are of particular interest both to the neurosurgeon and to the pathologist. Some are primary, i.e. they are directly due to injury and occur at the time of impact; others are secondary to brain displacement which, in turn, may be due to post-traumatic intracranial haemorrhage or brain oedema. Secondary lesions develop within a few minutes, hours or even days after the injury and are theoretically preventable. Primary lesions may be complicated by the onset of secondary lesions.

Brain stem lesions may be quite obvious to the naked eye. They are found as a rule in the midbrain and upper pons. They are rarer in the lower pons and quite exceptional in the medulla of those patients who survive long enough to reach hospital alive; when found in the medulla, they are almost invariably associated with fractures in the region of the foramen magnum. Visible brain stem lesions are haemorrhagic, usually multiple, of variable size and tend to lie centrally in the tegmentum either in a cluster or distributed in the mid-line in a linear fashion running anteroposteriorly (Fig. 12.6). In some cases a narrow zone of petechial haemorrhages may be seen in one or other lateral border of the midbrain and may also involve the cerebral peduncles. On rare occasions, the lesions are found anteriorly in the stem immediately beneath the pia. Lacerations or total rupture of the stem are seen occasionally in those who have died immediately at the roadside. Such gross injuries are always due to severe fracture dislocation involving the posterior fossa and atlantoaxial joints.

Not all stem lesions are haemorrhagic. Although the stem may appear macroscopically normal, histological examination in patients who survive 12 hours or longer will often disclose microscopic lesions resembling infarcts; these tend to be perivascular and are possibly the forerunners of the gross haemorrhages.

Primary stem lesions
Several different types are recognized; namely:

1. Those caused by local injury, usually associated with fracture of the basisphenoid and basiocciput and often characterized by gross laceration of the stem.
2. Those caused by the contre coup mechanism, which are usually

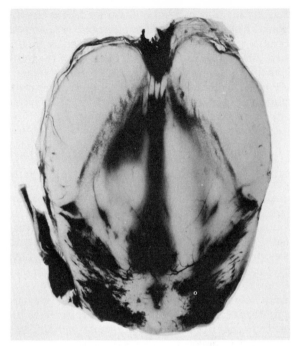

Fig. 12.6   Cleared preparation of midbrain, showing severe secondary stem haemorrhages.

found when the patient falls on the back of the head, fracturing the occipital bone; in such cases the stem haemorrhages are often arranged in a mid-sagittal line in the tegmental portion of the midbrain.

3. Those caused by lateral dislocation of the brain. If the head moving in a lateral direction is suddenly arrested against a solid object, not only may contusions be noted at the site of impact on the lateral aspect of the cerebral hemisphere, but the stem may impinge against the free edge of the tentorium on the same side. Le Count and Apfelbach[17] described this mechanism as: 'stretching the brain (cerebral hemisphere) away from the brain stem because the former is more movable'.

Secondary stem lesions
Secondary stem lesions commonly complicate severe head injury and may occur in any circumstance in which an intracranial, usually supratentorial, space-occupying lesion develops. Quite apart from any local effect on the brain, such an expanding lesion within the skull will eventually cause a rise in intracranial pressure, with distortion and displacement of brain tissue. Displacement may be in any direction but, in the event of a supratentorial space-occupying mass, it is believed that movements in the lateral and/or downward direction are of major significance. The space-occupying lesion following violence may be haemorrhage (extradural, subdural, subarachnoid or intracerebral) or

brain oedema or both of these. The sequence of events which accompanies an expanding extradural haematoma offers a convenient example. As the underlying cerebral convexity is compressed, the ipsilateral ventricle is also compressed and is bodily displaced towards the opposite side along with the third ventricle and other mid-line structures. The contralateral ventricle may dilate if its drainage into the third ventricle becomes occluded. The slender perforating branches of the circle of Willis which supply the basal ganglia, thalamus and hypothalamus are compressed or stretched; small ischaemic or haemorrhagic foci of necrosis may develop in these areas, possibly on the basis of vascular spasm consequent upon the mechanical distortion. The cingulate gyrus on the side of the extradural haemorrhage becomes displaced towards the opposite side, passes under the falx and carries with it the anterior cerebral arteries. The midbrain may also be thrust against the free edge of the tentorium, giving rise to a shallow, linear indentation on its contralateral cerebral peduncle; this is the so-called Kernohan's notch and, on section, subpial petechial haemorrhages are found at this site.[13] It must be remembered that similar laterally placed haemorrhages in the midbrain without grooving may result from

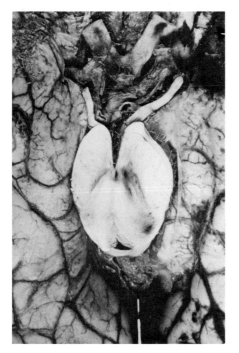

Fig. 12.7 Base of brain, showing severe herniation of the whole of the left parahippocampal gyrus and distortion of midbrain, in which small secondary haemorrhages are seen. The left oculomotor nerve is stretched, flattened and indented.

damage at the time of initial injury due to the lateral dislocation of the stem against the tentorium. The development of Kernohan's notch is of clinical importance for it may give rise to ipsilateral (i.e. on the side of injury) hemiparesis. In addition to lateral displacement of midline structures, there is a tendency for the supratentorial contents to be forced downwards. The brain stem moves caudally and the uncus, or even the whole of the parahippocampal gyrus on the side of the extradural haematoma, is squeezed against the midbrain and is also crowded through the tentorial opening (Fig. 12.7). The midbrain is compressed from side to side, elongated anteroposteriorly and to some extent rotated about its long axis. A deep groove may be seen on the inferior surface of the temporal lobe as far as 1·0 cm lateral to the herniated uncus or parahippocampal gyrus; the hernia, which can extend the whole length of the gyrus, may eventually undergo haemorrhagic infarction. Depending upon its rate of onset and its magnitude, this downward shift may affect the blood supply, certain cranial nerves, the cerebrospinal fluid circulation and the brain stem.

Blood supply
The circle of Willis can be considered as being anchored at four points— where the internal carotid arteries pierce the dura beside the anterior clinoid processes and where the posterior cerebral arteries pass upwards through the incisura and turn over the free edge of the tentorium to run posteriorly towards the occipital poles. Caudal displacement of the stem and herniation of the temporal lobe produces the secondary stem lesions by stretching and compressing the perforating and circumferential vessels of the midbrain and upper pons. Although some of the haemorrhages may be venous in origin, the majority are arteriolar and capillary,[12] and are probably preceded by small foci of ischaemic necrosis. Haemorrhagic infarction of the ipsilateral calcarine cortex is also encountered in some cases and is believed to be due to compression of the posterior cerebral artery between the edge of the tentorium and herniated parahippocampal gyrus; for some reason, this lesion has become much less common of recent years.

Cranial nerves
Uncal herniation is frequently associated clinically with dilatation of the pupil on the same side; this is due to interference with the parasympathetic fibres of the third nerve (Fig. 12.7) as a result of compression and stretching. Small haemorrhages can be seen on the surface of the nerve in some cases. It is uncertain whether the nerve is actually compressed against the tentorium by the uncus or is trapped between the superior cerebellar and posterior cerebral arteries. The sixth cranial nerve has a long intradural course which is almost parallel to the long axis of the stem and is therefore liable to be stretched by caudal displacement of the brain stem. As either or both sixth nerves may be involved in any given case, lateral rectus paresis, unlike pupillary dilatation, has no value as a lateralizing sign.

Cerebrospinal fluid circulation
Interference with cerebrospinal fluid circulation may occur as a result of compression of the aqueduct, obstruction of the subarachnoid space by the herniated uncus or occlusion of the roof foramina of the fourth ventricle by cerebellar coning (see below).

Lower stem
If the downward shift is severe enough, the cerebellar tonsils may be driven down into the foramen magnum. This is referred to as cerebellar coning, tonsillar herniation or foraminal impaction. In normal circumstances, some brains show at post mortem a shallow or even quite deep groove which divides the medial portion of the cerebellar cortex alongside the medulla from the remainder of the interior aspect of the cerebellar hemisphere and which corresponds in outline to the margin of the foramen magnum. This groove is much deeper in the presence of tonsillar herniation; the herniated cerebellar tonsils may be stippled with petechial haemorrhages and undergo necrosis. The medulla in such cases may show no evidence of ischaemic damage, presumably because death has usually occurred too rapidly. If, however, the patient has been maintained on a ventilator in the presence of foraminal impaction, diffuse nerve cell necrosis may occur in the medulla with minimal cellular inflammatory reaction. This is part of the spectrum of change seen in the deanimated brain syndrome.[15,25]

Infratentorial space-occupying lesions
A clinically significant haematoma in the posterior fossa without associated supratentorial brain damage is uncommon following blunt head injury but the lesion is of extreme importance. Because of the relatively small size of the subtentorial compartment, quite a small haematoma, especially one of extradural type, may produce severe secondary effects due to displacement. In addition to the cerebellar coning, which may be unilateral, with its associated risk of acute medullary failure, the superior vermis may herniate upwards through the tentorial notch. Both displacements give rise to acute hydrocephalus.

Prevention and differentiation of stem injuries
Primary stem lesions occur in a high proportion of fatal deceleration head injuries, particularly in those following impact to the back of the head, and the only method of reducing their incidence lies in accident prevention.

Secondary stem haemorrhages, on the other hand, should theoretically not be allowed to occur and will not do so if blood clots are treated before they become large enough to cause brain displacement and if brain oedema can be adequately controlled. It is therefore of considerable medicolegal importance for the pathologist to endeavour to establish whether stem lesions are of primary or secondary type. The major problem is that many head injuries are complicated by raised

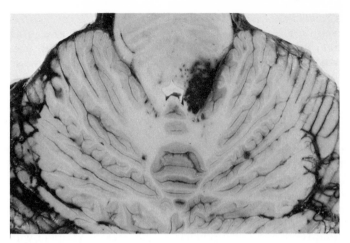

Fig. 12.8   Upper pons and cerebellum. Primary stem lesion in right superior cerebellar peduncle.

intracranial pressure and that consequently secondary stem lesions may mask primary lesions. According to Crompton,[3] the primary lesions are areas of ischaemic necrosis, small or microhaemorrhages and foci of shearing and degeneration of axons, which may be found anywhere from the subthalamic region to the medulla but are least common in the pons. In an undistorted brain stem, lesions localized to one side of the tegmentum, the periaqueductal grey matter or superior cerebellar peduncles (Fig. 12.8), are said to be fairly typical of primary injury. Crompton also noted neuronal degeneration in the vestibular and inferior olivary nuclei of the medulla in a number of cases. The secondary stem lesions which accompany cerebral shifts are gross uni- or bilateral paramedian liner zones of haemorrhagic necrosis or rounded lesions centrally placed in the tegmentum of the midbrain and upper pons.

The particular difficulty in establishing the presence or absence of primary stem injury is considerable both clinically and pathologically—clinically, because the term is applied to signs and symptoms of brain stem dysfunction which, while they may indeed be caused by focal trauma to the stem, may equally be due to lesions at a higher level; pathologically, because there is so often evidence of brain shifts and distortion of the upper brain stem by the time a head-injured patient dies. Continuous monitoring of intraventricular pressure following blunt head injury is now carried out in some centres; studies by Mitchell and Adams[20] in fatal cases, in whom the intraventricular pressure had never been raised, have demonstrated the special characteristics of primary stem lesions. These workers emphasized the regular occurrence of focal lesions in the corpus callosum, the inconstant presence of lesions in the region of the superior cerebellar peduncles and the presence of axonal retraction balls or microglial stars in the brain stem which are unrelated to infarcts or haematomas.

In the absence of intracranial pressure monitoring, a knowledge of the clinical state of the patient from the time of injury to death may assist the pathologist to reach a decision as to the type of a given stem lesion. If lesions are present in a patient who was rendered unconsious immediately after accident, remained deeply unconscious and died within a short time without cerebral swelling or clots then it is a fairly safe deduction that they are primary. This view is corroborated if fractures of the skull base are present, though it must be emphasized that no fracture of the skull is found in many of these cases. It is considered unlikely in our present state of knowledge that a conscious patient can have a gross stem lesion; thus, if an individual recovers consciousness or the conscious level improves significantly following accident, only to deteriorate after some hours or days, if the brain is swollen or clots are present and if shifts are noted at necropsy then it is probable that the stem lesions are secondary. In one study[19] of 173 fatal head injuries, brain stem lesions were found in 83 cases. Applying the above clinicopathological criteria, it was considered that approximately one-quarter of the stem lesions were primary, one-quarter were secondary and no opinion could be given in the remainder. The survival time of these brain stem cases was generally short; 60 died within a few hours or days, 11 more had died within 4 weeks and only 12 survived for longer than 1 month.

Ischaemic brain damage in fatal head injuries
Foci of ischaemic necrosis may be found in the brain quite apart from those lesions which may be directly ascribed to the primary injury, those due to brain displacement and to rare cases of fat embolism.[6] Such lesions are either within major arterial distribution territories or in the so-called watershed boundary zones between them. They are seldom due to local arterial occlusion and are generally ascribed to inadequacy of cerebral perfusion as a result of raised intracranial pressure and/or systemic hypotension.

Long-term survivors

The majority of persons sustaining fatal head injuries die shortly after the accident. In the Maloney and Whatmore series,[19] 41 per cent died within hours of hospital admission, a further 34 per cent survived less than 1 week and 13 per cent less than 1 month; 12 per cent survived 1 or more months. Among the long-term survivors is a small but interesting group of patients in whom the clinical and pathological findings are remarkably constant. These patients are usually young people who have been rendered immediately unconscious by a blunt closed head injury sustained in a road traffic accident. Skull fractures are often absent. Initially decerebrate, they eventually recover to a state of akinetic mutism without clinical evidence of raised intracranial pressure and they may remain in this condition for months or even years before dying from some intercurrent infection. At autopsy evidence of gross brain damage is slight and is easily missed on casual inspection. A typical case shows slight haemosiderin staining of the meninges, a few scattered, small, healed contusions in the cortex and small softenings, which often show rusty discoloration, in the corpus callosum, in the white matter close to cortex or in the basal ganglia, periaqueductal grey matter and superior cerebellar peduncles. The ventricular system is slightly dilated. Histological examination, however, reveals most striking changes which have been fully documented.[21, 24] In essence, these consist of widespread diffuse degeneration of white matter which, in so far as both axons and myelin sheaths are affected, appears to be Wallerian in type. Strich[24] found no obvious focal lesions which could have explained the interruption of nerve fibres and she presented evidence which strongly suggests that the degeneration is secondary to the tearing or stretching of individual nerve fibres throughout the brain consequent on shear stresses caused by rotational acceleration or deceleration of the head at the time of injury. Similar widespread damage to nerve fibres must obviously occur in the majority of cases which die acutely after severe head injury but is rarely sought, being overshadowed by the gross contusions, lacerations and haematomas to which death is usually ascribed.

References

1. Adams, J. H. (1975). The neuropathology of head injuries. In: *Handbook of Clinical Neurology*, Vol. 23, Part 1, Chap. 3. Eds. P. J. Vinken and G. W. Bruyn. Amsterdam: North Holland Publishing Co.
2. Courville, C. B. (1950). *Pathology of the Central Nervous System*, 3rd edn., pp. 296–301. California: Pacific Press Publishing Assoc.
3. Crompton, M. R. (1971). Brain stem lesions due to closed head injury. *Lancet* i, 669.
4. Freytag, E. (1963). Autopsy findings in head injuries from blunt forces: statistical evaluation of 1367 cases. *Arch. Path.* 75, 402.
5. Gallacher, J. P. and Browder, E. J. (1968). Extradural haematoma: experience with 167 patients. *J. Neurosurg.* 29, 1.
6. Graham, D. I. and Adams, J. H. (1971). Ischaemic brain damage in fatal head injuries. *Lancet* i, 265.
7. Graham, D. I. and Adams, J. H. (1972). The pathology of blunt head injuries. In: *Scientific Foundations of Neurology*, Section X, Chap. 6. Eds. M. Critchley, J. L. O'Leary and B. Jennett. London: Heinemann Medical.
8. Greenfield, J. G. and Russell, D. S. (1963). Traumatic lesions of the central and peripheral nervous systems. In: *Greenfield's Neuropathology*, 2nd edn., Chap. 7. Eds. W. Blackwood, W. H. McMenemey, A. Meyer, R. M. Norman and D. S. Russell. London: Edward Arnold.
9. Gurdjian, E. S. (1971). Mechanisms of impact injury of the head. In: *Head Injuries*, Proceedings of an International Symposium held

in Edinburgh and Madrid, Section I. *Prevention of Head Injury*, p. 17. Edinburgh and London: Churchill Livingstone.

10. Holbourn, A. H. S. (1945). The mechanics of brain injuries. *Brit. med. Bull.* **3**, 147.
11. Jamieson, K. G. and Yelland, J. D. N. (1968). Extradural haematoma: report of 167 cases. *J. Neurosurg.* **29**, 13.
12. Johnson, R. T. and Yates, P. O. (1956). Brain stem haemorrhages in expanding supratentorial conditions. *Acta radiol. (Stockh.)* **46**, 250.
13. Kernohan, J. W. and Waltman, H. W. (1929). Incisura of the crus due to contralateral brain tumour. *Arch. Neurol. Psychiat.* **21**, 274.
14. Klatzo, I. (1967). Neuropathological aspects of brain edema. *J. Neuropath. exp. Neurol.* **26**, 1.
15. Kramer, W. (1963). From reanimation to deanimation. *Acta neurol. scand.* **39**, 139.
16. Langfitt, T. W. (1971). The microcirculation in mechanical brain injury. In: *Head Injuries*, Proceedings of an International Symposium held in Edinburgh and Madrid, Section IX. *Pathophysiological Basis for the Management of Head Injuries*, p. 221. Edinburgh and London: Churchill Livingstone.
17. Le Count, E. R. and Apfelbach, C. W. (1920). Pathologic anatomy of traumatic fractures of cranial bones and concomitant brain injuries. *J. Amer. med. Ass.* **74**, 501.
18. Lindenberg, R., Fisher, R. S., Durlacher, S. H., Lovitt, W. V. and Freytag, E. (1955). Lesions of the corpus callosum following blunt mechanical trauma to the head. *Amer. J. Path.* **31**, 297.
19. Maloney, A. F. J. and Whatmore, W. J. (1969). Clinical and pathological observations in fatal head injuries: a 5 year survey of 173 cases. *Brit. J. Surg.* **56**, 23.
20. Mitchell, D. E. and Adams, J. H. (1973). Primary focal impact damage to the brain stem in blunt head injuries. Does it exist? *Lancet* **ii**, 215.
21. Oppenheimer, D. R. (1968). Microscopic lesions in the brain following head injury. *J. Neurol. Neurosurg. Psychiat.* **31**, 299.
22. Pudenz, R. H. and Shelden, C. H. (1946). The lucite calvarium—a method for direct observation of the brain. Part II. Cranial trauma and brain movement. *J. Neurosurg.* **3**, 487.
23. Rowbotham, G. F. (1964). *Acute Injuries of the Head*, 4th edn., pp. 72, 76. Edinburgh and London: Churchill Livingstone.
24. Strich, S. J. (1961). Shearing of nerve fibres as a cause of brain damage due to head injury. A pathological study of 20 cases. *Lancet* **ii**, 443.
25. Walker, A. E., Diamond, E. L., Moseley, J. (1975). The neuropathological findings in irreversible coma. A critique of the 'respiratory brain'. *J. Neuropath. exp. Neurol.* **34**, 295.

13

Violence in the home

Introduction

Almost one-third of all serious assaults occur in the home of the victim and are made by a close relative.[32] Doctors with an interest in legal medicine have known this for many years but it has come to the attention of the general public only recently.

The reaction has been the same as to any unpleasant truth—denial, hysteria and eventual acceptance. Denial has led, in some instances, to death after repeated violence which could have been prevented if first reports of assaults had been believed and acted upon.[38] Hysteria has caused emotional and misleading terms to be attached to various forms of violence—'battered babies', 'wife battering' and even 'granny bashing'; battering is neither the only nor necessarily the most dangerous form of infant assault.[5] However, the term 'battered child', which was coined by Kempe in 1962,[30] served to stimulate widespread interest in the subject. This has slowly led to the acceptance of the facts of violence in the home and to more sociological and psychiatric research into its causes and associations.[14]

Violence to children

Gil[19] has defined child abuse as 'non-accidental physical attack or physical injury, including minimal as well as fatal injury, inflicted upon children by persons caring for them'. While this definition would nowadays be extended to include wilful neglect and deprivation,[28] we are mainly concerned in this chapter with traumatic injury. This is of two main types. The first occurs as a single incident; the other, which is more frequently seen by doctors, involves many assaults often of bizarre type. While one may be a precursor of the other, it is often found that different parental behaviour is associated with each type. Violence in the first results from a single outburst of rage that is instantly regretted, promptly reported and seldom repeated. Death may, however, result and an attempt to disguise the true nature of the case is therefore likely to be made. The family background of the second type is discussed below.

As about half of non-accidental traumatic deaths occur in the first year of life (Table 13.1), there is potential confusion with infanticide or

Table 13.1 Characteristics of parents and children in different series of non-accidental violence to children

	Birmingham[46]	San Francisco[31]	National British Survey[44]	National American Survey[19]	Fatal cases only[14]
Age of mother	60% aged 20–25	Average age 22½	Average age 23	80% aged 20–25	Average age 22
Age of child	50% under 1½	63% under 2	78% under 2 56% under 1	25% under 2 25% aged 2–6	61% under 2
Siblings also injured	19%	53%	7%	} 60%	} 76%
Previous injury to child	33%	44%	40%		
Further injury after hospitalization	69%		60%		
Parents themselves injured as children				21%	40%
Parents with criminal record: Mother	11% (2% violence)		9% } 12% violence		
Father*	29% (14% violence)		45% }	15% fathers only. All crimes	66% (27% violence)
Parents with severe psychopathic personality disorder: Mother	13% (50% aggressive)		14% } habitually		
Father*	33% (90% aggressive)		33% } aggressive		
Parents with neurosis:[1] Mother	48%				
Father*	10%				0%
Parents' IQ:[49] Mother	80 (Controls 95)				} 1 parent less
Father*	92 (Controls 102)				} than 80
Mortality	8%	4%	5%		0%

* 'Father' includes natural father or cohabiting spouse.

its Scottish equivalent, child murder. The Infanticide Act 1938 allows substitution of a charge of manslaughter for murder if a mother, by wilful act or omission, kills her child, under 1 year old, while her mind was unbalanced by the effects of childbirth or lactation. In practice, the majority of true infanticides relate to death within 48 hours of parturition and they frequently turn on whether the child was ever alive, in the legal sense, rather than on the precise cause of death. A charge of infanticide may also be proffered for those cases with a truly isolated injury, usually to the head, which have been mentioned above. Smith[45] did not feel that there was any psychiatric difference between women charged under the Infanticide Act and those who killed their children when they were over 12 months old but his cases were, inevitably, few in number.

Incidence of child abuse
Many assaults remain undiscovered but, even so, it has been estimated that up to 4500 children may be 'battered' each year in the United Kingdom; some 30 per cent of these will sustain brain damage and permanent handicap, and about 15 per cent will die.[48] Kempe[28] concluded that non-accidental injury represented 10–15 per cent of all childhood trauma seen in casualty departments and that it had a mortality of about 10 per cent.

Family background
The social and psychiatric background of families who abuse their children have been reported in several large series but in only a few have control populations been studied in a similar way.[31,46] Data summarized from some of these investigations are presented in Table 13.1.

Medical history
Often the first clue that one is dealing with a case of child abuse is a discrepancy between the proffered history and the physical findings. Typical stories are 'it fell' or 'I tripped while carrying the child'. These will be incompatible with the location, multiplicity and severity of the injuries. Cameron[6] has given a comprehensive list of excuses compared with the probable explanation in each case.

There is a characteristic delay in reporting injuries, which is usually of several hours or occasionally of days. This will never occur after a genuine accident and the discrepancy may only become apparent when the stated time of the injury is compared with its appearance. Other types of inappropriate behaviour by the parent or guardian are also diagnostic. They may appear totally 'ignorant' of injuries, bringing the child to the clinic for some trivial reason—this may be a 'cry for help'.[28,44] Sometimes children are left unattended in the clinic for long periods. When multiple injuries are pointed out, parental reaction is often very casual or they will be at great pains to ascribe them all to a single incident. Other subtle indications of the likelihood of child abuse have been discussed by Kempe.[29] Many parents are by now well aware of the sudden death in infancy syndrome; we have discovered 4 instances in 74 'cot deaths' where parents gave a typical history of this condition in an attempt to conceal violence to the child.

Examination of the living

The doctor's first duty is to treat the injuries but it is equally important to protect the child from further assaults; success in this will depend upon the quality of the evidence offered at the now common 'case conference'. A particularly thorough examination is necessary. *The clothing* should be personally inspected by the examining doctor who should remain present as it is removed. Its cleanliness and quality may well provide evidence of deprivation. *Radiography* of the skull, chest, abdomen and full skeleton is essential, not only to discover the extent of the acute injuries but also to disclose the presence of healed lesions and to exclude natural disease such as scurvy or osteogenesis imperfecta.[8] The radiologist must be fully informed of the nature of the examination so that appropriate lateral and oblique views may be taken; he should also be made aware of the likelihood of his findings being produced in Court and reviewed by a radiologist for the defence.

Careful inspection of the entire body surface is the most important part of the examination. *Photographs* provide an invaluable adjunct to the written description. If photography is not available, simple *line drawings* on pre-prepared whole body diagrams are an excellent substitute; being selective, they often have more clarity. We find them particularly helpful in preparing a detailed and concise report while photographs are being processed but Polaroid photography may be useful for this purpose.[24] The report should include the height, weight and head circumference. The size, position and colour of all injuries must be described, with particular reference to bruises in which the contrast between the blue/black colour of a recent bruise and the yellowy tinge of an older one provides evidence of repeated injury. Arthur and his colleagues[3] recommend that a practising police surgeon should be directly involved in the clinical examination. Police surgeons are usually more practised in giving evidence in the witness box and, in addition, they will not be influenced by having to continue caring for the parents and children involved when a case is over.

Regional examination

Head, neck and scalp Bruising of the scalp is often more easily felt than seen; typically, there will be a tender, slightly fluctuant swelling. The inside of the lips must be carefully examined for bruises, lacerations and a torn frenulum which has been described as an almost pathognomonic sign of deliberate violence to a child.[10] Particular attention should be paid to the conjunctivae and sclerae for the presence of haemorrhage; retinal damage is not uncommon and preferably should be sought by an ophthalmologist.

Trunk and limbs Very recent injury, particularly of the ribs and long bones, may not show as a bruise but will be tender to palpation. Cameron has recommended examination under ultraviolet light, which may reveal inconspicuous older bruises in more detail.[9] There may be no visible or palpable evidence of some chronic bony injuries which will, nevertheless, reveal themselves by limited voluntary movement of the affected part. The genitalia should not be ignored. *Burns* are common, the alleged incidence varying from 6 to 20 per cent in different series. [19,31,44,46]

Re-examination

The examination should be repeated after a day or two, by which time alterations in the size, colour or even position of bruises can be startling. More importantly, bruising from injuries sustained just prior to the original examination may now be apparent.

Similarly, radiology should be repeated after a week or ten days. Fresh undisplaced hair-line fractures will now show visible callus or elevation of the periosteum. For an excellent account of the radiology of this condition the reader is referred to Cameron and Rae.[8]

Autopsy examination[11]

A detailed examination with full photography (Fig. 13.1) and radiography (Fig. 13.2) applies equally to autopsy as to clinical examination. The autopsy should start with an examination of the clothing while still on the body and the clothing must also be preserved.

The brain should be the first organ removed so that blood drains from the body. This minimizes artefactual 'bruising' of the soft tissues,

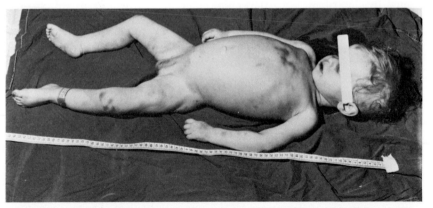

Fig. 13.1   Typical external features suspicious of child abuse. Multiple bruises can be seen on the face, chest, left forearm and wrist, and left knee joint. The pattern of bruising on the left forearm is strongly suggestive of gripping. The abdomen is distended. The mother asked her general practitioner to call because 'she went to check her daughter at 8.45 p.m. and found her unconscious'. (Reproduced by kind permission of the Crown Office.)

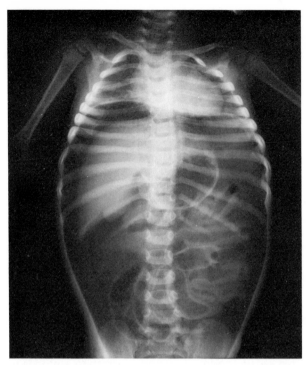

Fig. 13.2   A plain anteroposterior radiograph of the case shown in Fig. 13.1.
A pneumoperitoneum has raised the diaphragm on both sides, separating it
from the upper surface of the liver. There is a fracture of the right clavicle.
(Reproduced by courtesy of Dr. G. M. A. Hendry, Consultant Radiologist,
Royal Hospital for Sick Children, Edinburgh.)

especially in the neck, due to extravasation of blood during their
removal. The dural venous sinuses must be inspected and the middle
ears opened.

The tongue must be completely removed and examined for bruises
or bites. Epileptic convulsions, which may be associated with bruising
of unusual distribution, have explained some infant deaths.

All bruises should be incised so that their depth and extent can be
measured and photographed and also blocks taken for microscopic assessment of their age from the extent of vital reaction.[37]

Particular note should be made of the gastric content to compare
with the common story of 'collapsing just after a feed'.

As much blood as is feasible should be taken for identification of
blood stains and in case of any dispute as to paternity. In addition, it is
as well to preserve blood and urine for toxicological analysis; some
toxicologists will require liver samples.

Selected fracture sites should be removed *en bloc* for microscopic
confirmation of their varying ages.

Natural disease must be rigorously excluded.[42, 48] Blocks of all organs, including bone marrow, should be taken for microscopy. Bacteriology should include culture of blood as a routine[20] and other organs and fluids (e.g. meninges, cerebrospinal fluid, airways, intestines, etc.) as appearances indicate.

Pathological findings

Injuries to the head and neck

Facial bruises. These have been well illustrated and discussed in detail by Hall.[21] Their commonest cause is probably gripping across the mouth to stop the child crying, rather than striking by the hand. The pathognomonic feature of this type of 'fingertip' bruising is a solitary bruise in the region of the right temple caused by the thumb with a series of bruises in a vertical line on the other side due to the fingers. These may merge with time. Fingertip bruising causes none of the swelling or skin damage associated with a blow or fall. Bilateral facial bruising is inconsistent with a single fall.

Black eyes are produced by blows into the orbit. By contrast, falling on to a flat solid surface produces periorbital bruising unless the bones of the orbital walls, usually the roof, are fractured. In a total of 30 cases with ocular damage,[23, 34] 19 had retinal haemorrhages; there were cases with complete retinal detachment and others with subluxation of the lens. Twenty had permanent visual impairment.

Scalp bruising is usually due to blows but may also be produced by forceful pulling of the hair.[29]

Neck bruising is often seen but Scott[41] attributed death to asphyxia in only 1 of his 29 fatal cases.

Abrasions and lacerations are usually the result of direct impact. Only a small proportion are inflicted by weapons[31, 41, 46] and these will often leave a tell-tale imprint. Stab wounds are rare in most series. The most serious injuries must be at least carefully photographed but should preferably be removed *en bloc* for subsequent comparison with weapons suspected of having caused them; such specimens must also be available to the defence.

Several causes of a torn frenulum of the upper lip have been postulated—ramming a feeding bottle against the lips, forcing the teeth open with a spoon, a forceful grip to prevent crying or a direct blow. Parents or counsel may suggest that this injury, as well as others, such as broken ribs, may have been caused by efforts to resuscitate. In most instances, the differences in ages of the rib fractures will rule this out and, as Simpson has indicated,[42] injuries to the lips are almost never seen in cases where vigorous resuscitative efforts, even by the unskilled, are known to have been tried. Nevertheless, a careful history of such procedures should be obtained.

Intracranial haemorrhage

Subdural haemorrhage with limb fractures was known for some time as 'Caffey's syndrome'[4] before it was realized that both were caused by non-accidental violence.

The common finding is of multifocal recent subdural and/or subarachnoid haemorrhage with or without cerebral contusion. Extradural and chronic subdural haemorrhages are rare.

While some intracranial haemorrhages may be caused by direct blows, many are due to a sudden rise in venous pressure caused by compression of the body, swinging by the feet or violent shaking.[5] This may explain why these haemorrhages are so often multifocal;[42] the same applies to retinal haemorrhages, which are frequently bilateral.[18,23,34] It is worth emphasizing that severe internal injuries may be associated with trivial external signs; this applies particularly in the home where heavy impact against soft furnishings may leave no mark on the skin. In Smith's series,[46] 15 per cent of cases with intracranial haemorrhage showed no bruising of the scalp.

Skull fractures
The skull is the commonest site of fracture due to non-accidental injury. Such fractures can clearly be caused by genuine accidents but then they will usually be isolated injuries and will almost certainly be reported immediately. Non-accidental fractures of the jaw are most unusual.[42]

Injuries to the chest
Again, firm gripping often explains many superficial bruises, the single thumb mark on each scapula with a pattern of bruises over the costal margins being characteristic of gripping the child from behind with both hands. These marks may be at different levels on each side, consistent with adjusting the grip during violent shaking.[21]

Multiple rib fractures, the majority posterior, with varying degrees of vital reaction, are classical and probably result from compression. Single fractures suggest a blow.[8] Pulmonary contusion and traumatic rupture of the heart and major vessels are rare. Pleural, epicardial and thymic petechial haemorrhages should be sought but interpreted with care.[12] Their significance as a pathognomonic sign of asphyxia is doubtful and, certainly, most pathologists would agree with Camps[11] that they are not a measure of the severity of the asphyxiating injury.

Limbs
Bruises due to gripping are often clustered around joints. Fractures may occur at any site and, in the diaphyses, will seldom be missed radiologically. Avulsions of small fragments of the ends of the metaphyses are more difficult to detect; these are probably caused by indirect traction rather than direct blows.[5] Joint effusions may be evident on radiographs. Widespread focal aseptic necrosis of bone following traumatic pancreatic injury has recently been reported.[27]

Abdomen
Lacerations of the liver, bowel (especially the duodenum) and pancreas are all common (Fig. 13.3). Again, bruising of the skin or muscles of

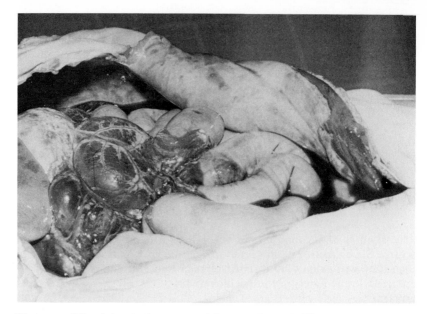

Fig. 13.3   The abdominal contents of the case shown in Figs. 13.1 and 13.2. Fresh blood is present in the peritoneal cavity and the greater omentum is distended with air. The duodenum was completely torn across the junction of the second and third parts. (Reproduced by kind permission of the Crown Office.)

the abdominal wall may be slight or absent. Many of these injuries are probably the result of compression caused, for instance, by kneeling on the child. This will both crush mid-line structures against the spine and also puncture hollow viscera as a result of raised intraluminal pressure —most perforations are on the antimesenteric border. Lacerations due to deceleration commonly involve supporting mesenteric structures at fixed points as in the adult.[22] Haemorrhage from abdominal injuries was the second commonest cause of death in one series.[41]

The genitalia are not often injured, attesting to the fact there is seldom a sadistic sexual element in these attacks.[28,46] A patulous anus is a common post-mortem artefact (Fig. 13.4). Occasionally, a ligature mark is reported around the penis which has presumably been tied in an attempt to prevent bed-wetting.

Bites[47]

These consist of a pair of roughly linear, interrupted, almost semi-circular bruises which can, in some instances, be matched with dental impressions.[43] Unlike many other skin lesions found in child abuse, characteristic bite marks cannot be confused with or misrepresented as being due to disease or accident. Bites from other children should be considered, as should bites which are self-inflicted, possibly in an effort

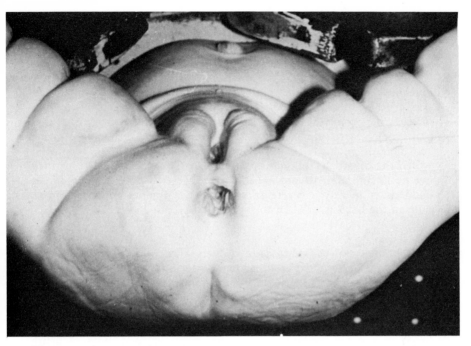

Fig. 13.4 An unusually patulous anus in a child aged 9 months. There is no evidence of injury.

by the child to restrain its own screams.[2] Self-inflicted bites will obviously appear only on accessible parts of the arms.

Burns
Non-accidental burns are usually circumscribed and localized to one side or part of the body, being caused by thrusting that part or throwing the infant directly against the heat source. All reports speak of the frequency of thermal injury to the buttocks and perineum. Keen and his colleagues have described the typical appearances in detail,[26] and have suggested that burns inflicted by cigarette ends or by a hot poker are more readily attributable to calculated, premeditated assault than are the more common injuries which may be due to outbursts of temper. True accidental burns are usually more widespread and diffuse and they will be reported immediately. Burns from cigarette ends, pokers, etc., will leave scars which may be difficult to distinguish from those due to localized chickenpox.[42] The safest method of distinguishing accidental from non-accidental burns is to seek evidence of the other types of non-accidental trauma.

Poisoning
The increase in screening of children with unexplained illnesses or failure to thrive for the features of non-accidental injury will inevitably

lead to more and more new types of injury being added to the syndrome. One of the most recent is poisoning. Rogers et al. have described six cases of non-accidental poisoning.[40] The drugs involved were barbiturates, salicylates, amitriptyline, codeine, oral hypoglycaemics, diuretics and even 6 g of table salt. It appears that parents may give their children any of the drugs they themselves happen to be taking. Rogers has recommended that doctors should take careful notes of medicines prescribed to the parents of infants presenting with unexplained or bizarre symptoms and should always save specimens of urine and blood in such cases. We have seen one case of fatal child abuse in which the blood alcohol was 22·8 mmol/l (105 mg/100 ml). This may not be uncommon, though whether it represents deliberate injury to children or merely a reversion to Victorian practice of using gin to quieten the baby is difficult to say.

Immersion
A preliminary survey of cases of drowning in childhood has revealed several with quite unexpected signs of typical non-accidental injury.[35] The authors suggested that the circumstances of these cases were distinct from those of true accidental drowning. In accidental cases there had been an unexpected diversion of parental attention, leaving the child, usually the youngest, unattended in the bath with other siblings; in non-accidental cases, the mother was in a state of acute anxiety and the child, usually the eldest, was alone in the bath. In one of our drowning cases, the presence of thumb bruising over the sacrum and between the scapulae strongly suggested the aetiology (Fig. 13.5).

Neglect
Although starvation, anaemia and severe nappy rash are encountered from time to time, it is a surprising fact that most of the children involved are well nourished and looked after. Only 16 per cent of Smith's fatal cases were physically neglected. It is the apparent anomaly of a well-nourished child with gross physical injuries which may account for the initial reluctance of social workers, doctors, etc., to believe that such infants could have been abused.

Summary of non-accidental injury in children
The 'typical' findings are that the victims are young (less than 2 years old) and the parents are in their early twenties. Child abuse is rare in single-parent families. Reporting of injuries is delayed, the story is inconsistent with the clinical findings and parental behaviour is inappropriate in other ways. Injuries are multiple in distribution, age and mode of infliction. Failure of diagnosis and treatment leads almost inevitably to repeated acts of violence. These are not limited to heavy blows; violent pulling and tugging of children's limbs, together with vigorous shaking of the body are equally prevalent and just as damaging, especially to the brain. Burning, drowning, poisoning and serious neglect can also occur.

The majority of parents have neither serious character disorder nor psychotic mental illness, though both are found in most series (see Table 13.1). No social class is exempt, so non-accidental injury should never be excluded by virtue of a prosperous appearance in the parents.

The family background appears identical for both major and minor degrees of injury, with or without neglect.[41] A subgroup of cases

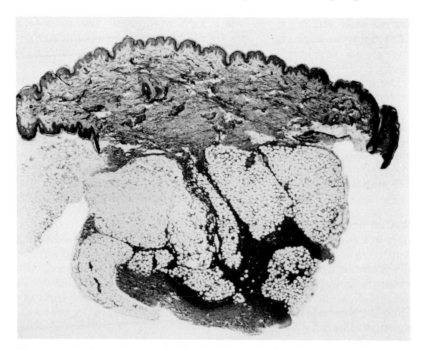

Fig. 13.5 A photomicrograph of a deep bruise in the subcutaneous tissue from the back of a boy found drowned at home in the bath. Post-mortem hypostasis may mimic bruising in this area but histology in this case reveals undoubted extravasation of blood into adipose tissue. This bruise, because of its depth, produced only a faint external mark, illustrating the value of incising and taking sections of all lesions suspicious of bruising. (H & E, × 19)

presenting with bizarre injuries (e.g. cigarette burns) seems worth separating because they are most resistant to management;[46] the parents generally show severe psychopathy and there is a high incidence of repetition and escalation of violence. Otherwise, incidents become progressively less frequent as the children grow up. Co-operative management by general practitioners, hospital services, social services and police is essential, the objectives being to protect the child while at the same time increasing parental confidence and competence in child-rearing. Although the most important concern must be for the safety of the child, there is increasing feeling among criminologists that rehabilitation is preferable to punitive imprisonment.[17]

Violence to wives

Whereas violence to infants by their parents was disbelieved at first but is now a well recognized syndrome, violence to wives by their husbands has been acknowledged and accepted without question for centuries—as the Select Committee on Violence in Marriage[39] has observed: 'Some people, even in high places, [ask] is it not a husband's right to beat his wife? Might she not even enjoy being beaten?' Insistence on a wife's right to escape and shelter from a husband who assaults her has only grown significantly in the wake of the women's liberation movement.[36]

There are very few factual surveys on 'battered wives'—defined as women who have suffered serious or repeated physical injury from the men with whom they live[39]—and the populations which have been studied are often not strictly comparable. The Select Committee, noting the inadequacy of the information available, quoted the possibility of there being 5000 battered wives each year in Wales out of a population of 680 000 married women.[39] Gayford[15] has reviewed the literature and has given details of the injuries and circumstances of 100 wives voluntarily seeking shelter from their husbands.

Physical findings and implications[15]
All had been punched, 60 per cent kicked, 42 per cent assaulted with a weapon (mostly sharp instruments but including belts and buckles) and 19 per cent had been strangled. Large deep bruises predominated, with clustering around the scalp and eyes, the sides of the body, the tops of the shoulders, the front of the chest and the lower back. Forty-four per cent had sustained lacerations and 32 per cent fractures; 9 per cent were admitted to hospital unconscious.

All assaults took the form of multiple severe blows on numerous occasions over at least a year before shelter was sought. Forty-two per cent of the wives had made suicidal gestures. Curiously, few bore a grudge against their husbands; a quarter even admitted to assaults prior to their living together. As with assault on children, there was little evidence of sado-masochism.

The implications for the pathologist and clinician are clear. 'Premonitory' visits to surgeries and clinics with trivial injuries inadequately explained are frequent and should alert suspicion. In the presence of an apparently isolated severe injury, others must be presumed to be present until proved otherwise.

The clinician, however, is in a far more delicate ethical position with regard to divulging evidence of injury to married women than he is in the case of children. The latter are in need of protection; the former can, at least in theory, defend themselves through the processes of law. Unfortunately, practice in this respect is generally far removed from theory, not least because the police are often unwilling to intervene in marital disputes.[36, 39] Differences in the law, including the need for the corroboration of evidence, make the woman's position particularly vul-

Table 13.2 Characteristics of husbands* in non-accidental violence in the home

	Husbands who assault their wives†		Husbands who assault their children	
	Husbands interviewed in prison[13]	Information from wives in shelter[15]	Fatal and non-fatal cases[46]	Fatal cases only[41]
Mean age	33	39	25	27
Regular heavy drinkers		51%	No association	4%
Injured in childhood by their own parents		50%		40%
Aggressive personality disorder	4%		30%‡	
Neurotic symptoms	24%		10%	0%
Previous convictions for violence	12%	33%	14%	27%
Previous episodes of similar assault	60%	76%	33%	76%

* Husband includes married or cohabiting spouse.
† Husbands also assaulting children[16] 54%.
‡ Most of these also assaulted their wives.

nerable in Scotland;[39] Lord Hunter recently indicated that the passage of the Divorce (Scotland) Act 1976 may open the door to improvements in the situation[25]—for example, by allowing sheriffs to issue exclusion orders.

Social circumstances (see also Chapter 21)
Table 13.2 compares some of the features of husbands who assault their wives with those who assault their children. Assaults on wives tend to occur at a later age. The husbands have more neurotic symptoms than do fathers but they show fewer severe personality defects. Violence is frequently associated with alcoholism. Intramarital violence seems to spill over to other members of the household—as many as 37 per cent of the assaulted mothers admitted violence towards their own children.

Violence to other members of the family

Some elderly people living with their adult children are probably as vulnerable and defenceless as are the very young. The presence of grandparents in the home can become intolerable and there may, in addition, be financial incentives to hasten their death. Cameron[7] believes that, with 7 million people aged over 65 in Great Britain, violence to the aged will become more prevalent, but there is as yet no objective data about this.

It is particularly difficult to differentiate between non-accidental and accidental injuries in this age group because the latter are so frequent. The aged bruise more easily and potentially serious pathology, such as subdural haematoma, can follow the most trivial, even unnoticed, injury.

Similarities and contrasts in the social circumstances of parents who assault each other, their children and other relatives have been discussed by Gibbens[17] and More.[33] Distinctive profiles of the different types of violence in the home are emerging but the current impression is that violence, once established, has an ominous tendency to spread to all occupants of the home and repeat itself in the next generation.

The common pathological features of all types of non-accidental violence in the family will be multiple injuries of varying aetiology, both recent and old, the most extreme occurring more often after a 'crescendo of violence'[28] than as isolated outbursts.

Violence in the home should be seen in perspective. Approximately 4500 children and probably as many wives will be maltreated each year in Great Britain; 97 000 people will be killed or injured on the roads.

References

1. American Psychiatric Association (1952). *Diagnostic and Statistical Manual for Mental Disorders*. Washington, DC: APA.

2. Anderson, W. R. and Hudson, R. P. (1976). Self-inflicted bite marks in battered child syndrome. *Forensic Sci.* 7, 71.
3. Arthur, L. J. H., Moncrieff, M. W., Milburn, W., Bayliss, P. W. and Heath, J. (1976). Non-accidental injury in children: what we do in Derby. *Brit. med. J.* 1, 1363.
4. Caffey, J. (1946). Multiple fractures in the long bones of infants suffering from chronic subdural hematoma. *Amer. J. Roentgenol.* 56, 163.
5. Caffey, J. (1972). On the theory and practice of shaking infants. *Amer. J. Dis. Child.* 124, 161.
6. Cameron, J. M. (1976). The fetus, neonate, infants and children. In: *Gradwohl's Legal Medicine*, 3rd edn., Chap. 24. Ed. by F. E. Camps, A. E. Robinson and B. G. B. Lucas. Bristol: John Wright.
7. Cameron, J. M. (1977). Personal communication.
8. Cameron, J. M. and Rae, L. J. (1974). *An Atlas of the Battered Baby Syndrome*. Edinburgh and London: Churchill Livingstone.
9. Cameron, J. M., Grant, J. H. and Ruddick, R. (1973). Ultra-violet photography in forensic medicine. *J. forensic Photog.* 2, No. 3, 9.
10. Cameron, J. M., Johnson, H. R. M. and Camps, F. E. (1966). The battered baby syndrome. *Med. Sci. Law* 6, 2.
11. Camps, F. E. (Ed.) (1969). Injuries sustained by children from violence. In: *Recent Advances in Forensic Pathology*, Chap. 6. Edinburgh and London: Churchill Livingstone.
12. Editorial Comment (1955). Tardieu spots in asphyxia. *J. forensic Med.* 2, 1.
13. Faulk, M. (1973). Men who assault their wives. *Med. Sci. Law* 14, 181.
14. *First International Congress of Child Abuse* (1977). In Press. Ed. by C. H. Kempe. *Int. J. Child Abuse Neglect 1.1*. Oxford: Pergamon.
15. Gayford, J. J. (1975). Battered wives. *Med. Sci. Law* 15, 237.
16. Gayford, J. J. (1975). Wife battering: a preliminary survey of 100 cases. *Brit. med. J.* 1, 194.
17. Gibbens, T. C. N. (1975). Violence in the family. *Med.-leg. J.* 43, 77.
18. Gilks, M. J. and Mann, T. P. (1967). Fundi of battered babies. *Lancet* ii, 468.
19. Gil, D. G. (1969). Physical abuse of children: findings and implications of a nationwide survey. *Pediatrics* 44, 857.
20. Gresham, G. A. (1975). *A Colour Atlas of Forensic Pathology*. London: Wolfe Medical.
21. Hall, M. H. (1975). A view from the emergency and accident department. In: *Concerning Child Abuse*, Chap. 2. Ed. A. W. Franklin. Edinburgh and London: Churchill Livingstone.
22. Haller, J. A. (1966). Injuries of the gastro-intestinal tract in children. Notes on recognition and management. *Clin. Pediat. (Phila.)* 5, 476.
23. Harcourt, B. and Hopkins, D. (1977). Ophthalmic manifestations of the battered baby syndrome. *Brit. med. J.* 2, 398.

24. Hunt, A. C. (1967). Instant photography in forensic medicine. *Med. Sci. Law* **7**, 216.
25. Hunter, Lord (1977). *The Scotsman* Feb. 3rd, p. 11.
26. Keen, J. H., Lendrum, J. and Wolman, B. (1975). Inflicted burns and scalds in children. *Brit. med. J.* **4**, 268.
27. Keeney, R. E. (1976). Enlarging on the child abuse injury spectrum. *Amer. J. Dis. Child.* **130**, 902.
28. Kempe, C. H. (1971). Pediatric implications of the battered child syndrome. *Arch. Dis. Child.* **46**, 28.
29. Kempe, C. H. (1975). Uncommon manifestations of the battered child syndrome. *Amer. J. Dis. Child.* **129**, 1275.
30. Kempe, C. H., Silverman, F. N., Steele, E. F., Drougemueller, W. and Silver, H. K. (1962). The battered child syndrome. *J. Amer. med. Ass.* **181**, 17.
31. Lauer, B., Broeck, E. T. and Grossman, M. (1974). Battered child syndrome: review of 130 patients with controls. *Pediatrics* **54**, 67.
32. McClintock, F. H. (1974). The phenomenological and contextual analyses of criminal violence. In: *Violence in Society: Collected Studies in Criminological Research*, Vol. 11. Strasbourg: Council of Europe.
33. More, J. G. (1974). *A Study of 23 Violent Matrimonial Cases*. London: NSPCC.
34. Mushin, A. A. (1971). Ocular damage in the battered child syndrome. *Brit. med. J.* **2**, 402.
35. Nixon, J. and Pearn, J. (1977). Non-accidental immersion in bath water: another aspect of child abuse. *Brit. med. J.* **1**, 271.
36. Pizzey, E. (1974). *Scream Quietly or the Neighbours will Hear*. Harmondsworth, Middx: Penguin.
37. Pullar, P. (1973). The histopathology of wounds. In: *Modern Trends in Forensic Medicine—3*, Chap. 4. Ed. A. K. Mant. London and Boston, Mass: Butterworths.
38. *Report of the Committee of Inquiry into the Care and Supervision Provided in Relation to Maria Colwell* (1974). London: HMSO
39. *Report from the Select Committee on Violence in Marriage* (1975). Vol. 1, HC 553–i, London: HMSO.
40. Rogers, A., Trip, J., Bentovim, A., Robinson, A., Berry, D. and Goulding, R. (1976). Non-accidental poisoning: an extended syndrome of child abuse. *Brit. med. J.* **1**, 793.
41. Scott, P. D. (1973). Fatal battered baby cases. *Med. Sci. Law* **13**, 197.
42. Simpson, K. (1973). Child abuse—the battered baby. In: *Modern Trends in Forensic Medicine—3*, Chap. 2. Ed. A. K. Mant. London and Boston, Mass: Butterworths.
43. Sims, B. G., Grant, J. H. and Cameron, J. M. (1973). Bite marks in the battered baby syndrome. *Med. Sci. Law* **13**, 207.
44. Skinner, A. E. and Castle, R. L. (1969). *78 Battered Children: A Retrospective Survey*. London: NSPCC.
45. Smith, S. M. (1975). Personal communication.

46. Smith, S. M. and Hanson, R. (1974). 134 battered children: a medical and psychological study. *Brit. med. J.* **4**, 664.
47. Sognnaes, R. D. (1977). Forensic stomatology. *New Engl. J. Med.* **296**, 197.
48. Webb, J., Cooper, C., Jackson, H., Colvin, I., Rogeroft, A. and Wilson, D. (1973). Non-accidental injury in children. A guide on management. *Brit. med. J.* **4**, 657.
49. Wechsler, D. (1955). *Manual for the Wechsler Adult Intelligence Scale.* New York: The Psychological Corpn.

14

Robbery with violence

This chapter is written without intent of establishing moral issues. We have no desire to debate the arming of law enforcement officers, the different views taken of gun control laws or the movement to arm householders and shopkeepers. Rather, it is an effort to detail the experience of two Americans involved in the large modern medicolegal investigation system located in Dallas County, Texas, which covers an area of nearly 900 square miles with a population of approximately 1·5 million. Much of the county is urban; some sections are quite rural.

The Dallas County Medical Examiner's Office is involved in the scientific investigation of death. Much of the detail in this chapter will thus deal with the 'ultimate' expression of violence occurring in relationship to robbery—that is, murder. Some attention will be devoted to non-lethal forms of violence associated with robbery, of which there are many. Robbery, like rape, may be an expression of internal hostility suddenly focused and directed at the victim and, in some instances, at society in general. Not all robberies are associated with violence, unless the act of robbery itself is defined as one of violence. In so far as this chapter is concerned, the simple act of threatening the victim and then causing him to deliver valuables to the robber is not considered to be 'robbery with violence'. It is when the robber goes further than is necessary to extort—when he inflicts bodily harm, when he loosens internal damaging emotional drives directed towards the specific victim or to society in general—that 'robbery with violence' is involved. In a sense, 'robbery with violence' represents a failure of the normal inhibitions which are usually carried into the robbery event by the perpetrator.

Robbery with murder

Robbery with murder is the ultimate of robbery with violence, provided that the robber dispatches the robbery victim or some other individual who is, perhaps, only remotely related to the incident. Thus, the bank teller is slain or a shopper is killed during the robbery.

There is another side to the coin, however—the robber himself may be the victim. This killing may be carried out by an intended victim of robbery, such as another clerk in the target store, by a bystander or by a law enforcement officer. A lawman may be present to protect the premises in which case his slaying of the robber may be an example of excusable homicide. The law enforcement officer may be present in a 'stakeout' situation when an attractive target is kept under surveillance during maximum danger times and the lawmen anticipate contact with the thieves; such arrangements may be made in areas where there have been repeated robberies. Another possibility exists—the lawman is an off-duty police officer who is present at the scene only by inadvertance. Thus, it may be that the robber is the recipient of his own intended (or non-intended) violence.

The victim is killed

A wide spectrum of possibilities exists here which is outlined in Table 14.1. The possibilities include homicide during a robbery carried out apparently as a part of the internal, hostile emotional thrust of the robber towards the robbery victim; deliberate elimination of the robbery victim to avoid subsequent identification (both of these being so-called cold-blooded killings); killing as part of a show of force for the

Table 14.1   The robbery victim is killed

---

1. As part of the explosion of violent emotions within robber:
   (*a*) Directed to the individual, specific victim;
   (*b*) Directed to society generally.

2. To prevent the robbery victim from becoming an identifying witness:
   (*a*) At the scene;
   (*b*) As part of kidnap/extortion scheme.

3. As part of the show of force/extortion action:
   (*a*) At the scene;
   (*b*) Kidnapped, dispatched later:
      (i) deliberate:
            no ransom forthcoming;
            victim becomes unresolvable logistic problem;
      (ii) inadvertent.

4. As a result of sudden reaction to show of force by victim: spontaneous alarm response.

5. Inadvertently by trauma:
   (*a*) Smothered by gag while bound or restrained;
   (*b*) Smoke inhalation and/or burns during robbery with arson;
   (*c*) Wild shot or ricochet bullet during robber/third party confrontation.

6. As a result of minor force:
   (*a*) Combined with pre-existing disease;
   (*b*) In combination with stress, fear.

---

purpose of extortion; inadvertent death as may result from suffocation by a gag; and death due to minor force superimposed upon pre-existing disease.

   1. *The victim dies because of emotional upheaval within the robber.* The intense emotional thrust of the perpetrator here is directed either towards society in general or to the victim specifically. The robber is hostile. Indeed, robbery may be the excuse rather than the true underlying motive and the real objective is the search for a release of pent up anger and frustration.

   Because of the sudden breakthrough of the extreme emotional wave, killing of the robbery victim may appear to be of an apparently uncalculated, unplanned type. No predetermined method is obvious to those who examine the scene or the body of the victim. The murder has not taken place out of sight or out of earshot of passers-by. No immediately fatal wound has been inflicted. The death situation appears entirely haphazard.

   One possible hallmark is 'overkill'; there are too many fatal wounds—more than necessary—an indication that the victim was a handy target not only for the killer to eliminate as a witness but for him to attack over and over again in release of volatile emotions and tensions. This type of robbery with violence leaves a lifeless victim who resembles the rape/murder victim.

   The effect of drugs (including alcohol) in decreasing the robber's inhibitions has not been well studied. The difficulties of such research are obvious. The assailant would have to be caught redhanded at the scene and specimens of blood and urine would need to be collected immediately for extensive toxicological analysis. Even the best toxicology laboratory which was provided with quite adequate samples of blood and urine could only report meaningless qualitative and quantitative findings. Drugs do not affect each individual to the same degree and in the same manner. Even ethyl alcohol, perhaps the best studied of all the chemicals introduced by man into himself, affects different persons in different ways. The effect of combinations of drugs in modifying behaviour has been little explored. Some drugs may cause changes in behaviour when taken in very small quantities and the amounts may be so small that the drugs can be detected by toxicological techniques used only in special research laboratories.

   Perhaps the best subjects to study from the point of view of the detection of drugs present would be the lifeless bodies of those robbers who failed to leave the scene alive. These would include those who were killed during the robbery attempt or who committed suicide immediately following apprehension or who died in a motor-car crash during the escape attempt. Intensive toxicological study of the body fluids and tissues collected from these individuals might yield information which, when correlated with other similar findings, might be subject to meaningful interpretation. But, to date, such individual studies are few, scattered and buried, perhaps even unrecognized, in the files of medicolegal investigative offices the world over. Attempts to find 'similar cases' are hampered by many differences in language, systems, philosophies and by political considerations. All who have attempted such correlative studies find themselves blocked and frustrated.

But what about the study of the behavioural aspects of the robber whose emotional turmoil overcomes whatever inhibitions may be present and causes mayhem and murder? If the perpetrator can be identified and his behaviour pattern studied, knowledge will perhaps be forthcoming as to how better to identify, modify or control such aberrant behaviour. Such research can be conducted in a prospective manner by psychiatrists and psychologists upon the imprisoned individual or in a retrospective manner by exploring the criminal, social and medical histories of the person involved; a combination of the two methods may be possible. The result of such studies—and many have been conducted—will, at best, help to identify problem personalities; the attempted modification of the behaviour patterns of such persons has been non-productive in all but a few instances.

Illustrative case 1. A 23-year-old healthy man was apprehended at about midnight by the police who responded to a report of an apparent robbery of a small store located in a predominantly residential district of Dallas. Because the suspect was unable to explain his presence, he was taken to the city jail and booked for breaking and entering the store. His behaviour was abnormal in that he was unusually nervous, tense, hyperactive and very bellicose. He was found dead in a jail cell shortly after he was placed in it. He had tied his shirt to the bars of the cell and was partially suspended by the neck from the garment. Death was obviously due to hanging.

Toxicological examination revealed a blood alcohol level of 40 mmol/l (186 mg/100 ml) blood and a propylhexedrine level of 16 μmol/l (0.25 mg/100 ml) blood. The effect of the combination of the two substances has not been studied; it can only be surmised that the combination of the toxic substances and the pressures surrounding the breaking and entering, apprehension and jailing led to a suicidal solution to the situation.

2. *The victim is killed to prevent identification of the robber.* This type of slaying has many forms. The two common patterns are, first, the on-the-spot killing of a shopkeeper and, second, the execution of the kidnap victim. Both situations are encountered frequently and both are often recognized by examination of the scene or body, sometimes by a combination of both, which can be incorporated into the development of the circumstances surrounding the case (see below—'Convenience store robberies' and 'Service booth robberies').

3. *Death is part of the show of force/extortion action.* The robbery victim may be dispatched at the scene as part of the force exhibition of the robber or the victim may be removed to another location and killed later. Planned kidnapping may or may not be part of the crime. Death may be due to deliberate action on the part of the robber or, possibly, the bound and gagged victim may smother inadvertently.

4. *Death is a result of a sudden reaction to a show of force by the victim: a spontaneous alarm response.* The robber, armed with a firearm and making a show of force, is suddenly confronted with counter-force, perhaps in the form of the victim reaching for a weapon. The reaction of the robber may well be to discharge his weapon. There can be no doubt but that force begets force. The sudden reaction to unexpected counter-force is a nearly automatic escalation of force and the robbery victim is left dead or, at best, wounded.

5. *Inadvertent death by trauma.* An occasional robbery victim, left bound and gagged, may smother as a result of the airway being shut off. The robber may set the premises afire; the victim, lying unconscious as a result of pistol-whipping or other injury, may die from the inhalation of carbon-monoxide-laden smoke or he may sustain lethal burns. It has happened that the robbery was discovered while in progress and that shots exchanged between the robber and the third party resulted in the unplanned death of the victim. Other possibilities exist and the inadvertent death of the victim by trauma is not rare.

6. *Death results from minor force.* The courts of many jurisdictions in the United States of America have ruled that 'you must take your victim as you find him'. If the robber's victim has extreme heart disease and, following closely upon the use of relatively minor force by the robber, he collapses and dies as a result of that disease, the natural disease death becomes a homicidal death in the eyes of the law. Other disease states may be so involved; the rupture of a congenital aneurysm at the base of the brain with resultant massive subarachnoid haemorrhage or the precipitation of an intracerebral haemorrhage in an individual with hypertensive cardiovascular disease are two examples.

Illustrative case 2. A 48-year-old man was found dead behind the counter of his small convenience store. The money drawer of the cash register was open and empty. The proprietor was obviously the victim of a robbery. Much blood covered the face of the victim and had been splashed on the floor and cabinets of the store. It appeared as if he had been shot in the face. However, examination at the Medical Examiner's Office revealed multiple marks of pistol-whipping (blunt injury due to the employment of the muzzle and barrel of a firearm as a bludgeon) on the face and head. Despite the extensive bleeding, the wounds were minor. Death was due to the rupture of a congenital aneurysm of the right middle cerebral artery with massive subarachnoid haemorrhage.

It may be that minor force in combination with marked fear and stress may precipitate death in an individual with no apparent natural disease. Perhaps this type of death falls into the category of 'instantaneous physiological death'. Although much has been written regarding this condition, few factual data have been gathered.[6] It should be obvious that any robbery victim who dies must become the subject of a complete autopsy examination performed under good conditions by a skilled pathologist. There is no substitute for this. The embalmed body is, in our opinion, not suitable for ideal examination. Worse still is the exhumed body, buried in haste by the grieving relatives with the tacit permission of the authorities only to be later unearthed in an attempt to answer questions which should have been posed at the time of the death.

Convenience store and service booth victims
Two special situations are encountered in most areas of North America and possibly in other countries. These are: slaying of convenience store operators and of service booth operators.

The first of these, convenience stores, present a special hazard to the operators because of their small size and the employment of only one or two clerks associated with the hours of operation which are around-the-clock or, at least, until very late at night (Fig. 14.1). The service booth operators are engaged in a hazardous situation because of their geographic isolation from other stores and from prompt help.

Convenience store robberies
Although the convenience store is an attractive target for robbery with force, it has its drawbacks from the point of view of the robber. The late operating hours and the single operator or very small working crew make the store robbery a reasonable 'calculated risk'. However, the expected one-to-one confrontation presents a real hazard to the robber—his ready identification if he is later apprehended. Disguise is one strategy to avoid later 'fingering' of the robber. Execution of the convenience store operator

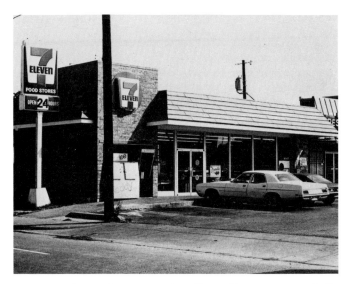

Fig. 14.1 Convenience store. Area for parking motor-cars in front. Somewhat isolated location, small, vulnerable to robbery by a determined individual. Such stores sell food, dry goods, soft drinks, ice-cream and some non-prescription drugs.

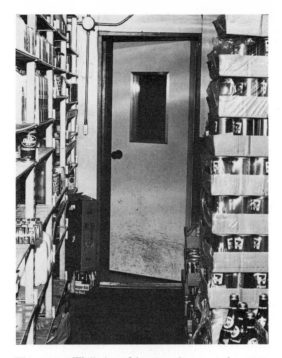

Fig. 14.2 Walk-in refrigerator in convenience store. The photograph shows the interior of the refrigerator and the entrance door, heavily insulated and affording a 'sound-proof' area, useful for execution by firearm.

presents a more effective and permanent method. Such deaths are encountered with considerable frequency.

Murder of the store operator so as to eliminate a potential witness may be detected in four ways: (1) by eyewitnesses; (2) by confession of the perpetrator; (3) by examination of the scene; and (4) by examination of the body.

Frequently the scene examination, coupled with the examination of the body, is most productive in the diagnosis of slaying for the purpose of witness-elimination:

1. Tell-tales at the scene:
   a. The body is in a back room or walk-in refrigerator (Fig. 14.2);
   b. There are no signs of active resistance to the robbery;
   c. There are no witnesses;
   d. There has actually been a robbery with removal of cash and/or valuables;
2. Tell-tales on the body:
   a. Gunshot wound:
      i. location—head, occipital area, immediately behind the ear (Fig. 14.3), forehead;
      ii. range—firm or loose contact, very short range;

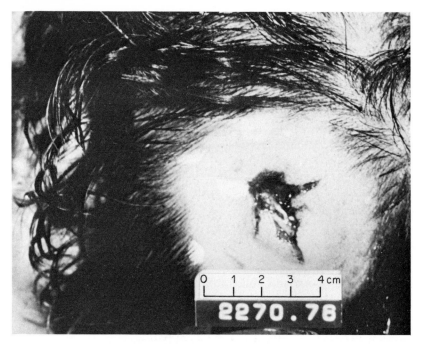

Fig. 14.3 Contact gunshot wound of back of head. The victim was a convenience store operator and was executed by the robber to silence the witness.

   b. Firearm residues:
      i. on the back of the hands—from a 'hands on the head' position;
     ii. on the palmar surfaces of the hands—imploring mercy.

In summary, the victim is dispatched in an out-of-sight location, often without having offered resistance and usually neither bound nor secured, with the firearm wound inflicted at point-blank range in an area apt to cause rapid unconsciousness and death. Not all of the tell-tales of execution of a potential witness are necessarily present in a given case. More than one victim may be so slain in a single convenience store.

Service booth robberies
'Shopping centres' are a hallmark of urban and bedroom communities in the United States of America. Many shopping centre parking areas have included with them one or more very small, single-storey structures so situated as to allow vehicles to drive alongside and where purchases can be made from the motor-car. Stores offering service for the amateur photographer frequently conform to the service booth design (Fig. 14.4).

    Isolated in the parking area, easily screened from view on one side by the robber's vehicle, the attendant—who often is a young, inexper-

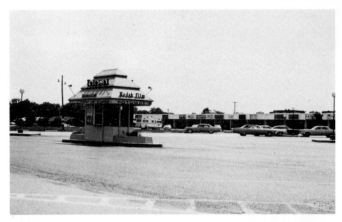

Fig. 14.4   A shopping centre service booth. Note how isolated the booth is from other stores in the shopping centre. With many motor-cars parked in close proximity to the service booth, concealment of the robber is well afforded.

ienced girl—is alone and vulnerable. She may be shot by the robber who is intent upon elimination of the only possible witness to his crime or, perhaps worse, kidnap/extortion may become an offshoot of what began as a robbery. The victim is forced at gunpoint to join the perpetrator in the vehicle, she now becomes kidnapped and is later killed when she becomes a logistic problem.

Drive-in bank teller windows, sometimes located at a considerable distance from the mother bank, are a special example of the service booth (Fig. 14.5). These are much better protected booths with 'bullet-

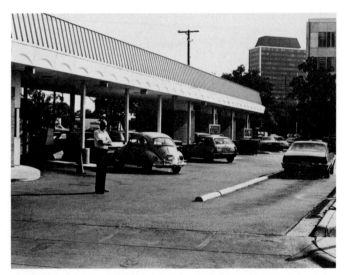

Fig. 14.5   Drive-in bank 'windows'. An example of a special type of service booth. Note the armed guard who roves about the premises.

proof' glass, alarm systems and, sometimes, roving guards nearby. Vulnerability is lessened as protection increases, but the apparent vulnerability continues to entice robbers and causes many deaths, of both booth operators and robbers alike.

The robber is killed

Sometimes the tables are turned and the robber who uses force to accomplish his mission is left dead; Table 14.2 lists several different circumstances which may so result. Usually, death is at the hands of the robbery victim or a third party, who may be a law enforcement officer. Family members, fellow workers and bystanders have slain robbers at the scene.

1. *The robber is killed by a law enforcement officer.* In many areas, lawmen are considered to be always on duty. Thus, the so-called off-duty police officer who is a customer in a store when the robbery takes place may be armed (in the United States of America and perhaps in other countries) and may very properly take action to prevent the crime or to apprehend the robber; indeed, such an 'off-duty' lawman could be criticized for failing to take action. When it is considered that one-half

Table 14.2   The robber is killed

1. By the intended victim.

2. By a third party present:
   (*a*) family member;
   (*b*) fellow worker;
   (*c*) bystander.

3. By a law enforcement officer:
   (*a*) At time of robbery:
      (i) happenstance presence;
      (ii) stakeout;
      (iii) response;
   (*b*) During the search for suspect;
   (*c*) During the chase following robbery.

4. Inadvertent death:
   (*a*) Combination of pre-existing disease and minor injury;
   (*b*) Combination of pre-existing disease and drugs and/or fear;
   (*c*) Accidental during getaway and chase:
      (i) motor vehicle crash;
      (ii) falling off building, etc.

5. By robber himself (suicide):
   (*a*) When in hopeless situation:
      (i) surrounded;
      (ii) having dispatched victim, faced with enormity of crime;
   (*b*) Confusion, paranoia, irrational behaviour as a result of drugs.

to two-thirds of a police force is in 'off-duty' status at any one time, there is a reasonable opportunity that such an individual may be present at the time of an attempted robbery. Such is the experience in all large urban areas.

On-duty police officers may be present at the scene for a variety of reasons. Response to a burglar alarm is one encountered situation. It may be that the store is an attractive and tempting target and, because of previous robberies, the law enforcement agency has established a watch or 'stakeout'. The target is kept under observation and the armed police officers move in to apprehend the perpetrator when a robbery attempt commences. Tension is high, surprise is nearly certain and a shoot-out may result. The robber may well be wounded or killed by the great firepower of the 'stakeout squad'. Because of the variety of weapons employed, the death can sometimes easily be categorized at autopsy by X-ray examination of the body; a combination of revolver and carbine bullets and shot-gun pellets is practically diagnostic of a 'stakeout' death (Fig. 14.6).

Death of the robber as a result of confrontation with a police officer may take place at the scene of the robbery as described but a good possibility exists for the confrontation to occur either during the chase

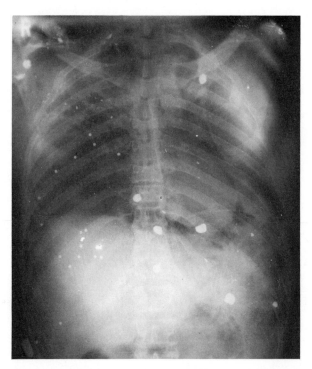

Fig. 14.6 X-ray film of a robber killed by police during a stakeout. Note bullet, buckshot and birdshot, attesting to the multiple types of firearms used.

after the robbery or attempted robbery or during the search for the suspected perpetrator.

2. *The robber dies an inadvertent death which is somehow associated with the robbery.* As is the case with the victim of the robbery, the combination of pre-existing disease and minor injury may cause the death of the robber. Since most robbers are young and shopkeepers may be middle-aged or older, the natural disease/minor trauma association leading to death is found more often among the latter than among the former. The same is true of the combination of pre-existing disease and fear.

Drugs in combination with pre-existing disease, and with the emotions of fear and anxiety added, may cause death. Since drugs would be expected more frequently in the robber than in the victim, extensive toxicological examination of the unexpectedly dead robber may produce information of great value (see Illustrative case 1). Propylhexedrine, certain volatiles such as freon, amphetamines and drugs with similar actions, cocaine and other drugs may be detected; in the absence of an overt cause of death, a reasonable suspicion of the drug/disease/fear triangle may ensue.

Accidental death of the robber, usually during the retreat from the scene, can and does occur. Thus, fatal falls from buildings and death in the accidentally crashed getaway vehicle are occasionally recorded.

3. *The robber kills himself (suicide).* Such deaths are often confusing, particularly if they occur when the robber is engaged in a shoot-out with surrounding law enforcement officers. He may feel that the situation is hopeless or that, having killed the robbery victim, he has committed a greater crime than he had intended (with greater penalties probable). He may be labouring under a great drug burden with resultant confusion, paranoia and irrational behaviour.

Illustrative case 3.   The police were notified of the planned burglary of a large supermarket grocery store. On the day and at the time of the anticipated burglary, officers were posted so as to intercept the individual after he had robbed the store. Plans went awry when shooting broke out as the robber left the store and, after a fusillade, he was left dead in front of the store. The informer, who was present at the scene, accused the officers of having shot the robber.

Examination revealed a gunshot wound in the region of the right temple. This was surrounded by a 2 cm radial, concentric zone of soot deposit, the hallmark of a very short range of fire. The bullet of 0·32 calibre was recovered from the brain of the victim. It was compared with bullets fired from the victim's own revolver and was proven to have been fired by that weapon. No weapon of this calibre was carried by any police officer at the 'stakeout'.

The death was certified to be of a suicidal type. Despite many rounds discharged by the police officers, only the robber's bullet found its mark.

The necessity for preservation of the body without destruction, alteration or obscuring trace evidence may be obvious to the coroner or pathologist (or medical examiner) but may not be so easily recognized by those at the scene of the killing. Preliminary and sometimes very inexpert examination of the body at the scene, well intentioned to be sure, may make proper documentation and interpretation of the wound very difficult, if not impossible. Soot deposit expected in very short-range firearm wounds of suicidal nature is easily wiped away and one tell-tale of a suicidal inflicted wound is thus removed; the very proof of suicide is thereby eliminated when the bullet has exited. Unfortunately, much confusion surrounds many such robber/police officer confrontations and these are the very situations where a plethora of officials and investigating officers may well hamper the ideal death investigation.

Other deaths associated with robbery with violence

Other deaths associated with robbery are outlined in Table 14.3. Little further needs to be added. There are all manner of innocent victims of violence associated with robbery. Bystanders, women, children, even the unborn have died as true sacrifices to the direct approach to unearned and illegal gain.

Table 14.3   Other deaths associated with robbery with violence

---

1. Fellow workers
2. Family, friends
3. Bystanders
4. Law enforcement officers:
    (*a*) On duty:
        response to call;
        stakeout;
        inadvertent presence
    (*b*) Off duty

Increase in the incidence of violence

There is no doubt but that, in the past two decades, there has been an increase in the recorded violence in many, if not all, countries in the world. There are some variable arguments regarding the better reporting of crime, more attention being paid to violence because of better and faster communication, and more visible statistical information becoming available because of computer storage and retrieval of information. But there has been a real increase in reported violence and the trends have been clearly marked by agencies of many different countries.

The increase in violence has been most observable in the urban areas. Because of this apparent relationship to population concentrations, explanations have been based upon overcrowding, ageing of the cities, violence mirroring that seen on television, etc. Many theories have been proposed and rejected and the subject is discussed in detail in Chapter 21.

The effects of this explosion of violence are seen, at least in the United States of America, on every hand—the increase in the size and scope of action of local police forces; the fear of citizens to walk in town at night; the development of security forces by industry, retail stores and universities; the employment of private neighbourhood patrol forces by householders to supplement municipal police; the growth of business devoted primarily to the production, installation and operation of private household burglar alarm systems. There are many others. The arming of householders and shopkeepers has been advocated by some individuals and groups. There are those who feel that force begets force and that the situation is very similar to arms races between nations with what might be termed an escalation of the capability for violence.

Statistics regarding murder and non-negligent manslaughter, forcible rape, robbery and aggravated assault for standard metropolitan areas and for cities in the United States of America are readily available.[2,3,4,5] These are based upon the so-called Uniform Crime Reports made by all reporting agencies and sent to the Federal Bureau of Investigation. This agency is charged with aggregating, collating and placing these data in usable form. Because of the rigid definitions and strictly applied parameters, perusal of such statistical information does not reward the searcher with quantitative details regarding 'robbery with violence'. Table 14.4 has been derived from the Index of Crime compiled by the Federal Bureau of Investigation and this indicates the upward trend in crime for the years 1960, 1965, 1970 and 1975. But how many robberies with violence are contained in these figures? No reasonable assessment appears to be at hand.

Murder associated with robbery can be examined by means of specific studies. One such is the excellent work of Block dealing with homicide in the city of Chicago.[1] The period covered in his study was 1965–73. He noted that there was a marked increase in the absolute number of homicides recorded. Of particular interest is his finding that homicide based upon robbery increased more rapidly than did homicide of all types.

Table 14.4 Number of reported instances of certain violent crimes, entire United States of America

	1960	*1965*	*1970*	*1975*
Murder and non-negligent manslaughter	9 110	9 960	16 000	20 510
Forcible rape	17 190	23 410	37 990	56 090
Aggravated assault	154 320	215 330	334 970	484 710

Table 14.5 Homicides in Dallas
County, Texas (January through
April 1977)

Domestic, victim and assailant related	57
Hit-and-run victims (failure to stop and render aid)	5
Battered babies	5
Drug 'related'	9
Associated with robbery	17
Total	93

A review of the homicides recorded in the first four months of 1977 in Dallas County, Texas, yields an overview of the reasons for, or the structures of, homicide. This is not a statistical review; the study is of a short time period. Perhaps more investigation of these recent cases will reveal details which might cause reclassification of individual cases. But the pattern is there to be seen. Nearly 20 per cent of the homicide victims were somehow associated with robbery attempts (Tables 14.5 and 14.6). Not all of the categories of death noted in Tables 14.1, 14.2 and 14.3 are found. However, a good idea of the spectrum to be encountered can be gained from an examination of Table 14.7.

Table 14.6 Robbery-associated
homicides in Dallas County,
Texas (January through
April 1977)

Weapon employed:	
Firearm	16
Smothered (gag)	1
Total	17
Death of:	
Robbery victim	13
Robber	3
Other	1
Total	17

Non-lethal violence associated with robbery

Mention has been made of the general increase in violence as indicated by the statistics of murder, forcible rape, robbery and aggravated assault, and also of the fact that these figures cannot be used to quantify the association between robbery and violence. Since all forms of

Table 14.7   Basic details of robbery-associated homicides in Dallas
County, Texas (January through April 1977)

Sex and age (years)	Weapon	Circumstances
Robbery victims		
1. Male, 62	Shotgun	Shot while resisting robbery in convenience store
2. Male, 78	0·22 magnum revolver	Robbed and shot at residence
3. Male, 39	0·38 revolver	Robbed, shot, dumped in alley
4. Male, 64	Gagging and ligature strangulation	Bound and gagged in residence robbery
5. Male, 27	0·38 revolver	Manager of radio shop, shot during robbery
6. Male, 36	Shotgun	Robbed, shot, body dumped by roadway
7. Male, 57	0·22 hand-gun	Owner of store shot while resisting robbery
8. Female, 42	0·22 revolver	Robbery victim shot by robber to eliminate witness
9. Male, 41	0·22 revolver	Shot during robbery of home–office
10. Male, 58	0·25 auto-loading pistol	Robbed, shot, and dumped in vacant house
11. Female, 62	0·38 revolver	Ice-cream store operator, executed to eliminate witness
12. Male, 24	0·38 revolver	Robbed and shot in his motel room
13. Male, 69	0·38 revolver	Shot while resisting robbery of bicycle shop
Robbers		
1. Male, 51	0·41 magnum revolver	Suspected robber of store shot by police when resisted arrest
2. Male, 29	Shotgun	Shot by police while fleeing from robbing restaurant
3. Male, 23	0·25 auto-loading pistol	Customer in convenience store shot robber
Other		
1. Female, 28	0·38 revolver	Third party shot during confrontation between robber and victim

reported violence have increased in frequency, it would seem that robbery associated with violence has likewise escalated.

There are different categories of non-lethal violence associated with
robbery. The most common of these carries different names: aggravated assault seems to be the official name of what is termed by

Table 14.8   Aggravated assault and other
forms of violence in Dallas City, 1976

Aggravated assault:	
With firearm	1325
With knife or cutting instrument	954
With other dangerous weapon	632
Hands, feet, etc.	704
Total	3615
Robbery:	
Armed with any weapon	2544
'Strong-arm'—no weapon	891
Total	3435
Murder	239
Rape	735
Other assaults	4992

many as 'mugging'—this being defined in Webster's Dictionary as 'the
act of strong-arming a robbery victim from behind; *also*: a street assault
or beating esp. when robbery is involved'. Table 14.8 gives the number
of aggravated assaults reported during the year 1976 to the Dallas City
Police Department, which represents a population of approximately
900 000—the largest population concentration within Dallas County.
There were about 35 assaults of different types in each 24-hour period.
These raw figures give some idea of the assault activity in a large USA city.

Aggravated assault involves the forcible removal of property from an
individual. There are many ways to accomplish this and several illustrative cases, taken from the Dallas City Police Department files, follow.

Illustrative case 4. The victim said that the man approached him and
asked for the time. When he raised his arm to look at his watch the
man tried to jerk the watch from his wrist. When he failed to get the
watch he struck the victim repeatedly in the face and head, causing a
cut on the bridge of the nose and black eyes.

Illustrative case 5. A 46-year-old woman had just walked out of the
grocery store and was approaching her automobile when she was
struck on the head from behind and forced to the ground. She was
then struck on the head again and again. The assailant removed her
money from her pocket and fled.

Illustrative case 6. A 33-year-old woman was preparing breakfast in her
home when there was a knock at the door. Upon opening the door, a man

entered and seized her by the arm and ordered her to get her purse and to give it to him. When she hesitated, he began beating her on the face.

Illustrative case 7. A 16-year-old boy was on the street waiting for a bus. Two youths approached him and proceeded to pummel him on the sides of his rib cage. This was extremely painful. They forced him to surrender his wallet.

These four cases of aggravated assault were chosen to illustrate 'mugging' without a weapon. Cases of robbery with dangerous weapons (firearms, knives, clubs, etc.) are legion. Regardless of the name applied, robbery with violence is implied.

Kidnapping with intent to extort is another example of robbery with violence but is, however, rarely encountered. As in murder with poison, much advance planning is essential for kidnapping and many problems are encountered which are hard to resolve—where to hold the victim, how to arrange for non-traceable communications, etc. Although many robberies require planning, the act itself is short-lived in contrast to the prolonged action of kidnapping. Occasionally, the kidnap victim is subjected to violence well beyond that required for simple security and restraint. Unusual holding devices (a coffin buried in earth was used in a recent American case) or actual deliberate torture of the victim may be encountered. Of course, these are expressions of the emotional, sometimes psychotic, state of the perpetrator, perhaps aided by the actions or personality of the victim. Hostages held by terrorists—a recent international explosion—may suffer similarly.

The implications of violence in the act of robbery have emotional overtones which must belong in the areas of neuroses, psychopathic (sociopathic) personality and, in some instances, psychoses. Failure of the robbers to find valuables upon the person of the victim may provoke an outburst of violence far beyond that necessary to subdue the victim. The burglar failing to find the cache of money in the home may turn to destruction with smashing of household goods and burning of draperies, other inflammables and, perhaps, the entire dwelling. The hostile internal turmoil of the perpetrators is thus revealed. The authors are neither psychiatrists nor psychologists but one need not be a behavioural scientist to be aware of this sequence of events.

References

1. Block, R. (1976). Homicide in Chicago: a nine-year study (1965–1973). *J. Crim. Law Criminol.* **66,** 496.
2. Hoover, J. E. (1961). *Crime in the United States 1960.* Uniform Crime Reports, 141 pp. Washington DC: US Government Printing Office.
3. Hoover, J. E. (1966). *Crime in the United States 1965,* Uniform Crime Reports, 192 pp. Washington DC: US Government Printing Office.

4. Hoover, J. E. (1971). *Crime in the United States 1970*, Uniform Crime Reports, 208 pp. Washington DC: US Government Printing Office.
5. Kelley, C. M. (1976). *Crime in the United States 1975*, Uniform Crime Reports, 297 pp. Washington DC: US Government Printing Office.
6. Petty, C. S. (1977). Instantaneous 'physiologic' death. In: *Forensic Pathology*, p. 126. Eds. R. S. Fisher and C. S. Petty. Washington DC: US Government Printing Office.

15

Injury and sudden death in sport

The range of leisure activities is greater and more widely available in times of prosperity. Deaths and injuries result from such activities but it is difficult to obtain a reliable estimate of their number.

The Registrar General's Report for 1973[34] records 105 deaths in 'places of recognised sporting activity' but this figure is doubly misleading in that it includes both spectators and participants and takes no account of the numerous outdoor sports in the countryside, on the coasts and on the waterways. In the same year, for example, the Royal Life Saving Society reported over 300 'recreational' drownings.[37]

The majority of sport-associated deaths are, in fact, natural. Every golf club loses elderly members due to ischaemic heart disease. Squash-rackets is notorious for the high incidence of sudden cardiac death in middle-age players, not only during the game but also in the changing room afterwards. Some clubs actively discourage those over 40 years old from taking up the sport. Many others emphasize the need of prior training sessions and 'warming up' before beginning competitive play.

Occasionally, young athletes suddenly collapse and die. Such deaths, although taxing to the pathologist, are outside the scope of this chapter and will be mentioned only briefly. The majority are due to unsuspected ischaemic heart disease which may occur even in the 20–24-year age group. Others are due to unsuspected congenital cardiac anomalies—for example, an atrial septal defect or hypertrophic obstructive cardiomyopathy. A small minority are associated with viral respiratory infections and, rarely, myocarditis is found at autopsy.

The majority of injuries and traumatic deaths during sport are remarkable only for the circumstances in which they occur and are of no special interest to the pathologist. This chapter is therefore confined to unusual and specific sequelae of selected sporting activities.

Combat sports

Boxing
This, the 'noble art', has been a popular attraction since Greek and Roman times. It revived in the United Kingdom at the end of the eighteenth century, when bare knuckle contests extending over as many as 75 rounds attracted national interest and enormous wagers. So

intense was national boxing mania at this time that reports of the storming of the Bastille were relegated to the back pages of the London papers—the event clashed with a heavyweight contest at Chalk Farm. The sport remained popular until the Second World War but, now, only about 7000 bouts are staged in the United Kingdom per year, and death and injury are becoming increasingly rare.

In the first quarter of this century there was little or no medical supervision. The 'punch drunk' syndrome was first described in 1928,[26] since when both public and medical concern have mounted. All boxers, whether amateur or professional, must now have regular medical examinations throughout their careers. A further examination is carried out before each contest. Any boxer who is 'knocked out', or who is stopped 'to prevent further punishment', must be fully examined, with an electroencephalogram for professionals, within 28 days. His licence to box is suspended until a new certificate of fitness is submitted to his licensing body. Although this system of surveillance is less than perfect, there have been only 10 deaths following professional contests in the United Kingdom since 1946. One of these was due to an undetected congenital cardiac lesion and 2 were in boxers from overseas who had not been subject to British Boxing Board of Control Regulations[6] prior to the fatal bout. There have been no deaths in amateur contests during the same period. The incidence of punch drunkenness or 'pugilistic encephalopathy', which reached a peak in boxers who had been fighting between 1920 and 1940, is also declining.

Minor soft tissue injuries are common in boxers. Cuts over the eye occur frequently and many promising boxers have abandoned their career because of their susceptibility to such injuries. 'Cauliflower ear', due to necrosis of the auricular cartilage following a haematoma of the pinna, is rare nowadays because prompt medical treatment is usually available. Fractures of the nasal septum are not uncommon; maxillofacial and mandibular injuries occur less frequently. This improvement is due both to insistence upon efficient gum shielding and to the use of heavier gloves. The preliminary binding of the hands is now carried out, by regulation, with either zinc oxide adhesive plaster or with cotton bandage in place of the heavy crepe bandage which used to be applied. This has led not only to a further decline in facial skeletal injury but also to a reduction in the incidence of fractures and displacement of the metacarpal bones.

Death due to acute injury
This is nearly always due to intracranial bleeding.[30] Subdural haemorrhage, usually into one of the middle cranial fossae, has been the most common in the cases personally studied. For many years it was generally held that this type of bleeding was caused by a single blow to the point of the jaw with transmission of force through the temporomandibular joints. A similar mechanism is seen in road traffic accidents where a single facial impact may produce a fracture across the middle cranial and pituitary fossae. The view which is now more commonly

held is that prolonged battering is the causative factor. The repeated deceleration forces within the skull lead to tearing of dural emissary veins but contusion of the under-surface of the temporal lobes is not as prominent as it is in single-impact injuries. This view of causation is shared by officials of the Amateur Boxing Association[2] who have, for many years, restricted amateur bouts to a maximum of five rounds.* They are satisfied that this has played a major part in the reduction of both acute head injuries and their chronic sequelae. The professional Board, however, retains ten- to fifteen-round contests 'because of public demand'.

Pathology of fatal head injury in boxers
Old and recent facial injuries are generally to be found at autopsy. The meninges are usually tense, the brain swollen and its convolutions flattened. There is a thin film of traumatic subarachnoid bleeding over the cerebral hemispheres and, less commonly, there are small surface contusions of the parietal lobes near to the vertex. Subdural haemorrhage is at first dark red, mainly solid and readily washed or peeled away from the overlying dura mater. It becomes firmly adherent within 36 hours and, after 4 days, is overlain by a 'neomembrane' which consists of a layer of fibrin incorporating leucocytes, macrophages and fibroblasts. This membrane is 3–4 cells thick; the fibroblasts begin to invade the clot over the next few days. By 6 days, the red cells are beginning to lose their sharp contours, the centre of the clot liquefies and an abundance of pigment-laden macrophages is seen. Over the next 3 weeks, the fibroblasts further invade the haematoma forming loculi, the contents liquefy further and the neomembrane becomes as thick as the associated dura. The membrane and dura are stained yellow/brown due to haemosiderin deposition. When survival is prolonged, further episodes of bleeding may occur into the cystic spaces, with concomitant variations in the patient's clinical condition.

If death occurs soon after injury, the brain shows little naked eye or microscopic change. In the event of survival for some time, generalized brain swelling and compression by the subdural haemorrhage may lead to compression of the brain stem in the foramen magnum (coning) and nipping of the cerebral peduncles by the free edges of the tentorium cerebelli. Minor surface contusions may be present on the under-surfaces of the temporal lobes. Rarely, petechial haemorrhages are seen in the white matter and some intraventricular bleeding may occur. The changes are discussed in greater detail in Chapter 12.

Histologically, there is distension of the perivascular and pericellular spaces and the capillaries show congestion with endothelial swelling (Fig. 15.1). The axons are swollen and stain poorly, the astrocytes appear swollen and the nerve cells show chromatolysis and cytoplasmic vacuolation.

* In practice, very few amateur bouts exceed three rounds, and this applies at international level.

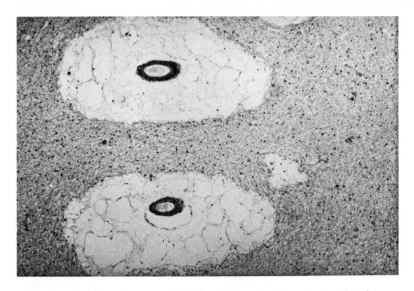

Fig. 15.1 Section of temporal lobe from 66-year-old ex-boxer, showing dilated perivascular spaces and thickened arteries (H & E, × 2·4) (Courtesy of Dr. D. G. F. Harriman.)

Chronic sequelae—'traumatic encephalopathy'
The first description of the late effects of boxing upon the central nervous system was published in 1954.[5] Among the best known papers which followed are those by Spillane[40] and Mawdsley.[28] In 1969, the Royal College of Physicians[36] published the report of their committee on boxing. These findings were subsequently incorporated in a monograph.[35] Corsellis et al.[8] reported the neuropathological findings in 15 retired boxers, with an extensive review of previous observations.

The clinical 'punch drunk' syndrome is well known. The victim suffers progressive dementia, is dysarthric, ataxic and often parkinsonian. The mood is labile, the tolerance of alcohol poor and air studies show progressive ventricular dilatation. The pathological findings may be summarized as:

    1. Abnormalities of the septum pellucidum.
    2. Cerebellar and other scarring.
    3. Regional occurrence of neurofibrillary tangles similar to those seen in Alzheimer's disease.
    4. Degeneration and depigmentation of the substantia nigra.

The normal septum pellucidum consists of two leaves or thin sheets of tissue, which are usually contiguous or fused. Separation of the two leaves is seen in only 20 per cent of the general population; the condition is known as 'cavum septum pellucidum'. Fenestration of the leaves is seen only very rarely. In boxers, a cavum septum is the rule rather than the exception and its average width is three times that seen in non-boxers. The septal leaves in Corsellis' series were all grossly fenestrated. The lateral ventricles are widely dilated and the corpus callosum is thinned. The mechanism of production of fenestrated cavum septum is uncertain. Repeated straining of the septum, movement of the corpus callosum on the rigidly fixed fornices, enlargement of the lateral ventricles due to cortical thinning and direct shearing forces all may play their part. Whatever the mode of its production, the presence of a fenestrated cavum septum is conclusive proof of brain damage and nervous tissue loss (Fig. 15.2).

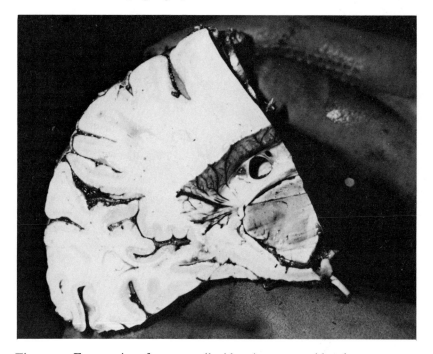

Fig. 15.2 Fenestration of septum pellucidum in 54-year-old ex-boxer.

There is a loss of Purkinje cells which is three times greater on the ventral surface of the cerebellum than it is on its dorsum. Small areas of scarring may also be found in the cerebellar tonsils and in the medulla oblongata. Scarring of the cerebral hemispheres is seldom seen but patchy loss of myelin has been reported. The reduction in brain weight, ventricular dilatation and thinning of the corpus callosum are specific to boxers as opposed to the generalized thinning of the mantle cortex which is caused by age alone.

Alzheimer's neurofibrillary tangles are found in many elderly people *but they are nearly always accompanied by senile plaques.* In a few rare conditions (e.g. postencephalitic parkinsonism) similar tangles without plaques occur mainly in the pons and midbrain. Such tangles show a completely different distribution in boxers. Vast numbers are seen throughout the cerebral cortex and in the brain stem but senile plaques are present only occasionally. The intensity of the change is much greater than is seen in the conditions noted above and is well demonstrated by silver impregnation methods, by Congo red and by viewing with polarized light (Fig. 15.3).

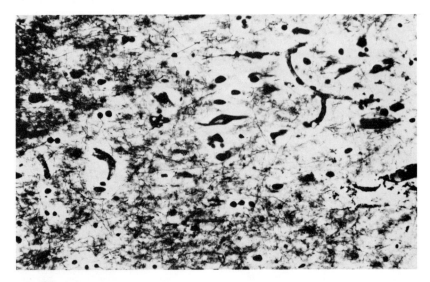

Fig. 15.3   Neurofibrillary tangles in temporal lobe of 66-year-old ex-boxer (von Bielschowsky, × 3·6). (Courtesy of Dr. D. G. F. Harriman.)

Loss of pigmented nerve cells in the substantia nigra is the major concomitant of parkinsonism. Depigmentation is frequently seen naked eye in those boxers who had parkinsonian symptoms during life and, in most others, microscopic examination shows widespread loss of the pigmented cells, with neurofibrillary change in the survivors. Lewy bodies are absent. Similar depigmentation may be seen in the locus coeruleus.

Wrestling
Wrestling is one of the oldest known sports. Both free-style and Graeco–Roman style are practised in the international amateur field. In Graeco–Roman wrestling, no holds are allowed below the waist and the use of the legs is not permitted. Free-style wrestling derives from 'catch-as-catch-can'; any fair hold is allowed and a detailed code of rules protects the competitors from injury. The competitors must be freshly shaven, the hair must be short and no grease or lubricant may be used on the body. Pulling of hair, ears or genitals, twisting of the

digits, brawling, blows with the fist and kicking are all forbidden. An opponent must always be thrown sideways and some part of the body other than the head must touch the mat first. Injury to the cervical spine is a well known hazard of the sport and all wrestlers in training practice 'bridging' exercises to strengthen the neck muscles (Fig. 15.4). If a wrestler forms a 'bridge' during a contest his opponent must refrain from any action which places the head and neck in jeopardy.

Local medical control follows guide-lines laid down by the controlling bodies. Each contestant must have a medical examination immediately before a fight; a 5 minute rest period must be allowed after any fall on to the head or any sign of bleeding from the nose. The contest is then stopped if the victim has not made a complete recovery.

Professional 'all-in' wrestling is a more spectacular sport in which no holds are barred and blows with the forearm or the flat of the foot are permitted. Despite its apparently violent nature there have only been 2 deaths in the United Kingdom in the last 40 years. One of these was a competitor in his early fifties who died of a myocardial infarction a few hours after a bout. In the second case, a young contestant died of intracranial haemorrhage after being thrown out of the ring and falling heavily among the spectators.

Death and serious injury are rare in amateur wrestling in the Western world but this does not seem to be the experience in Eastern Europe and the USSR. Gabashvili[19] reported 4 deaths due to cervical spinal injury in the Soviet Republic of Georgia in 1 year. This may be

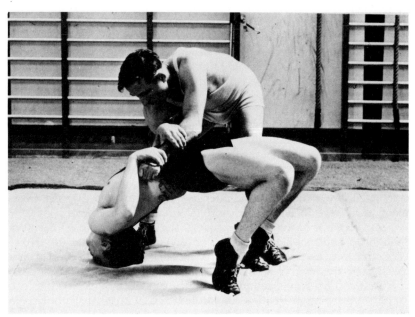

Fig. 15.4 A wrestler practising 'bridging'. The risk of cervical injury is obvious. (Courtesy of E. P. Publishing Ltd.)

because certain holds which are barred in the West are still permitted in the Soviet Union.

Chronic disabling injuries are more common. Knee injuries—usually meniscus or ligament tears—are frequent and follow forcible hyperextension and rotation of the leg. Injuries of the shoulder joint and rotator cuff result from twisting of the trunk and upper arm. Facial injuries and 'mat burns' are common, but these produce only transient disability. There have been no reports of long-term cerebral damage in wrestlers, many of whom continue to compete into the fourth and fifth decades of life.

Contact games

Association, Rugby Union and Rugby League football
The national bodies involved in these sports keep no detailed records of deaths and serious injuries. The author has been largely dependent on advice or publications from club and team medical officers. Walkden[42] estimated that, in England alone, over 200 000 males play Rugby Union regularly; possibly more than twice that number play Association Football and a smaller number regularly play Rugby League.

Death is rare on the rugby field. Only 1 fatality has been investigated by the Leeds Department in the last 12 years. This was due to extradural haemorrhage following a head-on collision between two players, one of whom sustained a fracture of the squamous temporal bone. Non-fatal head injuries requiring overnight hospital admission make up 6·5 per cent of Walkden's series, and similar incidences are reported in earlier studies. Fracture dislocation of the cervical spine is rare but, when it occurs, usually produces life-long disability. Other injuries are less serious but it is estimated that, in a 30 match season, 1 in 10 regular players will be sufficiently badly injured to leave a game.

The few deaths of Association Football players which have been traced have all been due to pre-existing natural disease. Only 2 serious non-fatal injuries have been discovered. One player developed gas gangrene following a compound fracture of the tibia, and a goalkeeper dislocated his cervical spine after collision with a goal post.

Non-fatal but disabling injury among professional soccer players seems to be on the increase. There are pressures on these highly paid stars to return to duty quickly; intensive physiotherapy, diapulse treatment and local injections of steroids are not infrequently given.[11] Repeated trauma to high-risk areas (e.g. the knees and ankles) has been thought to lead to a high incidence of osteoarthrosis in later life. However, this was not the experience of Adams[1] in his studies of a first division professional football team.

Harris and Murray[20] found radiological evidence of osteitis pubis in 19 of 26 Association Footballers studied, and of chronic sacroileitis in 20 out of 37. It has been suggested that the increased incidence of these conditions is due to the use of lighter boots which expose the player to the risk of a sideways skid which twists the pelvis and sacrum. These pelvic conditions require total rest for periods of up to 3 months and arthrodesis of the symphysis pubis and sacro-iliac joints becomes necessary in the few cases in which instability persists.

American football
This, 'the most dangerous game in the world', is played by over 50 000 school and college students in the USA. In the course of an average season, 1 player in 5 can expect to be carried off the field and 1 in 12 will require hospital admission.

In contrast to the rules of Rugby football, high tackles are permitted and the use of the head and shoulder in charging is common. Four 'downs'—either by tackle or by charge—are permitted in each advance of 10 yards. In Canadian football, which is played on a slightly larger field, only three 'downs' are permitted in each 10 yard advance and the incidence of injury is therefore somewhat lower.

Each player wears a full suit of protective clothing with a carefully fitted helmet and face guard, padding over the shoulders, loins and thighs and shin pads. Coaches insist on high standards of physical training and fitness and the player should, ideally, be of heavy build; players weighing under 80 kg (12 stone) are likely to be poorly placed in the frequent forceful collisions.

Non-fatal injuries are very common. Injury to the knee is the most frequent cause of permanent disability. No part of the knee joint and its surrounding ligaments is spared, but perhaps the most serious injuries are those involving the medial ligament, the anterior cruciate ligament or the medial meniscus. Chronic ligamentous and soft tissue lesions about the neck and shoulders also lead to many premature retirements. Fractures or dislocations of the shoulder and elbow result from falls on to the extended arm or 'straight-arming' a charging opponent. Other soft tissue injuries include laceration of the face and chin, which occur when an ill-fitting helmet is jerked backwards or pushed down on to the bridge of the nose. Tears of the muscles of the trunk and thighs give rise to the painful haematoma known as 'charley horse' (painstaking research has failed to disclose the origin of this expression!). Internal injuries are rare but haematuria following bruising of the kidney may occur, and ruptured spleen—often in a college boy suffering from infectious mononucleosis—is seen from time to time. Recent improvements in the design of face bars have dramatically reduced the incidence of facial fractures.

Injuries to the head and neck account for nearly all fatalities. Fractures of the skull are less common than formerly (due to improved helmet design) but temporal fractures with injury to the middle meningeal artery are still seen. Concussion with brain stem injury often follows a frontal impact, leading to prolonged coma and death; the mortality rate is high. In other incidents, temporal lobe lacerations may be found with or without middle cranial fossa subdural haemorrhage. The football player has little protection to his cervical spine. Indeed, the added weight of his helmet and face guard may increase the risk of cervical injury following an accelerated fall. Fracture-dislocations of the upper cervical vertebrae all too frequently lead to quadriplegia and death.

Other fatal injuries are rare. A direct blow to the sternum by the helmet of a charging opponent has been known to cause myocardial rupture or infarction. Prompt diagnosis and treatment has reduced the incidence of fatalities following ruptures of the abdominal viscera.

Aquatic sports

Sub-aqua diving

The British Sub-Aqua Club (BSAC) has over 20 000 members in the United Kingdom and exerts stringent control over the activities and training schedules of its affiliated clubs. Unfortunately, the safety standards of many non-affiliated clubs vary widely. Any member of the public can buy the basic equipment and then dive without supervision, previous instruction or awareness of the dangers to which he is exposed. There were 16 deaths among amateur recreational divers in the United Kingdom in 1973;[7] numerous sports divers have died in Australia[3] and in 1972 there were 120 scuba deaths in the United States.[23] A good review of the hazards of scuba diving is given by Dueker.[10]

The scuba diver carries compressed air or a mixture of oxygen and nitrogen in bottles on his back, the air being fed through a pressure reduction system. A neoprene foam wet suit is usually worn but, as the dive becomes deeper, this becomes increasingly compressed and is a poor insulator. The use of an undergarment covered by a dry suit partly overcomes this problem, the suit being inflated from an auxiliary gas bottle. Some form of water or electric heating is now frequently used.

The principal risks to which the diver is exposed relate to sudden changes in pressure. The atmospheric pressure is doubled at 10 m (33 ft) and is increased by a further 101 kPa (1 atm) for every 10 m (33 ft) of depth. Thus, at 6 m (20 ft), a diver needs twice the volume of air to fill his lungs that he requires at the surface, with a fourfold increase in volume requirement at 33 m (100 ft). The rapid decrease in atmospheric pressure which occurs during an uncontrollable ascent therefore results in over-distension of the lungs and of the air-containing body cavities—for example, the paranasal sinuses and the middle ears.

At constant temperature, the amount of gas which dissolves in a liquid with which it is in contact is proportional to the partial pressure of the gas (Henry's law). Nitrogen has a partial pressure of 80 kPa (600 mm Hg) at normal atmospheric pressure. Thus, the amount of nitrogen dissolved in the blood and tissue fluids is increased in proportion when the atmospheric pressure is doubled.[29] This can, of itself, produce toxic symptoms—the so-called nitrogen narcosis. This condition was named 'ivresse de la profonde' by Jacques Cousteau and is usually translated as 'raptures of the deep'. This author prefers the more literal translation 'drunkenness' which the early symptoms so closely resemble (see Chapter 17).

A sudden reduction in partial pressure releases the nitrogen from solution; bubbles form in the small vessels and produce the varied manifestations of 'the bends'. In addition to these pressure effects, darkness, cold and psychiatric instability may lead to the diver's losing control of his situation. Pain due to the exacerbation of pre-existing local disease—most commonly otitis media, dental caries or sinusitis—may also precipitate disaster.

During ascent, the diver must allow sufficient time for the nitrogen to pass out of solution and also slowly re-establish normal gas volumes in his lungs, nasal sinuses and ears. Too rapid an ascent may cause the painful sinus or the more severe pulmonary barotrauma. A tear of the lung substance which involves pulmonary capillaries may allow air at high pressure to enter the circulation and produce systemic air embolism. A large cerebral embolus may cause paralysis, convulsions or blindness. The spinal cord is a particularly tragic, and surprisingly common, site for embolism; paraplegia or quadriplegia may result.

Pulmonary barotrauma
This most commonly occurs when the diver holds his breath or develops laryngeal spasm during ascent. As the atmospheric pressure falls, the lungs are distended to their full capacity; blood is displaced from the pulmonary capillary bed with resulting hypoxia; breaks in the continuity of the alveolar membranes occur. Subpleural bullae, which may rupture into the pleural cavities, are formed as the intrapulmonary pressure increases. On reaching the surface the victim exhales, reopens the capillary bed and air may then enter torn capillaries, leading to systemic air embolism. More commonly, no systemic ill-effects occur but the victim has chest pain, haemoptysis and, sometimes, interstitial emphysema of the chest wall, neck and face.

The role of over-distension in the production of pulmonary barotrauma has been confirmed experimentally[24] and in studies using human cadavers.[25]

'The bends'
The protean manifestations of this syndrome result from the release of nitrogen bubbles into the circulation during decompression. The bubbles lodge in capillaries, producing ischaemia and pain, large joints being the classical sites. The victim adopts a semi-flexed position—whence the name. Involvement of the skin capillaries produces pruritis and erythema—the 'prickles' or the 'creeps'; vertigo—the 'staggers'—may occur; and laryngopharyngeal involvement, compounded by pulmonary over-distension, produces the 'chokes'.

Many of the acute problems of decompression are avoided by the application of adequate decompression routines. These ensure that the pressure for a diver is reduced in steps so that sufficient time is allowed for previously dissolved gases to be removed by the blood stream and lungs. The accumulation of gas bubbles in peripheral tissues or the sudden expansion of gas in closed spaces are, thus, avoided. The importance of decompression tables becomes more evident in industrial and military diving. (See Chapter 17.)

Repeated exposure to compression and rapid decompression produces aseptic necrosis of bone ('Caisson disease') but no cases are known to this author to have occurred in amateur divers.

Nitrogen narcosis (drunkenness of the deep)
The first symptoms of nitrogen toxicity are euphoria, irresponsibility, joviality and garrulousness. The experienced diver—like the experienced drinker—can suppress some of these early behaviour disturbances but his response to signals and commands is slowed, his judgement is progressively impaired and he becomes increasingly inco-ordinated. The condition is more of a commercial than a sporting hazard and is considered in detail in Chapter 17.

Acute oxygen toxicity
Bert[4] observed convulsions in small experimental animals exposed to high oxygen pressures; Thomson first reported the syndrome in man.[41] There is wide variation in tolerance to high oxygen tensions, not only between individuals but in the same individual from day to day. The onset of symptoms is usually noticed after about 50 minutes at 404 kPa (4 atm) pressure but may be accelerated by the performance of physical work. Again, it is essentially an industrial problem and is discussed in Chapter 17.

Latent hypoxia and hyperventilation
This is a risk peculiar to the skin diver who deliberately overbreathes before diving to wash out CO_2 and, thereby, increase his breath-holding time. A hard swim of 46 m (50 yards) requires upwards of 3 litres of oxygen—more than the lungs can contain. At the end of such an effort, therefore, the diver has a low arterial Po_2 but his deliberately reduced Pco_2 delays the onset of respiratory efforts. Peripheral pooling of blood occurs when the exertion ceases and the cardiac output falls; an already hypoxic brain is thus subjected to further oxygen deprivation. Unconsciousness and drowning quickly follow.

The situation is further aggravated at depths greater than 18 m (60 ft) because the alveolar oxygen partial pressure falls as the lung re-expands during ascent. Many swimmers have lost consciousness on the way to the surface after an apparently uneventful dive, and international convention now limits skin diving to depths of less than 15 m (50 ft).

Autopsy technique in diving fatalities
Any pathologist is likely to encounter such a case as death may occur in lakes, inland waterways and swimming pools. Much helpful information is usually volunteered by the deceased's fellow divers and their

conclusions are correct in the vast majority of cases. The deceased's previous medical record should also be obtained and particular attention should be paid to any recent attacks of middle ear or sinus infection.

Special techniques are required in the post-mortem examination of diving fatalities and these are described in detail in Chapter 17.

As regards sports diving, Miles[29] has concluded that asphyxia, anoxia, pulmonary barotrauma and illness in the water are common causes of death. Hypothermia is unlikely to cause death in the amateur diver although chilling can precipitate errors of judgement. Indeed, all these conditions are generally only the precursors of drowning which accounts for most recreational diving deaths.

The biochemical basis of drowning is covered in standard textbooks on forensic medicine. It is sufficient here to mention the need for collection of blood from the right and left heart and from peripheral veins for measurement of sodium and chloride concentrations and of specific gravities—and to emphasize the need for caution in the interpretation of such results. The value of diatom studies in suspected drowning, especially in decomposed bodies, is well reviewed elsewhere.[33] A demonstration of the equipment in use at the time is often of great help and local clubs or the police underwater search team will always willingly give of their time and expertise.

Association with subatmospheric decompression
One further hazard threatens the unwary sports diver who returns from his holiday by air. The slightly reduced cabin pressure in commercial aircraft is normally of no significance but symptoms of decompression may arise if compression has occurred within the previous 24 hours. These are usually minor—earache, etc.—but classical and fatal attacks of 'the bends' have occurred in flight. The BSAC now advises its members not to dive within 24 hours of a projected flight.

Water-skiing
This sport enjoys increasing popularity, being limited mainly by adverse climatic conditions. It has been estimated that there are over 3000 regular skiers on the Hawkesbury River (New South Wales) alone.[31] Speeds in excess of 40 km/h (25 m.p.h.) are regularly attained. The present Australian 'barefoot' record is 127·6 km/h (79·3 m.p.h.), and speeds of almost 160 km/h (100 m.p.h.) have been achieved in the USA. The incidence of serious injury is very low but strains and bruises due to heavy falls are common, as are ruptured eardrums, sinusitis and facial soft tissue injuries. Rope burns, usually of the legs, occur rarely. Cervical spinal injuries with quadriplegia are not unknown. Paterson[31] recorded 4 cases with permanent disabilities of varying degree. The 2 most serious cases both suffered fracture-dislocation of the fifth cervical vertebra. The two most typical water-skiing injuries are entirely preventable—these are power boat propeller injuries and 'douching'.

Propeller injuries
These are always due to contravention of regulations. Australian States' laws require that the tow-rope must be over 21 m (70 ft) in length, and that an adult observer must accompany the boat driver. Similar recommendations (although without the force of law) apply to clubs in the United Kingdom. The usual consequences of such mishaps are comminuted fractures or traumatic amputation of limbs—but severe head injury and drowning have also occurred. The cause of such injuries discovered in a water-skier is usually obvious.

Vaginal and rectal douches
These are due to a sudden 'squat' and can be prevented by wearing tightly fitting rubber pants. Skiers in cooler climates usually wear wet suits and are completely protected. The usual consequence of such douches is no more than mild discomfort but salpingitis and urethritis have been reported. The author has personal knowledge of one case where a urethral reconstruction operation was necessary following perineal lacerations in a young female. Rupture of the rectosigmoid junction with peritonitis is a rare but real risk. No fatalities have yet been reported.

Aerial sports

Sports parachuting
Parachuting 'is almost as safe as crossing a crowded street, and safer than playing army [Association] football'.[14] The British Sports Parachuting Association (BSPA) claim an average of less than 3 deaths per year. The Parachute Club of America (PCA) have recorded about 50 deaths per year over the past 5 years, but point out that the majority of the deceased were not Club members, nor were they participating in PCA-supervised events when the incidents took place. The wide safety margin of the standard type of sport parachute was recently demonstrated in Derbyshire (UK) when a trainee parachutist slipped on exit and became caught between the undercarriage and the fuselage of a Cessna 182 light aircraft; he pulled his reserve parachute before he could be freed. The canopy inflated successfully and pulled the aircraft, which was carrying three other passengers, into an inverted stall with the parachutist suspended between his canopy and the aircraft. The latter descended at a rate of 13.7 m s^{-1} (45 ft/sec). The most serious injury was a fractured femur.[17]

Over 90 per cent of such incidents are the result of acts of omission or of commission by the deceased. Such acts include failure to take corrective action following equipment malfunction—e.g. failure to deploy the reserve parachute. Only rarely is a medical reason found for such a failure. In one case known to the author, severe myocardial disease with a recent infarction was found in the victim, a 48-year-old medical practitioner. Another involved a man with a deformed hand; he could operate the main parachute but was physically incapable of releasing the D-ring which controlled the reserve parachute. The vast majority of such incidents are associated with panic.

The BSPA insists upon a full medical examination on entry to basic training and at least 10 hours of ground training before jumping is permitted. Experience is first gained in static line descents before free fall and aerobatic techniques are attempted.

The equipment most commonly used by sportsmen for static line descents consists of back-packed parachute, which is released without any action by the parachutist. When the static line is extended, it withdraws a small drogue from the pack which, in turn, initiates deployment of the main canopy; this is encased in a nylon sleeve to retard full development. Such controlled slow development reduces the risk of fouling of the rigging lines and almost completely eliminates the 'jerk' felt when a canopy opens rapidly—a deceleration of about 4G (42 m s^{-2}; 140 ft/sec^2). The main canopy has a vent at its apex which prevents oscillation of the parachute and a 'pendulum' landing. Descent takes place at 4 m s^{-1} (14 ft/sec).

The risk points in a descent are:

1. Exit and 'free fall'.
2. Parachute development.
3. Landing.

Risks of exit
Exit accidents are rare in sports parachuting. The side door of a light aircraft is usually removed completely and the parachutist is well clear of the fuselage and tailplane. Somersaulting and twisting are rare.

The risks of 'free fall' are somewhat greater. The parachutist may become disorientated, and ill-considered movements of arms and legs can lead to a rapid rotation of the trunk about its long axis—a so-called 'flat spin'.

Parachute deployment and development
Rope burns of the limbs and face are rare. Packing errors—e.g. incorrect knotting of the bridle cord, so that the sleeve fails to separate—are the commonest cause of equipment failure at this stage. Rarely, a canopy will split or foul, giving rise to a rapid descent with an impact speed of 53 m s^{-1} (120 m.p.h.). An unretarded deployment of the main canopy due to premature separation of the canopy sleeve sometimes produces perineal lacerations due to the deceleration forces transmitted through the harness.

The reserve parachute is carried in a ventral pack and is released by pulling a D-ring. The parachutist then pays out the exposed canopy slowly, keeping his arms fully extended as the rigging lines are deployed so as to avoid facial injury. Impact speed is slightly higher on the reserve parachute.

Hazards of landing

The correct technique is to land 'tucked up'. Extension of a leg or arm to save oneself almost always results in bony injury. Landing facing along the line of drift leads to pitching forward and maxillofacial injury.

The incidence and severity of landing injuries is directly related to body habitus. The ideal parachutist is short and stocky; the incidence of injury is greatly increased in those of powerful build, as it is in those who are tall and slim. Serious injury and death in sports parachuting are usually the result of high speed at impact. Multiple injuries are always present in fatal cases. They are widely dispersed in an uncontrolled fall. The injuries seen when the victim hits the ground feet first at a higher speed than normal are of particular interest. In such cases compression fractures of the tarsal bones are seen, with fractures through the ankle joints and fractures or dislocations of the heads of the fibulae. In other cases where the legs are firmly braced, the pelvis shows multiple fractures and the femoral heads are driven through the acetabula. Compression fractures of the spine are common, and the atlas may be driven through the base and foramen magnum—a so-called ring fracture. In extreme cases the sudden rise in intracranial pressure gives rise to a 'burst skull'.

There are usually multiple visceral injuries. The spleen is not only lacerated but detached from its pedicle, and the liver shows numerous lacerations. The heart and lungs may be detached from their vascular connections and the aorta is often torn across, usually just distal to the origin of the left subclavian artery.

An increasing number of sports parachutists are now wearing heavy crash helmets which weigh up to 2·3 kg (5 lb). This added weight increases the forward leverage of the head about the fulcrum of the cervical spine and one can expect, in the future, more civilian cases of the 'chin-sternum-heart syndrome'. This was first reported by Mason[27] in 1962 and later clarified by Simson.[39] It consists of laceration of the chin, fracture of the sternum and lacerations of the atria. The head jerks sharply forwards onto the chest; simultaneously, the chest contents are compressed upwards by the abdominal viscera with a concomitant rise in central venous pressure. Atrial rupture results. This triad of lesions was seen recently by the author in an 18-year-old girl.

Cervical spinal injuries are often associated with the chin-sternum-heart syndrome in Service parachutists. No doubt similar injuries will be found in civilian parachutists in the future.

From time to time an accident occurs due to 'an error of judgement' and it is suggested that hypoxia might be a contributory factor. The controlling bodies have recommended that descents should not be made from altitudes greater than 4575 m (15 000 ft) without supplementary oxygen apparatus. Descents from more than 2450 m (8000 ft) may be made only if the parachutist's total time at that altitude does not exceed 30 minutes. Laboratory experiments demonstrating impairment of mental and motor function after 2 hours at the equivalent of 3050 m (10 000 ft) confirm the wisdom of these restrictions.[9]

Hang gliding
The hang glider proper is basically a deltoid kite—Icarus updated, but employing cyanmethacrylate adhesives in place of beeswax. In its current form it consists of a delta-wing, of side 5–6 m (18–20 ft), made of Dacron with a rigid aluminium frame. The control bar hangs like a trapeze from the central transverse strut and the operator is suspended by a modified parachute harness. Control is effected by shifting the body weight forward or aft of the centre of the gravity. The novice usually adopts a sitting position but the expert stretches himself out prone.[21] There are over 10 000 regular hang gliders in the United States;[13] this figure is increasing monthly. The clothing requirements are simple—a motor-cycle-type crash-helmet, stout boots and shin-pads usually give adequate protection.

An average flight lasts about 1 minute and heights over 76 m (250 ft) are seldom reached. Experts can remain airborne for much longer periods. The world endurance record exceeds 10 hours and the altitude record is over 4200 m (14 000 ft). The US Federal Aviation Administration (FAA) exercises no formal control over the sport but issues a pamphlet of recommendation and guidance. National associations now exist in the USA, the United Kingdom and several European countries, and an International Commission of Hang Gliding has been recently established.

Four fatalities were reported in Colorado;[22] there were 2 deaths in the United Kingdom in the first 6 months of 1975.[12] All 4 of the Colorado cases sustained multiple injuries, including injuries to the head, thorax, abdominal viscera and one or more limbs. Three of the 4 victims flew in turbulent weather conditions. One had not only been drinking (blood alcohol = 50 mg/100 ml) but had also almost certainly been smoking marijuana.

Eight non-fatal but serious accidents in Colorado were also described.[22] Head and spinal injuries, with lasting disability, were the most common. The authors comment: 'Hang glider flying is a high risk sport. Because it is cheap, easy and unsupervised, those with little experience and poor judgement must perforce be at risk.' Their experience and that in the UK suggests, however, that seriously injured victims are most often those who, by virtue of experience and over-confidence, attempt flights in bad weather or, in particular, attempt a cliff take off, rather than the safer 'run down hill' technique. All the deaths so far reported have been due to error on the part of the sportsman rather than to equipment failure.

Sporting injuries due to firearms

Sporting injuries due to firearms are of three types—those due to air weapons, those due to small-bore pistols and rifles (usually on the firing range), and those due to shotguns either in the field or at clay-pigeon shooting.

Air weapons

The acquisition and possession of air weapons by minors is now governed by the Firearms Act 1968[15] and the muzzle energy of air weapons is restricted by the Firearms (Dangerous Air Weapons) Rules 1969.[16] Air rifles must have a muzzle energy less than 16 J (12 ft lbf), and air pistols a muzzle energy less than 8J (6 ft lbf).

Airguns are responsible for more than 60 per cent of all firearm injuries in England and Wales. Most are inflicted upon and by children and adolescents; they are usually the result of unsupervised irresponsibility but a few are malicious. At short ranges, say less than 6 m (20 ft), a 0·177 calibre slug fired from an air pistol can penetrate the skull and traverse the brain. Fatal wounds of the heart and great vessels are not uncommon at longer ranges. Direct or ricochet wounds of the eye are the most frequent non-fatal injuries resulting from the misuse of air weapons; blindness is all too often the sequel.

Pistols and small-bore rifles

Possession of these weapons is very strictly controlled by the 1968 Act and accidents due to them are, therefore, rare in the United Kingdom; the weapons are most commonly fired by club members under the strict supervision of experienced instructors and range officers. Only 1 fatal accident has been examined in the Leeds Department of Forensic Medicine in the last 10 years. This resulted from a novice marksman firing so high that he missed the stop butt completely. The spent 0·22 bullet struck a boy playing a considerable distance away from the range.

Shotguns

The commonest sporting shotguns in use in the United Kingdom are the 0·410 and the 12-bore. The 0·410 is usually single barrelled; many of these weapons are of inferior quality and are poorly maintained, having such a light trigger pressure that a sudden jar will produce accidental discharge.

The 12-bore is a more substantial, usually double-barrelled, weapon. The serious sportsman treats his gun and cartridges with respect; accidents due to poor maintenance are rare. Unfortunately, the use of reloaded casings is increasing and accidents can occur during the reloading operation. An excess loading of propellant may rupture an eardrum or may even burst a breech or barrel with consequent disfigurement or death. When confronted with a death due to a 'burst' the pathologist should consider the type of cartridge used as well as the age and condition of the weapon.

Accidents seldom occur in well organized small shooting parties but, at larger meetings, discipline is rather more lax with increased risks to fellow marksmen and beaters alike. Other accidents occur when a gun is used as a vaulting pole or as a club for despatching a wounded animal.

A significant proportion of accidents in the field are caused by badly disciplined dogs either tripping the hunter or knocking down a loaded, cocked piece.

Accident, suicide or homicide?

Homicide must be rare in the midst of a large shooting party—*pace* Hilaire Belloc!

The pathologist should carefully inspect the clothing and the entry wound. A wound inflicted at near contact range is usually almost circular and is only slightly larger than is the bore of the weapon. Cards and wadding are usually found in the depths of the wound. The wound and clothing are fouled by soot and unburned propellant grains. The nearby tissue is often bright pink due to carbon monoxide entering the blood. The site of the wound is of prime importance. Is it consistent with self-infliction? Multiple wounds do not always exclude suicide. In one case of the author's the deceased shot himself twice in the abdomen with a 12-bore shotgun and then walked into an adjacent room before blowing out his brains.

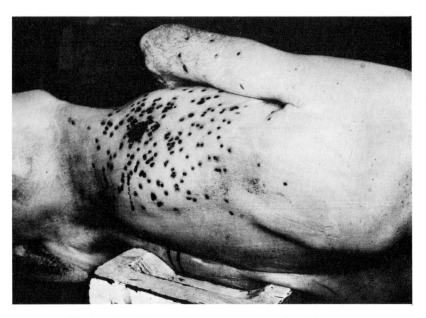

Fig. 15.5 Fatal 12-bore shot-gun injury, range 11 m (12 yd).

Shotgun wounds from distances greater than 1 m (3 ft) are always large, with a surrounding nebula of individual pellet wounds (Fig. 15.5). Fouling is absent. The distinction between accident and homicide in these cases must be made on circumstantial evidence at the scene rather than pathological examination. During the post mortem, swabs should be taken from around the wound for examination in the forensic science laboratory and samples of tissue should be taken for carboxyhaemoglobin estimation. The track of the wound should be followed and an attempt be made to assess the direction of the charge. The value of X-ray before autopsy in all types of firearm injury cannot be over-emphasized. It helps in the localization of a small missile such as a 0·22 round and, in shotgun injuries, the overall picture often gives a better idea of the track and of the amount of spread than does dissection alone.

Injuries to spectators

Crowds of up to 100 000 spectators frequently attend major sporting events and it is not surprising that accidents sometimes occur. Elderly spectators collapse, usually as a result of ischaemic heart disease, in extremes of temperature or at moments of excitement. Continuous ECG recordings taken from spectators at football matches have shown transient arrhythmias in such circumstances. There are 6 deaths yearly due to this cause at Leeds United Football Ground. Fainting is common but recovery is rapid when the patient is removed to less crowded conditions.

The risk of injury increases when disorder breaks out. Fights expose not only the participants to risk. Bystanders attempting to retreat from the incident may trigger off an uncontrollable stampede. The most dangerous situation arises at the end of the event when the crowd is leaving the stadium. The terraces are often steeply inclined, and a stumble or ill-judged push can cause those following to fall *en masse*.

Such a disaster occurred at a football match at Ibrox Park, Glasgow, in 1971. The game seemed destined to end in a goal-less draw and the disgruntled fans had started to leave. Then, in the closing minutes, a goal was scored and many of the departing crowd turned about, intent upon regaining their places. A crush barrier collapsed under the resulting pressure. Several hundred people tumbled down the steep terraces; 66 persons died and over 100 were seriously injured.

There have been several similar incidents, at other sports grounds, due to collapse of stands, stairways or barriers. Other disasters have been caused by inadequate provision of exits and gangways.

Many football clubs have voluntarily improved the standards of their premises, strengthened staircases and provided 'stream-splitting' exits. Such improvements are now mandatory,[38] safety certificates being required in respect of all stadia which accommodate more than 10 000 spectators. These certificates, issued by the local authority, lay down maximum numbers for each part of the ground, specify the number and design of corridors and exits, and control the siting and the strength of crush-barriers. The managers of the grounds are required to keep detailed records of attendances, of safety inspection and of maintenance of equipment. The local authority may issue such a certificate only after consultation with local police, fire and community health officers.

Crush asphyxia
Widely varied injuries, from minor abrasions to multiple fractures, may result from spectator disasters. The specific lesion—crush, or traumatic, asphyxia—was first described by Perthes.[32] The physical signs are basically those of asphyxia in general but all are greatly intensified. It has been estimated that sustained pressures in excess of 103 kPa (15 p.s.i.) are exerted upon the trunks of the victims. The external appearances of the fatal condition have been described in Chapter 8.

Internal examination
Multiple rib fractures are distributed symmetrically in the mid-axillary lines and at the costochondral junctions. Fractures of the necks of the ribs are less common but the body of the sternum may be broken. Fractures of the long bones are usually due to the initial fall rather than the sustained crushing. Fractures of the skull and intracranial haemorrhage have not been found in the cases personally studied. There are large petechiae in the temporal muscles, in the pericranium and in the oral and pharyngeal mucous membranes.

Recovery follows in 90 per cent of cases if the victim survives for more than 1 hour.[18] Those who die usually do so as a result of the multiple bony injuries and their complications. Crushing of large muscle masses occasionally produces the 'crush anuria' syndrome (see Chapter 19). Bronchopneumonia may be associated with reduced respiratory movement following multiple fractures of the chest in the elderly.

Other sports

It is quite impossible in a work of this length to detail the rare hazards of many minority interest sports. Riding accidents, although common, pose no special pathological difficulties in their interpretation, nor do the injuries sustained by fencers, pot-holers or climbers. When faced with such an unusual death, the pathologist can always obtain advice from the local office of the Sports Federation and the secretary or medical adviser to the appropriate local club.

References

1. Adams, I. (1975). Personal communication.
2. Amateur Boxing Association (1975). Personal communication.
3. Bayliss, G. J. A. (1969). Civilian diving deaths in Australia. *J. forensic Med.* **16**, 39.
4. Bert, P. (1878). *La Pression Barotraumatique*. Paris: Masson.
5. Brandenburg, W. and Hallevorden, J. (1954). Dementia Pugilistica mit anatomischem Befund. *Virchows Arch. path. Anat.* **325**, 680.
6. British Boxing Board of Control (1974). Revised Constitution and Regulations, London.
7. British Sub-Aqua Club (1973). Diving Officers' Conference Report, London.

8. Corsellis, J. A. N., Bruton, C. J. and Freeman-Browne, D. (1973). The aftermath of boxing. *Psychol. Med.* **3**, 270.
9. Courts, D. E. and Pierson, W. R. (1965). Sports parachuting and hypoxia. *Aerospace Med.* **36**, 372.
10. Dueker, C. W. (1970). *Medical Aspects of Sport Diving*. London: Thomas Yoseloff.
11. Editorial Comment (1974). The trainer's sponge. *Brit. med. J.* **4**, 488.
12. Editorial Comment (1975). Blowing in the wind. *Brit. med. J.* **3**, 266.
13. Eisman, B. (1975). Hang-gliding. *J. Amer. med. Ass.* **233**, 171.
14. Essex-Lopresti, P. (1946). The hazards of parachuting. *Brit. J. Surg.* **34**, 1.
15. Firearms Act (1968). London: HMSO.
16. Firearms (Dangerous Air Weapons) Regulations (1969). London: HMSO.
17. *Flight International* (1975). Private flight. 20th November, p. 748.
18. Fred, H. L. and Chandler, F. W. (1960). Traumatic asphyxia. *Amer. J. Med.* **29**, 508.
19. Gabashvili, I. (1971). Death of sportsmen in the Georgian SSR, 1955–70. In: *Abstracts of XVIIIth World Congress of Sports Medicine*, p. 57. London: BASM.
20. Harris, N. H. and Murray, R. O. (1974). Lesions of the symphysis in athletes. *Brit. med. J.* **4**, 211.
21. Jarrett, P. and Kent, D. (1973). Hang-gliding—the new sport. *Flight International*, 14th May, p. 593.
22. Kissoff, W. and Eiseman, B. (1975). Injuries associated with hang-gliding. *J. Amer. med. Ass.* **233**, 158.
23. McAniff, J. J. and Schenck, H. V. (1974). Investigation of scuba deaths. *J. Sports Med.* **2**, 199.
24. Malhotra, M. S. and Wright, H. C. (1960a). Air embolism during decompression underwater and its prevention. *J. Physiol. (Lond.)* **151**, 32.
25. Malhotra, M. S. and Wright, H. C. (1960b). *Air Embolism during Decompression Underwater and Its Prevention* (RNPRC). Rep. No. UPS 188. London: Medical Research Council.
26. Martland, H. S. (1928). Punch drunk. *J. Amer. med. Ass.* **91**, 1103.
27. Mason, J. K. (1962). *Aviation Accident Pathology*, p. 309. London: Butterworths.
28. Mawdsley, C. and Ferguson, S. R. (1963). Neurological disease in boxers. *Lancet* **ii**, 795.
29. Miles, S. (1969). *Underwater Medicine*, 3rd edn. London: Staples Press.
30. Moritz, A. R. (1954). *The Pathology of Trauma*, Chap. 9. London: Henry Kimpton.
31. Paterson, D. C. (1971). Water ski-ing injuries. *Practitioner* **206**, 655.
32. Perthes, G. (1900). Druckstauung. *Dtsch. Z. Chir.* **55**, 385.

33. Polson, C. J. and Gee, D. J. (1973). *The Essentials of Forensic Medicine*, 3rd edn., p. 442. Oxford: Pergamon.
34. Registrar General (1973). *Annual Report of Mortality Statistics.* London: HMSO.
35. Roberts, A. H. (1970). *Brain Damage in Boxers.* London: Pitman.
36. Royal College of Physicians of London (1969). *Report on the Medical Aspects of Boxing.* London.
37. Royal Life Saving Society (1973). *Analyses of Fatal Drowning Accidents.* London.
38. Safety of Sports Grounds Act (1975). London: HMSO.
39. Simson, L. R. (1971). Chin-sternum-heart syndrome—cardiac injury associated with parachuting mishaps. *Aerospace Med.* **42,** 1214.
40. Spillane, J. D. (1962). Five boxers. *Brit. med. J.* **2,** 1205.
41. Thomson, W. A. R. (1935). The physiology of deep sea diving. *Brit. med. J.* **2,** 208.
42. Walkden, L. (1975). The medical hazards of rugby football. *Practitioner* **205,** 201.

16

Kicking, karate and kung fu

Kicking

No organ or vital structure can be considered safe from kicks or from being stamped on or jumped on. Indeed, when inexplicable deep injuries are found following an assault, the possibility that the body has been kicked, or stamped on while lying on the ground, must be considered. The injuries to the body caused by kicking can be among the most significant seen in forensic medical practice. As well as producing obvious superficial injuries, which may be of a most severe nature, kicks directed against the body frequently produce extensive damage to the deeper placed structures and organs.[5]

Kicking as a means of attack is becoming increasingly common and is now ranked as third in order of frequency as a means of homicide in Great Britain. Only stabbing and manual strangulation are seen more frequently. It is not difficult to discover the reasons for the increase in the incidence of kicking. First, the greater use by the police of their powers to search a person for hidden offensive weapons may have had some effect in discouraging their use and, secondly, punishment is more severe on conviction for carrying offensive weapons. Potential criminals are, as a result, possibly more aware of their shod feet as ready-made instruments of violence.

Analysis of a kick
In most instances the kick is delivered in a standing position, with the weight of the body firmly placed over the fixed leg. The vertebral column and the pelvis are rotated laterally enabling the free swinging leg to be brought well back behind the body at the beginning of the swing. The lower leg is raised by flexion and the foot is also fully flexed. From the moment of the start of the delivery of the kick, the largest muscle groups of the body are co-ordinated to produce great power. There is more energy in a swinging foot than in a faster-moving, directionally controlled swinging hand. Although a kick is slow relative to a punch, there is a steady build-up of momentum, so that serious tissue damage may result from the relatively low velocity heavy impact. When the heavy footwear worn by some assailants is considered along with the kicking action, the degree of resulting damage is hardly surprising.

Kicks can be administered in other ways, a common method being the backward and downward jabbing motion using the heel and the back of the foot, similar to the 'heeling' movement used by rugby football players. Blows with the side of the foot are less effective because the sideways movement of the whole leg is relatively inefficient and lacks power. Such kicks prove to be more of annoyance value than disabling.

In association with the more conventional forward kick, it is becoming increasingly common to discover that the victim has also been jumped on or forcibly stamped on. The expression 'putting the boot in' as understood by both the police and the criminal classes frequently combines the two elements of kicking and stamping.

Types of footwear
The offence of kicking appears to be one committed mainly by youths and young adult males, and it would seem helpful to consider the types of footwear worn by the participants. Young people, being both gregarious and fashion-conscious, limit their footwear to a few styles.

One type of footwear frequently seen in kicking offences is a strong, heavy, blunt-ended boot or shoe, with a prominent welt, large heels and thick rubber or composite soles. Occasionally, the area of the toe-cap is strengthened and, together with a rather inflexible shoe as a whole, a hard toe-jab is easily delivered. A modification of this heavy-duty boot or shoe is seen in the industrial 'safety' shoe, which is designed to protect the toes from falling objects by incorporating a thin steel protective layer within the toe-cap. It is extremely easy with this type of footwear to deliver a powerful blow which may result in serious or lethal damage.

A second style of footwear, formerly quite popular and which may reappear on the fashion scene, incorporated the 'stiletto' heel. Found almost exclusively in women's shoes, the extremely thin but strengthened heel—with a weight-bearing surface area rarely more than 40 mm^2 ($\frac{1}{16}$ in^2)—could deliver a serious penetrating injury either by stamping or when held in the hand.

A third style of shoe, which is popular with young adult males, is known as a 'training shoe'. The shoes are soft and strong and have become widely acceptable in sports sessions and training programmes. It is fashionable to wear them as a soft shoe for everyday casual wear and, as such, are frequently found worn by young adult assailants.

The training shoe consists of a firm sole made from a pliable composite or plastic substance, while the upper part is made from thin soft leather, canvas or sometimes imitation leather. Toe-caps are occasionally present but they are not unduly strengthened.

It is clear, therefore, that the construction of this type of footwear makes it highly unlikely that the wearer of these shoes will be able to deliver a very serious blow of a conventional nature to a crouching body without, at the same time, causing some injury to his own feet. When a kick is made by an assailant wearing training shoes, it is made by means of the instep, the action being the same as in kicking a football. The impact on the body is spread over a wide area so that localizing injuries are seen less frequently. Nevertheless, stamping or jumping on a body can still be effected without injury to the attacker.

Training shoes, however, have a characteristic ribbed pattern to the soles. This enables a comparison of the shoe and patterned abrasions left on the skin to be made after the body has been stamped on. On more than one occasion the patterned shoe-prints left in blood stains on floor coverings and on exposed parts of the body have been responsible for assisting in the identification of young assailants following a homicide or a serious assault.

Sites for kicking

The victim is usually knocked or punched to the ground. He may have been tripped or kicked about the lower legs or the ankles. The result is that the victim is frequently found on the ground in a crouching or curled-up position when secondarily set-upon and kicked. The position adopted is an instinctive one to protect the face, abdomen and genitalia from further injury. If blows are delivered to these areas, serious or even disastrous results may follow. However, a kicking assailant frequently aims his blows indiscriminately against the head and upper part of the chest, often the neck, when the other areas are protected by arms and legs.

Because of its characteristic shape, the shod foot can deliver blows to areas which are relatively inaccessible or unlikely for attacks with a more orthodox blunt instrument. The sites where kicking injuries are usually seen are in the hollows and concavities of the body where the toe of the boot can be easily accommodated. They are frequently seen on the side of the neck, under the chin or lower jaw, especially the angle of the jaw, on either side of the nose and involving the eyes, behind the ears and in the nape of the neck (Fig. 16.1). Theoretically, any area can receive a kick but it is not common to find injuries on the vault of the skull, on the centre of the forehead or on the point of the chin. Elsewhere on the body, kicks are delivered to the loins and, if the body is outstretched, the genitals, the upper abdomen and lower chest.

Sites for stamping and jumping

Once the victim has been rendered defenceless and unconscious, through having received kicks about the head and neck, the assailant sometimes then engages in severe stamping with the heel or repeated jumping on the body. Such blows are commonly delivered to the chest and upper abdomen, probably because of the width and relative stability of these body areas. Stamping on the neck is seen occasionally. The face is less commonly assaulted in this way, probably because of the mobility of the tissues underfoot (Fig. 16.2). While kicks are frequently aimed at the genitalia, especially in sexual assaults, damage due to stamping or jumping on these organs is rarely seen because of the degree of protection provided by the thighs.

A particularly disagreeable form of stamping is that produced by a

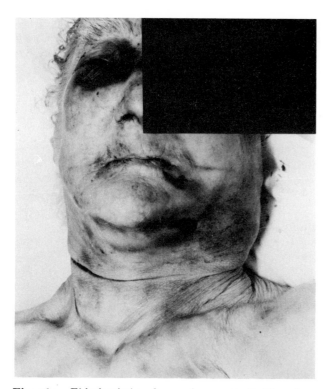

Fig. 16.1 Elderly victim of a murderous attack. There is massive swelling with superficial abrasion in the left neck region. The sternomastoid muscle beneath this was torn and there is no doubt that injury was due to a kick. The subject was also punched and strangled. (Reproduced by kind permission of the Crown Office.)

crushing or rolling motion by the foot on the nose, usually as part of some punishment; the result closely resembles the injuries produced by a downward stamping on the face.

Analysis of the injuries

The skin and subcutaneous tissues
The extent of the injury to the skin and subcutaneous tissues may be related to the physical properties and design of the footwear as well as to the velocity of the kick. The toe of the boot or shoe is usually rounded and this will result in a large area of skin compression. A contusion with marked intracutaneous and subcutaneous haemorrhage and swelling quickly develops. In addition—and this will depend largely on the flexibility of the skin at the point of impact—there is frequently a stretch laceration with considerable tearing of the skin and the underlying soft tissues. The laceration may be irregular and of

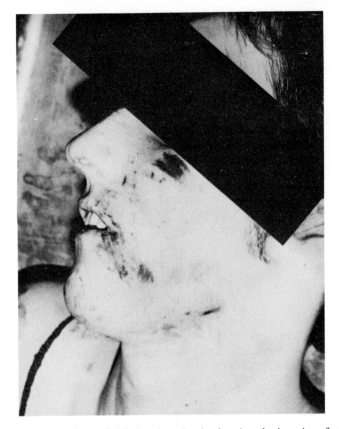

Fig. 16.2   Superficial abrasion clearly showing the imprint of a heel on the face of a victim of a stabbing incident. An abrasion in this position is more likely to be due to incidental treading during an affray rather than a deliberate stamping.

considerable size. As with lacerations from other causes, blood loss may be small. When the splitting of the skin occurs over a bony prominence, such as a cheekbone or the bridge of the nose, the injury may simulate an incised wound with relatively straight edges and without any protuberance of the underlying fatty tissue. Hair and debris may be carried into the wound. Over the skull, the stretch laceration may be so extensive as to expose a portion of bone.

The muscles
Because of the momentum conveyed by a swinging boot, the transfer of the force is not only to the skin and soft tissues but also to the underlying muscles. Haemorrhage within the more superficial muscle groups is often very extensive, an example of this being the haemorrhage into the

sternomastoid and strap muscles of the neck when a blow lands on the side of the neck. Not only is there frank haemorrhage but often there may be rupture of muscle bundles. Another common site for damage is on the side of the head, when the temporal muscles are involved. Damage following a kick is not confined to the superficial layers but, frequently, the deep muscles of the neck close to the vertebral column are injured. Haemorrhage is sometimes seen in the deep lumbar muscle groups when kicks are delivered to the renal areas, although actual tissue rupture is rare. Widespread damage is especially common with regard to the pectoral and intercostal muscles when the body is stamped or jumped upon. The muscular layers of the anterior abdominal wall are hardly ever spared during these attacks and, while haemorrhage may occur immediately below the site of the blow, it is sometimes seen in the flanks and towards the back. Unusual damage is found in the deep muscles of the perineum—in particular around the anus and rectum, which may be damaged following a severe kick in that region.

Deeper vital structures

A very hard kick delivered by a strong assailant wearing heavy boots can produce extensive damage to many internal organs. A blow aimed at the neck may result in a fracture of the laryngeal cartilages and the hyoid bone. The accompanying haemorrhage and oedema may cause death by asphyxia. The vessels of the neck and the vagus nerve are frequently injured at the same time.

Ruptures to solid abdominal organs such as the liver, spleen and kidneys easily follow a hard kick in these regions, while stamping or jumping on the abdomen often results in tears at the root of the mesentery, retroperitoneal haemorrhages and ruptures in the alimentary tract. Kicks and stampings about the thoracic cage may fracture the sternum and ribs, and bony fragments may secondarily produce pulmonary or, rarely, cardiac lesions.

Head injuries

Head injuries form a separate group for consideration. Apart from the obvious scalp lacerations, injuries to the skull and intracranial contents are frequently seen. Linear fractures usually extend from the point of impact towards the base of the skull. Depressed fractures are not uncommon. The effects of a severe kick on the brain include concussion, cerebral contusions, lacerations and haemorrhage. The first impact by the shod foot may result in concussion, which is an immediate transient brain dysfunction manifested by unconsciousness (see Chapter 12). Further blows, or the initial blow if it was particularly severe, will result in subarachnoid and possibly subdural or extradural haemorrhages. Intracerebral haematomas or multiple small haemorrhages throughout the brain are not unusual.

If the kick is received on the side of the neck, in the region of the base of the skull, a traumatic subarachnoid haemorrhage may result from rupture of the vertebral artery. This vessel takes a circuitous route around the transverse process of the first cervical vertebra before entering the cranial cavity. Rupture by a sudden stretching of the vessel in this site will produce a rapidly fatal basal subarachnoid haemorrhage. Occasionally, the transverse process of the first cervical vertebra is fractured by the blow. The subarachnoid haemorrhage is made more serious if, at the time, the victim is under the influence of alcohol, when muscular reflex activity and co-ordination are less pronounced.

Examination of the footwear of the accused

It is highly desirable that any item of footwear suspected of being the cause of the kicking be made available for examination before the post-mortem dissection is completed. The ideal situation is to have the boots or shoes present in the autopsy room, when an opinion as to the culpability of the footwear can often be decided on the spot. Unfortunately, however, the assailant is often not apprehended until some time later and opinions regarding his footwear are made in the laboratory. The examination of the boot or shoe should include a search for blood, body tissues and hair as a matter of routine but additional information regarding the weight of the boot and the degree of its rigidity, in particular of the toe-cap, can be most helpful.

Karate

Karate is one of the oriental martial arts of self-defence. It was introduced and developed by former inhabitants of Okinawa as a means of defending themselves at a time when they were prohibited the use of weapons. As practised today, it is known in two distinct forms: Karate-do, which is a philosophical way of life linked to the Zen religion, and Karate-sho, which is mainly concerned with spectacular physical skills ranging from rapid gymnastic movements to those involving the breaking of boards and housebricks and the killing of animals.

As a sport, karate makes its appeal through the development of very quick reflexes and a remarkably precise co-ordination of will, nerves and muscles. The result is a rapid release of enormous controlled energy. When there are added to this display colourful descriptions such as 'superpower', 'destructive' and 'terror tactics' with their overtones of mastery of an opponent, it is not altogether surprising that there have been many seeking instruction in this form of martial art in recent years. Leaders of organized clubs fully recognize the danger of admitting students whose reasons for receiving instruction is questionable and such who seek admittance are firmly discouraged. Nevertheless, as karate is the ultimate in weaponless self-defence, it is becoming increasingly popular as a sport in schools and athletic clubs, as well as being taught for a definite purpose to members of the armed forces and the law enforcement agencies.

Training manuals and illustrated textbooks on karate are at pains to stress the fact that, at the same time as the basic reflex actions are being developed, the danger also exists that a method of self-defence may instinctively turn to aggression and counter-attack—'a playful tap on the shoulder could be disastrous to the jester'.[3] The person who learns the finer techniques of the sport may acquire a pronounced aggressive attitude which is inseparably linked to his highly developed reactions. This, after all, is the basis of karate. But proper training teaches that the aggressive nature must be controlled and subdued. As all teachers of karate strongly emphasize, a partially trained or improperly trained person can be extremely dangerous, to himself as well as to others. For, in applying a rapid defensive manoeuvre, there exists a real danger that the person will instinctively convert it into an unprovoked and uncontrolled act of aggression. It can easily be seen, therefore, that a person with criminal intent and with some knowledge of karate can, under provocation, so augment his attack that it may end in death or serious permanent injury to the victim.

Methods used in self-defence and in attack
The actions involve thrusting, blocking and striking by means of the foot, knee, leg, hand, elbow and forearm. The karate student learns to turn aside very rapidly in order to parry or block the assailant's attack and then to counter-attack reflexly and powerfully. The supremacy and efficacy of karate over the other martial arts depends on ultra-fast thrusts and strikes achieved by bringing the entire power of the body into a single concentrated action which is both fast and strong. Having driven home the attack, there is a rapid withdrawal and immediate relaxation. In brief, the technique is a fast powerful blow followed by an equally fast withdrawal.

Foot strikes
The techniques involve striking an opponent's groin, stomach, armpit, neck or even the chin. The heel is used for striking the solar plexus, upper thighs, knees and other resistant areas while the ball of the foot is used to attack the softer regions, such as the neck. The flying front foot strikes are most spectacular and they can mete out considerable punishment. In effect, the action is an unusual form of high-kicking.

Hand strikes
The use of the hand is the technique best known to non-participants of karate. It can be used with the fingers rigidly outstretched, the so-called 'spear-hand strike', when the blow is aimed at the eyes, the front of the neck or the solar plexus. The side of the hand can also be used, as in a chopping action. The fingers and thumb are held straight and rigid and the outer side of the hand is slashed diagonally downwards. This form is known as the 'knife-hand strike' and a disabling blow can be delivered to the ear or the side or the back of the neck. A third form is a modified punch with the fist. It us known as the 'ridge-hand and fore-knuckle strike'. It is a very effective blow and in some ways more dangerous than the other two. It makes contact with the eyes, chin, neck or

ribs over a slightly larger area than does a knife-hand strike, and is a fast forward and powerful thrust.

All the hand strikes are described as dangerous, and students of karate are taught not to use them in actual self-defence unless it is absolutely necessary. Sportsmen are warned that these are precision movements and someone will definitely get hurt unless they are well learned before sparring.

Knee strikes

By bending the knee and either by raising it or by a forward thrust, heavy blows can be delivered over a short distance to the groin and genitalia as well as upwards into the region of the solar plexus.

Elbow strikes

As with the knee, similar powerful, short-distance blows can be made with the flexed elbow and these can be directed towards the solar plexus, face, ribs and the back of the neck.

Forensic medical aspects of karate

Karate is both a sport and a method of self-defence. It can be usefully included in a training programme for athletes in general as it helps to develop rapid reflex actions. However, from the standpoint of forensic medicine, karate can be the means of inflicting severe damage to an assault victim when certain vital structures are struck.

In a case reported by Camps,[1] the accused was convicted of the murder of a soldier by delivering a karate blow with the side of the hand to the front of the neck. This was an approved method of unarmed combat then used in the armed forces. The post-mortem examination revealed a vertical fracture of the thyroid cartilage, to the side of the mid-line, as well as several vertical tears in the carotid arteries.

At Irvine, Ayrshire, an autopsy was performed on a middle-aged male found tied up in a chair. Apart from a number of blows about the head and face, he had received a knife-hand strike on the left side of the neck, the assailant probably standing above and behind the seated victim. The karate blow produced a bruise in the soft tissues of the side of the neck at several levels, beneath which the left lamina of the thyroid cartilage was fractured into three separate fragments.

In conclusion, students of karate are taught to discourage an ordinary assailant by making their counter-attacks against certain vital points, thereby causing sharp pain and possible nerve shock. Nakayama and Draegar[4] say: 'This is the minimum form of punishment. A more severe punishment resulting in severe injury is possible by increasing the force of your attack or by attacking other vital points. A lethal attack is also possible if the karate technique is executed against certain vital points. The karate exponent therefore is able to deal out punishment in varying degrees. The seriousness of attacking vital points must be constantly in mind and your conduct in any situation must be based on the potential consequences. Karate used against an obstreperous person must of necessity be different from the method used against an assailant who is bent on taking your life.'

Kung fu

Kung fu is one of the earliest Chinese martial arts and is based on philosophies and techniques dating back several thousands of years. Taoism (Tao = the way) is one of the three main religious cultures of China and its precepts and spirituality underly the physical disciplines of the art of kung fu. It was from kung fu that some of the other well known martial arts, such as ju-jitsu, judo, aikido and several forms of karate, were later developed. A few of these later arts have received world-wide recognition and acceptance, even occasionally to Olympic status, but the basic essentials of kung fu have remained virtually unchanged and largely unknown. Recently it has received a totally unexpected stimulus in a rush of cinema and television films, with the result that kung fu has suddenly attracted many new adherents.

The main difference between kung fu and one of its derivatives, karate, is that the former has never been regarded as an aggressive sport, but rather as an exercise in the discipline of restraint by advocating the use of defensive manoeuvres.[2] Its philosophy runs completely contrary to the impression, formed quite incorrectly by many people, that kung fu encourages the use of violence. In fact, the training of this particular martial art seeks to increase control over one's natural aggressive tendencies when faced with a disagreeable and potentially dangerous situation.

The techniques which the students learn are essentially defensive movements by skillful use of the arms, elbows and fists. However, simply to ward off blows before the moment of impact is not always sufficient. Other techniques must be learned which can be used to counter dangerous attacks before they are executed. Whereas the defensive actions tend to involve the use of the upper limbs, the need to counter dangerous situations usually requires taking the initiative by using a variety of controlled kicks.

A back kick delivered with a straight raised leg can be effectively aimed at the abdomen or at an arm holding an offensive weapon while protecting one's face and front. Similar disarming actions can be effected by a sideways kick. Stampings and flying kicks, front kicks and circular kicks all form the counter-attacking programme. However, it must be remembered that such kicks are used to disarm an assailant and are not a means to disable him.

In the past kung fu may have been both an art and a code of defensive manoeuvres, but the practice today has been to retain the defensive techniques and to superimpose a competitive spirit with attacking movements. Instead of simply countering a blow or precluding its delivery the sport has been developing aggressive 'follow-up' body blows. The popular method appears to be based on the fist and the foot.

The clenched fist delivers strong blows, but without any outstanding speed, to the ribs, back, chin and side of head but avoiding the recognized 'vital' areas of the body. The foot is used as a flying kick, using the instep or the outer edge, or it is used as a forward-directed standing kick aimed mainly at the lower half of the body.

During the past few years there have been a number of television programmes, films and feature articles in magazines which have nurtured and encouraged a greater awareness of kung fu. In this enthusiasm, it is regrettable that there has been an inordinate concentration on modes of attack and counter-attack rather than on highlighting the sport as an art of self-defence. Kung fu has been made almost identical to karate. This is indeed unfortunate because there is no doubt that the art of kung fu remains a sport worthy of a separate identity.

It is incumbent on the followers of kung fu to see that the present trend of introducing the more dangerous and less philosophical elements of karate into kung fu is positively discouraged. They are two quite separate martial arts and should be kept so. In its present format kung fu is not a violent sport and is unlikely to be the means of inflicting real injury to a person but that will depend on a proper observance of its precepts.

References

1. Camps, F. E. (1959). The case of Emmett Dunne. *Med.-leg. J. (Camb.)* **27**, 156.
2. Harrington, A. P. (1975). *Defend Yourself with Kung Fu*. London: Stanley Paul.
3. Mattson, G. E. (1970). *The Way of Karate*. Rutland, Vt: Chas. E. Tuttle.
4. Nakayama, M. and Draegar, D. F. (1963). *Practical Karate*. Book I, *Fundamentals*. Tokyo and Rutland, Vt: Chas. E. Tuttle.
5. Teare, R. D. (1961). Blows with the shod foot. *Med. Sci. Law* **1**, 429.

17

The offshore scene and its hazards

The industrial activity presently concentrated in the northern North Sea employs approximately 10 000 offshore workers. These men work on drilling rigs and production platforms, on supply boats and on crane and pipe-laying barges. In addition to the general risks of a heavy industrial situation and the specific dangers of specialized employment such as diving, those who work offshore are exposed to the hazards of an often hostile environment.

There are three distinct but overlapping stages involved in the discovery and production of oil and gas reserves. These are

1. Exploration.
2. Development.
3. Production.

Exploration

When a suitable location has been indicated from seismic survey, a drilling rig is sited. Drilling rigs stand on the seabed if the water is less than 75 m (250 ft) deep. Semi-submersible rigs, which are kept in position by multiple anchors, are used in deeper water. In extremely deep water, drilling ships are employed which are maintained in position by a computer-controlled navigation system. Drilling is effected by the action of a table on the rig which rotates a column of drill pipe joined in 10 m (33 ft) lengths ending in a drilling bit.

Each drilling rig carries a crew of between 70 and 80 men. Of these, only 25 may be directly involved in drilling. The remainder are employed as crane drivers and communications engineers, as maintenance, marine and catering staff and as divers. Crew changes are carried out by helicopter. Each man usually works offshore for a 2-week period followed by a similar period of shore leave. When on the rig, a 12-hour shift is usual and all crew are on call in the event of an emergency.

Development

If the reservoir of oil or gas which has been found is considered an economic proposition, sufficient wells are drilled to produce a satisfactory flow and the oil or gas is conveyed to shore either by submarine pipeline or by tankers. Wells for production are drilled from permanent production platforms tethered to the seabed.

If a submarine pipeline is required to bring the oil or gas to land, barges of two types are employed. On pipe-laying barges (Fig. 17.1), 10 m (33 ft) lengths of large diameter pipe are welded into a continuous line which is then laid accurately on the seabed. Thereafter, pipe-burying barges draw water-jetting sleds along the pipe to make a trench

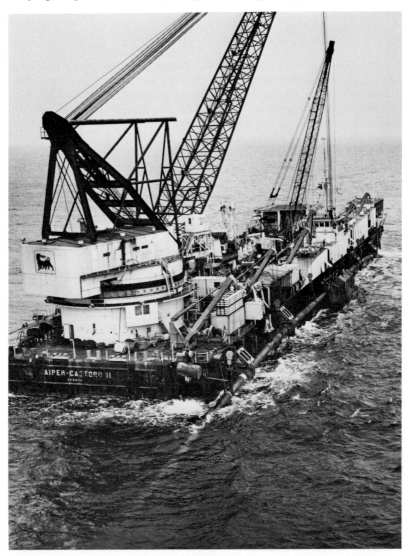

Fig. 17.1   Pipe-laying barge Castoro II at sea linking up sections of BP's 177 km (110 mile) submarine pipeline, connecting the Forties oilfield to land. (Photo by British Petroleum.)

in the seabed into which the pipe is lowered. Each of these types of barge carries a complement of 200–300 men and each is a self-contained unit.

Production

A production platform (Fig. 17.2) is tethered by large diameter piles driven several hundred metres into the seabed. Crane barges which can

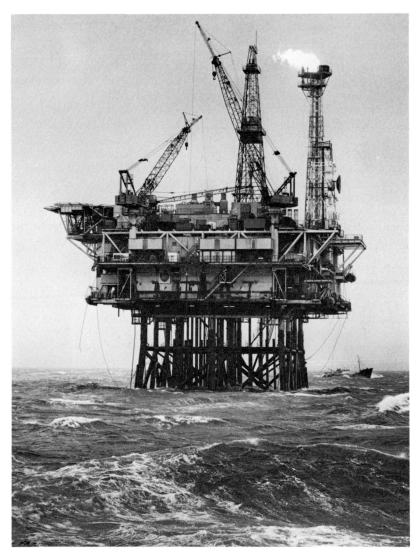

Figure 17.2   Production platform FA (Graythorp I) in BP's Forties oilfield in the North Sea. (Photo by British Petroleum.)

lift structural members weighing up to 2000 tons are used for this purpose. Although the crew of the completed platform will be about 120, the stage of installation of the modules requires a work-force in the region of 300 men.

Helicopters are employed to take men and minor supplies to and from the installations and barges at all stages of oil exploration. They also fulfil an essential role in the management and transportation of casualties. Because of the distance and time factors, the helicopter becomes, on occasion, a mobile intensive care facility.

Industrial accidents offshore

The attendances at the Casualty Department in Aberdeen Royal Infirmary in 1975 are shown in Tables 17.1–17.3. More than one-third of those men injured offshore during one year were in occupations confined to the drilling deck of an oil rig or drilling ship; this is, therefore, a high-risk phase in which the hazards are those of any industrial situation.

Many accidents occur during the handling of heavy equipment and materials, and the majority of injuries occur as the result of a worker being struck accidentally (Table 17.1). Crushing injuries of varying severity are also common, as are injuries resulting from falls. The role of the rig's crane drivers is important as misjudgement in a difficult situation may result in severe injuries to the deck crew; heavily loaded cranes have also toppled into the sea with the loss of drivers' lives.

Table 17.1 Causes of offshore accidents (Offshore workers attending the Casualty Department, Aberdeen Royal Infirmary, during 1975)

Struck by moving object	186
Struck by falling object	81
Crushing	178
Fall (including from a height)	151
Foreign body	28
Snapping cable/hawser	25
Twisting injury	21
Burn/scald/electricity	19
Cutting or penetrating	13

The hands and fingers are very often involved (Table 17.2); such injuries are particular to the actual drilling operation. A main task of the drilling crew is to connect and disconnect sections of drilling pipe; despite quick reactions and co-ordinated teamwork, hand and finger injuries are common. The lower limbs may be injured in varying degree by being trapped between sections of drill pipe on the deck of the rig.

Accidents which occur during development and construction of platforms or pipelines are again those encountered in any heavy industrial

Table 17.2 Site of injury
(Offshore workers attending the Casualty
Department, Aberdeen Royal Infirmary,
during 1975)

Hand/fingers/thumb	303
Upper limb excl. above	122
Foot/toes	75
Ankle	57
Lower limb excl. above	98
Head/skull/face	63
Spine	42
Eye	34

situation but the risks are exaggerated offshore because of the intensity and concentration of the operation. Many welders are employed and sustain a considerable number of minor injuries involving the eyes (Table 17.2).

Injuries on the barges are associated with the handling and lifting of heavy weights, the dangers being exacerbated by frequently adverse sea conditions. A particular hazard is produced by the movement of pipe lengths on deck, which can cause crushing injuries to the trunk and lower limbs. Hand injuries are again common and crushing injuries occur during transfer of heavy materials to installations and barges.

The nature of the injuries occurring in offshore work is analysed in Table 17.3. Out of a total of 684 attendances, 529 had only one injury, 157 had sustained multiple injuries and 5 patients were noted as having five distinct injuries on attendance. Both simple and complicated fractures are common.

Table 17.3 Nature of injury
(Offshore workers attending the Casualty
Department, Aberdeen Royal Infirmary,
during 1975)

Contusion/abrasion	384
Fracture	196
Sprain/strain	107
Laceration	102
Burn	26
Foreign body	20
Traumatic amputation	17
Dislocation	10
Tendon/nerve/major vessel	4
Haemo/pneumothorax	2

Fatal accidents offshore

There were 27 fatal accidents in the British sector of the North Sea between 1971 and 1975 inclusive. The fatalities can be divided into two groups—those which occurred on static installations, and those on mobile units such as barges and supply vessels.

Static installations (17 fatalities)
The fatalities listed in Table 17.4 showed no particular seasonal incidence.

Table 17.4   Fatal accidents on fixed installations

Falling from a height	5
Struck by falling object	4
Falling into the sea	3*
Crane pulled into sea	2*
Struck by cable	2
Explosion	1
Total	17 cases

* Bodies not recovered.

The commonest cause of death discovered is a fall from a height, such as from the derrick to the drilling floor or from the main deck into the sea, a distance of about 30 m (100 ft). The water impact injuries are probably such as are seen after precipitation from a high river bridge and include fractures of the thoracic cage and laceration of the heart and lungs;[16] the precise position of the body at impact may be critical.[42] Unfortunately, the extent of injuries in the 5 fatal cases in the North Sea is unknown because the bodies were not recovered. Heavy objects falling from a height, such as from the derrick or loading crane, constitute the other common cause of serious injury.

Barges and vessels (10 fatalities) (Table 17.5)
Of the nine fatal accidents which occurred on the drilling barges and supply vessels, 8 occurred in the months from October to February. The fact that 5 of the winter fatalities occurred on supply vessels shows

Table 17.5   Fatal accidents on barges and vessels

Injured by cable	4
Crushed on deck	3
Lost overboard	3*
Total	10 deaths

* One body not recovered.

that it is the men on smaller craft who are at greatest risk. Most of those killed on the mobile units were seamen.

The majority of these deaths can be attributed to rough weather which resulted in the loss of men overboard or in the movement of deck cargo or structures which crushed the victim against the guardrail. It is also during bad weather that mooring cables are likely to tauten or snap.

Fatal injuries

Only 5 of the 21 fatal casualties who were recovered survived long enough to reach hospital. Two died from brain damage, 1 after falling from a height and the other having been struck by a snapped cable. The third man sustained fracture of the arch of the atlas after falling 24 m (80 ft) from the derrick to the drilling rig floor, while the fourth was struck by a tautening anchor cable which ruptured the abdominal aorta. The last man died from burns occasioned by an explosion.

The 14 who died at the scene had suffered severe head, chest or abdominal injuries either in isolation or combination. The pattern of injury was that commonly seen from acceleration, deceleration or crush forces.

Three seamen were lost overboard and 2 of the bodies were recovered; death was due to drowning in both. One of them had survived for almost 1 hour in the water at $7°C$ $(44°F)$ and it is probable that cold injury played a major part in his death.

The hazards of diving

The hydrostatic pressure of water increases by 101 kPa (1 atm) for every 10 m (33 ft) of depth. The diver is therefore exposed to great physiological stress unless he is maintained in a submarine or other rigid casing. Diving techniques have been greatly advanced for the purposes of sport, research and industry. The first is covered in Chapter 15. During diving research programmes, men have been exposed to pressures of up to $61·1$ times atmospheric pressure in dry chambers corresponding to a depth of 610 m (2000 ft) of seawater. We are concerned here, however, with the implications of diving for industrial purposes.

The number of working divers has increased considerably in the last 5 years. There has also been an increase in the types of tasks and in the depths at which divers are expected to work routinely. Recent estimates suggest that, in 1976, there were 1000 divers employed in the North Sea alone. These operations are likely to yield an increase in the number of medical problems which will extend beyond those presently found in sports diving.

Introduction to diving techniques in operational use

Four diving techniques are used currently by commercial divers in the North Sea oil industry:

1. Self-Contained Underwater Breathing Apparatus (scuba) diving (Fig. 17.3).
2. Surface-orientated diving with surface decompression.
3. Bounce diving.
4. Saturation diving.

Deep bounce diving using oxygen/helium breathing mixtures and saturation diving on a commercial scale are almost exclusive to the industry. The 'standard diving suit' with its rigid copper helmet is not used.

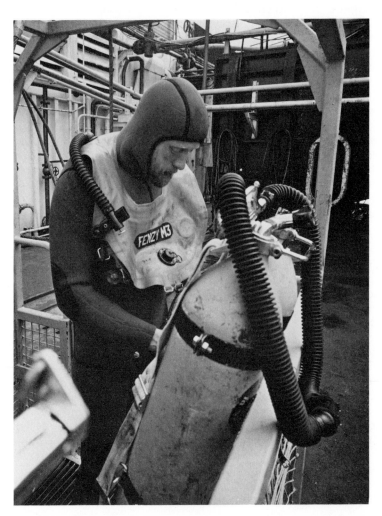

Fig. 17.3 Scuba diver on board BP's drilling platform Sea Quest. (Photo by British Petroleum.)

1. *Self-contained underwater breathing apparatus*
Apart from some applications during the laying of shallow underwater pipelines, scuba diving is little used in the oil industry. Its place in sports diving is described in Chapter 15.

2. *Surface-orientated diving with surface decompression*
The diver is connected to the surface by an 'umbilical' containing a gas line, a communication system and sometimes a heating line. His air or breathing mixture is supplied from the deck of the diving vessel. Like the scuba diver, he may wear a wet suit, but, more commonly, wears a dry suit with undergarment. It is now possible to heat the diver's breathing mixture before inspiration to prevent respiratory heat loss. Decompression stops (see below), if warranted, are carried out in a decompression chamber on the surface. The diver ascends fairly swiftly and must be recompressed in a deck-mounted chamber within about 5 minutes; this is followed by standard decompression according to accepted formulae. Surface decompression diving is limited by law in Britain to depths of less than 50 m (165 ft); the technique is widely used in the oil industry.

3. *Bounce diving*
The depth restrictions of diving using surface decompression have led to the development of the technique of bounce diving. The diver is lowered to his underwater work-site in a diving bell at atmospheric pressure. The gas pressure in the bell is increased to match the hydrostatic pressure outside when he is ready to begin work. The diver can then open the hatch and enter the water. Alternatively, a free-swimming diver can undertake a bounce dive without a bell or surface pressure chamber. After completing his time at maximum depth, he ascends in stages through the water. These 'wet stops' correspond to a decompression table.

The breathing mixture most commonly used is helium and oxygen. Helium replaces nitrogen in the mixture to avoid inert gas narcosis. The use of nitrogen/oxygen mixtures is not allowed on dives exceeding 50 m (165 ft) in British waters.

The time the diver can remain under pressure is limited if he is to avoid saturating his tissues with the gases in his breathing mixture. The greater the depth of the dive, the less time is available for working before he must return to atmospheric pressure. This can be done by gradual ascent through the water or, more usually, in the diving bell and, subsequently, the deck chamber.

Bounce diving can be carried out to depths of up to 100–200 m (330–660 ft) but the 'bottom time' at extreme depths is so short that the technique becomes uneconomic in a commercial operation.

4. *Saturation diving*
The saturation system comprises at least one deck-mounted living chamber, with full environmental control systems, and a diving bell

into which the divers transfer for transport to their underwater work-site. In larger saturation systems, the living chamber may remain pressurized for an entire diving season. Replacement of divers after their 2–3-week saturation period is accomplished in a smaller access chamber.

Although oxygen/nitrogen breathing mixtures can be used in shallow saturation systems, a helium/oxygen mixture is used in industrial situations which require diving to 500 m (1650 ft).

The pathology of pressure change

Pathological states may arise because pressure alters the physical properties of gases within the body. These states are of dysbarism, resulting from the expansion or compression of gases within closed spaces such as the chest, sinuses or middle ears, and of decompression sickness which results from escape of gases from solution in the body tissues and fluids as the ambient pressure falls.

With the possible exception of dysbaric osteonecrosis, there is no firm evidence that increased pressure itself causes adverse long-term effects. The pharmacological properties of oxygen and nitrogen do, however, become more marked at increased pressure, when oxygen can be toxic and nitrogen becomes increasingly narcotic (see p. 307).

The rapid growth of international commercial diving has, inevitably, led to confusion in medical terminology. The European Biomedical Society has recently issued a guide to the use of terms and these are included, with some additions, in Table 17.6.

1. *The effects of increased pressure*

(a) *Squeezes*
Skin squeezes are a relatively common form of mild dysbaric injury. They are caused by protrusion of the skin under pressure into folds of an uninflated dry suit with extravasation of red cells into the subcutaneous tissues. Divers may also experience a more severe form of squeeze in which a sudden increase in hydrostatic pressure tends to crush the chest; there is an equally sudden decrease in lung volume and distension of alveolar capillaries.

A fatal diving accident, presumed to be due to thoracic squeeze, has been reported.[43] The main lesion was intra-alveolar and interstitial pulmonary haemorrhage. The victim was a breath-hold diver who inadvertently exhaled at depth so that his total lung volume was insufficient to allow for further compression as he descended deeper in the water.

(b) *High-pressure nervous syndrome*
The aetiology of this is unknown. The symptoms are variously described as tremors, shakes, 'micro-sleeps' and nausea. The syndrome occurs almost exclusively during deep research dives in excess of 2 MPa (20 atm). Current theories suggest that it may be due either to a

Table 17.6

Term	Definition
Arterial gas or air embolism	A complication of pulmonary decompression baro-trauma in which gas or air ruptures centrally into the vascular system and passes out, notably to the central nervous system, by the arterial circulation.
Barotrauma	Mechanical damage to tissues as a direct result of change in environmental pressure. Includes both compression and decompression injuries.
Bends	This traditional term has been used for almost any manifestation of decompression sickness but should be used carefully to avoid ambiguity. Its most satisfactory use is as 'limb bends' to describe the musculoskeletal forms of acute decompression sickness.
Decompression barotrauma (pulmonary, otitic, sinus)	This occurs when the gases within a cavity expand during reduction of ambient pressure, with some obstruction preventing unrestricted venting of gases into the atmosphere. The chief sites of decompression barotrauma are intrathoracic, middle ear and sinuses.
Decompression disorders and the decompression illnesses	These terms cover both pulmonary decompression barotrauma, with its complications such as arterial gas or air embolism, and acute decompression sickness. They are particularly useful as they also include those not uncommon cases which seem to fall between the two major diagnostic categories.
Decompression sickness	The clinical syndrome resulting from a reduction of environmental pressure sufficient to cause the formation of bubbles from the gases which were previously dissolved in tissues and body fluids.
Type I and Type II decompression sickness	This classification of the clinical manifestations of decompression sickness is useful but arbitrary. Type I includes symptoms of musculoskeletal, cutaneous, lymphatic and minor general disorders such as fatigue. Type II includes all cases of a more serious nature with central nervous system, peripheral neuropathic or respiratory involvement.
Dysbarism	Any pathological condition arising from a change of pressure, compression or decompression, including, but not synonymous with, decompression sickness.

pharmacological effect of inert gases or to a direct effect of pressure on cell membranes. The condition can be prevented by using slower rates of compression; on some research dives to pressures of between 5 and 6 MPa (50 and 60 atm), it has been necessary to use compression routines lasting 3–4 days.

2. Decompression from pressure

(a) *Volume effects—ear and sinus barotrauma*
The mechanism underlying ear and sinus barotrauma is outlined in Chapter 15. Both are exaggerated by temporary or permanent obstruction to the normal venting of these spaces.

Although auditory damage due to diving has been attributed to aural barotrauma or aerotitis media, it now seems possible that some permanent inner ear damage with resulting neurosensory deafness may also occur. Similarly, it is now recognized that vestibular dysfunction is a common feature of deep diving accidents, although the mechanism for this is not yet entirely clear.

(b) *Volume effects—pulmonary barotrauma and gas or air embolism*
This condition, which was first recognized in 1932 by Polak and Adams,[38] must be clearly distinguished from decompression sickness although both may occur at the same time. Pulmonary barotrauma is occasionally seen in naval personnel undergoing submarine escape training[27] or in native pearl divers,[36] but all divers are at risk if they surface precipitately and there have been frequent accounts of its occurrence in recreational skin divers. Indeed, Chappell[5] is quoted as saying that it can occur in water as shallow as 2·1 m (7 ft) and could be a potential hazard even in swimming pools. The subject has, therefore, been introduced in Chapter 15.

The pathological consequences of rapid ascent without exhalation have been described by Shaefer *et al.*[39] Following rupture of the

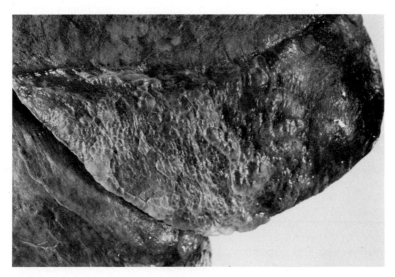

Fig. 17.4 Pulmonary interstitial emphysema. Subpleural 'bubbles' over middle lobe.

alveoli, air dissecting the connective tissues of the lung may give rise to pulmonary interstitial emphysema. Should the air track peripherally, it will present as glistening bubbles, up to 1 cm in size, under the visceral pleura (Fig. 17.4); rupture of one of these would lead to pneumothorax. Air reaching the hilum of the lung is free to spread to the other lung, or

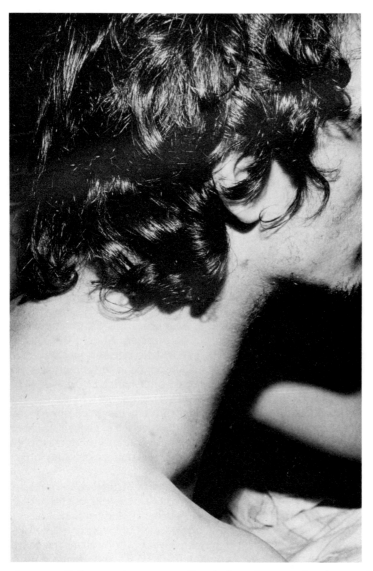

Fig. 17.5 Pulmonary barotrauma. Surgical emphysema of neck secondary to pneumomediastinum. The diver made a full recovery. (Dept. of Medical Illustration, Aberdeen University.)

upwards to appear in the subcutaneous tissues of the neck (Fig. 17.5), or downwards to reach the retroperitoneal tissues.

The subsequent production of systemic air embolism, of which cerebral air embolism is the most probable consequence in the erect posture, is described in Chapter 15; unconsciousness and convulsions followed by paresis may occur.[26] Coronary air embolism is a rare possibility although widespread myocardial infarction has been described in the autopsy of a youth who died 24 hours after collapse following a free ascent from a depth of 6 m (20 ft).[19]

Air trapping is a most important factor in pulmonary barotrauma.[29] This is a mechanical or functional obstruction to the escape of air from a segment of the lung, which results in a disproportionate gaseous expansion of the affected area during decompression. As the primary fault is pulmonary, this can occur even when normal diving procedures and techniques are being followed. The obstruction to the escape of air can be a stenosis, a valvular mechanism as in emphysema, or even bronchospasm due to a respiratory infection. Large bullae may form when air trapping is localized and these have been reported radiologically.[9] Chest radiography is essential whenever the possibility of lung damage is considered clinically; this applies equally in suspected cerebral air embolism because these cases, too, may be associated with a pulmonary lesion. It is now possible to diagnose pneumothorax accurately with the diver still under pressure.[6]

(c) *Decompression sickness*

The mechanisms inducing decompression sickness due to the release of gas from solution in the body tissues are described in Chapter 15. The longer a diver remains under pressure and the deeper his descent, the greater the degree of gas saturation of his tissues and the greater length of time he requires for subsequent decompression. Should this decompression be hurried or interrupted, gas will be released and will form bubbles, the formation and growth of which, both intravascularly and in cells and tissue spaces, is the essential abnormality in the pathogenesis of decompression sickness. Once in the venous circulation, the bubbles will behave as gas emboli. Recently, it has been appreciated that intravascular bubbles, acting as foreign particles, give rise to more serious complications such as platelet aggregation and the formation of lipid emboli; the pathophysiology of decompression sickness is, in fact, a complex subject.[13]

Details of the morbid anatomy of early cases of fatal decompression sickness in caisson workers have been collected and abstracted by Hoff.[24] Few additional cases have been reported during the last 50 years, but 2 more recent deaths of compressed air workers have been particularly well reported.[1, 41] There are even fewer published accounts of the autopsy findings in diving fatalities,[21, 34] and the possibility exists that the post-mortem appearances were modified by the simultaneous occurrence of gas or air embolism or by the effects of post-mortem decompression.

The fatal cases described fall into two categories. In the first, the deaths have been immediate, or within a few hours of the incident, and the findings include subcutaneous emphysema, generalized visceral congestion and the presence of gas bubbles. These are numerous in the veins and right heart chambers but scanty in the left heart and arteries. Extravascular bubbles and small haemorrhages may be seen in adipose tissue such as the mesentery and omenta. Petechiae are often to be seen in the white matter of the spinal cord. The second category includes deaths which occur after a lapse of several days or weeks, normally following a period of motor paralysis. The essential lesion in these cases is in the spinal cord where areas of degeneration and softening are found in the white matter. There is an almost exclusive involvement of the dorsal and lateral columns of the lower thoracic segments.[20] A 'swiss-cheese' appearance of the brain has recently been reported after an accident involving two scuba divers which was followed by post-mortem decompression[44] but we consider that this finding may well be a post-mortem change caused by gas-forming bacteria.

The histological appearances in experimental animals[3] include pulmonary haemorrhage, oedema, emphysema and atelectasis. Extravascular bubbles have been noted in adipose tissue, frequently in association with haemorrhage. When bubbles are present within fat cells they assume a foamy appearance and fat necrosis may develop subsequently. Gas bubbles have also been observed in the adrenal cortex. The selectivity of bubbles for lipid-containing cells is a result of the special solubility of gases, especially nitrogen, in fat.

Generalized fatty metamorphosis of the liver has been described,[41] as has centrilobular fatty change in 2 cases surviving for 6 and 5 hours respectively after the onset of symptoms.[1,44] Illustrations purporting to show gas dissolved in intracellular fat have been published[41,44] but their precise location is difficult to assess. We have examined material from a diver who died $1\frac{1}{2}$ hours after a precipitate ascent from 77 m (255 ft), where he had spent 45 minutes, and noted a patchy distribution of similar globules with slight fatty change of the adjacent liver cells. Our interpretation is that these globules are situated in the sinusoids and represent bubbles of gas coated with fat which have originated in the tissues drained by the portal vein and which constitute hepatic gas/fat emboli (Fig. 17.6). We did not see these hepatic globules, or fatty change, in material from 2 cases who died from pulmonary barotrauma during ascent but who had exceeded their depth/time limit and would have suffered from decompression sickness had they survived. It appears, therefore, that although their nature is uncertain, globules comprised of gas and fat are a not uncommon finding in those who die from decompression sickness after a short period of survival. It can be difficult to interpret the histological appearances in the tissues from a diving death when these have been modified by the liberation of gas during post-mortem decompression.

Fatty change in the liver has also been described in fatal subatmospheric decompression sickness. Fryer[15] discussed this topic at length

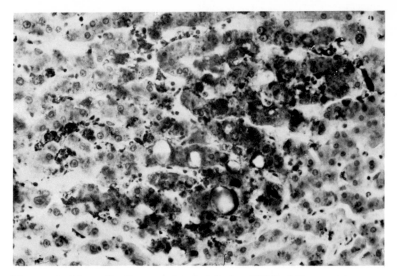

Fig. 17.6   Liver. Gas/fat vacuolated globules. (Oil Red O, × 207)

and concluded that the hepatic fatty change must have existed prior to
the exposure to altitude in almost all these fatalities but we believe it is
possible that the early onset of fatty change is related to hepatic gas/fat
emboli. Whatever its precise aetiology, fatty change in the liver may be
seen in fatal decompression disorders whether these occur after ascent
from depth or following exposure to altitude.

Fat embolism
Until recently, most of the interest in the occurrence of fat embolism in
decompression disorders has related to its role in post-descent shock
which was occasionally experienced by aviators after subatmospheric
decompression.[15] Pulmonary or systemic fat embolism was present to
some degree in 9 out of 17 fatal cases. Mason[31] commented that,
although the presence of fat embolism is by no means invariable, its
relationship to post-descent shock merits special consideration (see
Chapter 20).

Pulmonary fat and bone marrow emboli, and renal fat emboli, have
been reported in dogs which either died or were killed following an
experimental compression/decompression procedure.[7,8] In these experiments, the anaesthetized animals were compressed to 606 kPa (6
atm) for 1 hour before being decompressed to a simulated altitude of
4575 m (15 000 ft). Similar results with regard to lipid emboli in rabbits
were reported by Shim *et al.*[40] who also noted that the higher the temperature in the hyperbaric chamber, the more fat embolism was
observed in the lungs. When the temperature of the hyperbaric chamber was raised from 15·5° to 26·5°C (60° to 80°F) the number of fat
emboli in the lungs increased five times. These observations cannot be

directly related to the changes that might occur in man but, as an operational decompression chamber will be heated to around 35°C (95°F), the possible effect of ambient temperature should be kept in mind.

It is now being increasingly recognized that lipid emboli probably play an important role in the pathogenesis of post-compression decompression sickness. Fat embolism was first recorded as a complication in this condition by Muir.[35] Haymaker and Johnston[21] examined 3 diving fatalities. One of these who, despite repeated recompression, died 6 hours after a routine ascent from 72 m (236 ft) showed fat emboli in the lungs but only in a single renal glomerulus. The most detailed report[1] concerns the death of a compressed-air worker in whom many pulmonary fat emboli were found but none were seen in the kidney or brain.

We have recently examined 2 fatal cases of rapid decompression ('blow-up'). The first concerned a diver who surfaced rapidly, after spending 45 minutes at 77·7 m (255 ft), and died 1½ hours later. Numerous fat emboli were found in the lung sections and approximately 10 glomeruli per kidney section showed lipid embolism. Fat emboli were also noted in sections of brain and spinal cord. In the second case, a diver died on surfacing after a precipitate ascent from 78 m (256 ft), having spent 40 minutes at depth. Numerous fat emboli were found in lung sections, and from 1 to 3 glomeruli per kidney section showed lipid embolism. The brain, but not the spinal cord, was also involved. Pulmonary bone marrow emboli were seen but external cardiac massage had been performed.

For comparison, we have examined another 7 North Sea diving fatalities which occurred at pressure, but not as a result of a decompression disorder; the subjects were decompressed post mortem. With the exception of 1 man who died from heat stroke in a decompression chamber, pulmonary fat emboli were not found. No systemic fat emboli were demonstrated in these 'control' cases.

The true incidence of fat embolism in fatal decompression from pressure has yet to be assessed. Clearly, the diver must have spent sufficient time under pressure to be at risk from decompression, and it is likely that the degree of consequent fat embolism is roughly proportional to the extent and speed of the decompression. Presumably, fat emboli will be seen in the systemic circulation only when the subject survives for some time after his accident. One case has, however, been reported which should, on these criteria, have shown emboli but was, in fact, negative.[30, 41]

Vacuolated blood within the pulmonary arterioles was a conspicuous finding in the sections taken from our 2 cases of acute decompression. The vacuoles were seen to be at least partly sudanophil, indicating that they were composed of or surrounded by fat (Fig. 17.7). Occasional vacuoles were present in only 3 of our 7 'control' diving deaths. Our limited experience, therefore, relates the finding of gas vacuoles in the pulmonary arterioles in paraffin sections to the expected finding of fat emboli.

This supports the view that fat embolism in decompression disorder is the result of the redistribution of blood lipids. There is, indeed, mounting evidence of an interrelationship between the presence of intravascular bubbles, fat embolism and disseminated intravascular coagulation.[2, 17, 28, 37]

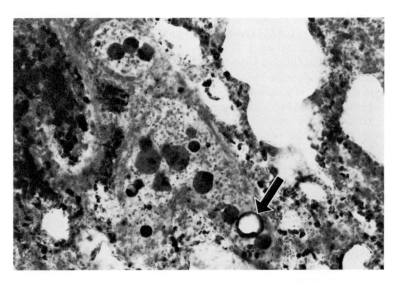

Fig. 17.7   Lung. Sudanophil globules in pulmonary arteriole, one showing vacuolation (arrow). (Oil Red O, × 83)

Alternatively, it has long been postulated that the source of fat embolism in decompression illnesses was adipose tissue disrupted by gas bubbles.[21] The most recent review of the origin of lipid emboli in dysbarism concludes only that the matter is still controversial.[31]

Whatever the origin, fat embolism may occur after decompression from pressure just as it does in post-descent shock and its presence is likely to be associated with other changes in the microcirculation. This information is of value both to the clinician and to the pathologist. From the therapeutic point of view it is now appreciated that, although recompression of a diving casualty can reduce the size of intravascular bubbles, it will do nothing to minimize the amount of circulating lipid or to correct other physicochemical changes in the blood. As far as the pathologist is concerned, the finding of fat emboli in tissue sections is of much help in confirming the presence of an ante mortem dysbaric lesion, provided, of course, that other causes have been excluded.

3. Dysbaric osteonecrosis
This occupational hazard is a form of aseptic bone necrosis which may develop insidiously several months or years after exposure to pressure. The aetiology of the condition is still unknown but it is held by many to

be the result of focal vascular obstruction, possibly produced by emboli of gas, fat or blood aggregates.

Radiologically and clinically, the lesions are divided into:

(a) Juxta-articular; and
(b) Head, neck and shaft lesions.

In each site, the severity of a lesion may vary from an area of increased density in bone, detectable only by radiology, to structural failure of an articular surface giving rise to considerable disability.

Dysbaric osteonecrosis presents initially in compressed-air workers or divers as a radiological but symptom-free lesion, usually discovered on routine examination. The commonest sites in which lesions are found are the neck of the humerus and femur and the upper end of the tibia. The process may begin after a single exposure to pressures of as little as 303–404 kPa (3–4 atm). The radiological abnormality may take years to manifest itself; the history of commercial diving in the North Sea is as yet too short to have revealed many cases with this condition.

The early diagnosis of cases may be difficult.[9, 14] Excellent accounts of the radiological appearances and histopathological changes in this condition have recently been given.[4, 10]

Disorders of the diving environment

1. *Oxygen toxicity*

Human cellular function is optimal within the P_{O_2} range of 80–200 mm Hg (10·7–26·7 kPa); dysfunction due to a raised arterial P_{O_2} is initially reversible. Oxygen poisoning is usually described as having two components. The first shows itself clinically following relatively short exposures to oxygen at pressures greater than 303 kPa (3 atm). Convulsions occur which may be fatal if a high P_{O_2} is maintained in the inspired air or gas mixture. No structural changes have been described in the nervous system following death from hyperoxic convulsions and it appears to be a biochemical phenomenon. Prolonged breathing of hyperoxic mixtures at ambient pressures of less than 303 kPa (3 atm) may cause pulmonary oxygen toxicity. Although not universally agreed, the consensus of present opinion suggests that the primary toxic effect is derived from a direct action of oxygen on the type 2 pneumocytes which produce surfactant. The initial lung lesion is characterized by the presence of an intra-alveolar fibrinous exudate, leading to hyaline membrane formation. If the subject continues to breathe a hyperoxic mixture, the microscopic picture changes to one of irreversible fibroblastic proliferation in the septa with hyperplasia of the alveolar lining. Death may then occur in paradoxical hyperoxic hypoxia.

Great care is taken to ensure that the partial pressure of inspired oxygen does not rise for long periods above the safe limit of about 80 kPa (600 mm Hg). When diving to more than about 50 m (165 ft), air is replaced as the breathing mixture by a composite of either oxygen and nitrogen or oxygen and helium. The oxygen level can be constantly monitored as in saturation diving systems.

The partial pressure of oxygen in breathing mixtures is sometimes deliberately raised to speed the process of inert gas elimination from a diver during decompression; oxygen pressures of about 200 kPa (2 atm) can be tolerated for short periods.

2. *Carbon dioxide effects*

Control of the level of carbon dioxide is critical in the confined atmosphere of a diving bell or chamber or in a closed-circuit breathing set. Two per cent carbon dioxide in the inspired air is unacceptable and the safe upper limit for arterial Pco_2 may be at around 6·7 kPa (50 mm Hg). Although a raised arterial Pco_2 normally stimulates ventilation and, thus, removal of carbon dioxide from the blood, this reflex may not always operate normally in divers. There may be increased tolerance or accommodation to a high level and, in such cases, inadequate stimulation to respiration may lead to hypoxia and possibly unconsciousness. The accumulation of carbon dioxide encourages heat loss and enhances the development of nitrogen narcosis.

Carbon dioxide retention tends to be cited as the cause of many diving accidents but evidence to support this is not easy to find; occasional cases of dizziness and unconsciousness may be due to a build-up of the gas in breathing sets or diving chambers. Carbon dioxide can be removed from the closed atmosphere by 'scrubbing' with a chemical absorbent such as soda lime.

3. *Inert gas narcosis*

Divers experience a sense of intoxication and loss of judgement with numbness, poor co-ordination, amnesia and other mental effects when breathing air at increased pressure. These are due to the narcotic action of the 80 per cent nitrogen component of air. Initially detectable at 30 m (99 ft) of seawater (400 kPa; 4 atm), the effects become exaggerated with increasing depth and air diving is not allowed to depths greater than 50 m (165 ft) in the North Sea. There is as yet no adequate explanation for the narcotic properties of nitrogen but divers do tend to become adapted to and less affected by narcosis.

Helium has no similar narcotic properties and can be used as the diluent for oxygen; helium, however, introduces problems of its own. Helium is six times less dense than air and this alters the velocity of sound, leading to 'Donald Duck' speech. This makes voice communication between divers in a helium/oxygen atmosphere almost impossible but the use of electronic voice unscramblers makes communication to the surface possible. The undesirable thermal effects of helium are discussed further below.

4. *Contaminants of breathing mixtures*

The dangers of contamination of breathing mixtures are due to hydrocarbons, carbon monoxide and other toxic substances introduced accidentally during preparation. Cylinders for self-contained under-water breathing apparatus (scuba) are recharged by compressors, and problems have arisen in the past because of contamination of the intake to these compressors by their own exhaust fumes. Most helium/oxygen breathing mixtures are prepared on site from stock cylinders of gases filled on shore.

As with all high-pressure gas supplies, valves and gauges must be lubricated with hydrocarbon-free silicones to avoid the risk of fire on contact with oxygen. Care must also be taken to clear gas supply systems of cleaning agents, such as Freon.

5. *Humidity and infection*

Control of humidity is a problem in some of the saturation diving systems used. Silica gel filtration may be inadequate and it has recently been reported that freshly ironed linen sheets are most effective absorbers of moisture when draped inside the chamber. Humidity and inadequate hygiene combine to give rise to troublesome infections by certain types of organism. Such infections occur particularly in the external auditory meatus and are even now occasionally responsible for the abandonment of saturation dives.

In the environmental conditions of the saturation chamber, the normally predominant gram-positive organisms in the external auditory canal are gradually replaced by a gram-negative flora which results in overt local infections. Particular difficulty arises with infections caused by *Pseudomonas aeruginosa* which flourishes in the conditions of the saturation chamber and readily becomes resistant to treatment. A diver developing a *Ps. aeruginosa* ear infection must be removed from the hyperbaric environment and await the return of gram-positive flora, a process which may take up to 8 months.

6. *Temperature*

The temperature of the water deep in the North Sea shows little variation and remains at about 5°C. A man falling into the water may require almost immediate rescue because of the dangers of cold exposure.[25] Due to compression of the neoprene foam, conduction of heat through a diver's wet suit is increased threefold by diving to 100 m (330 ft) and additional heat is lost by impregnation with helium, the thermal conductance of which is six times that of air. A dry suit protects the diver from direct contact with the sea but hot-water or electrically operated heating suits may soon become compulsory. During work at depths greater than about 182 m (600 ft), more heat may be lost through respiration than can be produced by metabolism, and heating of the normally cold breathing mixture becomes necessary below about 122 m (400 ft).

Diving bells have simple heating systems, but these are seldom adequate to maintain a comfortable working temperature. As in deck chambers, control of temperature is critical because the thermal conductance of helium increases even more under pressure.

Fatal diving accidents

The fatality rate for North Sea divers has recently been estimated as approximately 10 per 1000 employed per annum, which is a rate 8 times higher than that for near and middle water trawlermen, 33 times that of coal-miners, 50 times that of construction workers and 220 times that for factory employees.[32] During the years 1971–75 there were 24 fatal

Table 17.7   Fatal diving accidents

Date	Sector	Depth	Cause of death	Comments
Feb. '71	Norwegian	61 m (200 ft)	Drowning	No diving bell. Cold contributed
March '71	Norwegian	61 m (200 ft)	Decompression sickness	Suit over-inflated—'blow-up'. Umbilical broke off
Nov. '71	British	83·8 m (275 ft)	Acute decompression	Over-inflated suit to clear line; lost control—'blow-up'
May '72	British	13·4 m (44 ft)	Drowning	Big meal before dive. Vomited. Inadequate training. *Scuba diver*
Aug. '73	British	97·5 m (320 ft)	Pulmonary haemorrhage	Faulty equipment design
Dec. '73	British	18·3 m (60 ft)	Body not recovered	Air-line cut. Possibly panic
Jan. '74	Norwegian	76·2 m (250 ft)	Acute decompression ⎫	Bell accidentally surfaced. Winch brake malfunctioned—ballast
Jan. '74	Norwegian	76·2 m (250 ft)	Acute decompression ⎭	suddenly lost
April '74	British	91·4 m (300 ft)	Drowning	Umbilical entangled. Bellman cut lines in panic
June '74	British	61 m (200 ft)	Decompression sickness	Medically unfit
July '74	British	On deck	Tension pneumothorax	Onset at 27·4 m (90 ft) in decompression chamber. Diagnosed as pneumonia
Aug. '74	Norwegian	91·4 m (300 ft)	Anoxia	Pure helium provided in error. Communication failure
Oct. '74	British	Surface	Drowning/inhaled vomit	Also fractured ribs. Possibly struck underwater obstruction. *Scuba diver*
Oct. '74	Norwegian	61 m (300 ft)	Anoxia	Communication failure. Faulty gas supply
Dec. '74	Irish	80·8 m (265 ft)	Anoxia/drowning	Umbilical caught, then severed by heavy sea lifting bell
Dec. '74	British	30·5 m (100 ft)	Trapped in pipe	By suction. Valve on pipe knocked off
Feb. '75	Norwegian	42·7 m (140 ft)	Body not recovered	Detached life-line caught air-hose. Pulled mask off
March '75	British	140·2 m (460 ft)	?Hypoxia/cardiac irregularity	Hyperventilating? cold response. No suit heating
March '75	British	42·7 m (140 ft)	Natural causes	Cardiomyopathy
June '75	Norwegian	45·7 m (150 ft)	Body not recovered	Slipped life-line and failed to surface. *Scuba diver*
July '75	British	36·6 m (120 ft)	Asphyxia	Sucked into 0·9 m (36 in) pipe. Underwater accident
July '75	British	36·6 m (120 ft)	Drowning	Sucked into 0·9 m (36 in) pipe. Underwater accident
Sept. '75	British	On deck	Heat stroke ⎫	Chamber at 43·3°–48·9°C (110°–120°F). Pressure increased in error
Sept. '75	British	On deck	Heat stroke ⎭	from 94·5 to 182·9 m (310 to 600 ft) by rapidly adding helium

diving accidents in the North European area, 15 of which occurred in the British sector (Table 17.7). Although there has been a marked increase in the number of fatalities during the last 2 years, it must be remembered that there were 80 divers operating in 1971 and only 10 per cent were going deeper than 91 m (300 ft), whereas there were 1200 divers involved in 1975 and over 50 per cent were working at 91 m (300 ft) or deeper.

Surface-orientated diving

Table 17.7 shows that the majority of accidents involved surface-orientated divers and, in many of these, the circumstances are clear. The air-line was cut or severed in 3 instances, and in 2 cases the gas mixture was unsuitable to maintain life. One diver inadvertently freed his life-line from his belt which then caught the air-hose and accidentally removed his mask when he was being pulled up. On 4 occasions, a diver surfaced precipitately, either because he had over-inflated his suit ('blow-up') or because the diving bell had accidentally surfaced. Underwater accidents claimed 3 lives and 2 divers died in an unique accident in which the deck chamber, where they were decompressing, was over-heated as a result of sudden inadvertent compression. Faulty equipment, natural causes and a tension pneumothorax each accounted for 1 death. In the remaining 3 fatalities, however, the information is either vague or incomplete.

Few diving accidents result from a single diverse factor.[18] Vertigo, exhaustion, panic and hypothermia are among probable explanations, the last of these being regarded as a danger of the first order in the North Sea because it may insidiously lead to disorientation and irrational behaviour. Inadequate training and unsatisfactory techniques were encountered in the early days but these have now been eliminated by experience and legislation. Fatal communication errors occurred on two occasions while some accidents are pure misadventure as far as those involved are concerned, such as when a diving bell surfaces in error. The most mysterious and complex cases are those concerning divers who die or lose consciousness at depth. The survival of such a diver depends on the ability of his colleagues to bring him back swiftly and safely to the bell. Unfortunately, in most cases there is an unavoidable delay between the accident and rescue; inexperience, adverse environmental conditions and faulty equipment have been listed as important causal factors.[12]

Scuba diving

Three divers have died in the North Sea wearing scuba equipment (Table 17.7); death was due to drowning in all the bodies recovered.

It is most satisfactory that there have been so few scuba diver fatalities in the North Sea when so many have been recorded elsewhere, particularly in relation to recreation.[33] Major causes of scuba diving deaths are discussed in Chapter 15.

Diving autopsy procedure

The effects of decompression are not frequently seen in the post-mortem room and the examiner may be misled either by unfamiliar appearances or by artefactual changes.

A full account of the general lines along which a diving autopsy should be conducted has recently been given[18] where particular attention has been drawn to the doubtful significance of the location, or even the presence, of gas bubbles in the body of a diver who has died under pressure. Dissolved gas is liberated on post-mortem decompression and will appear in the body fluids and tissues. It has been suggested that the bodies of those dying in pressure chambers should be decompressed slowly to reduce this effect but any theoretical advantage in this practice is offset by the promotion of putrefaction, the temperature of a decompression chamber normally being around 35°C (95°F) after a dive. The suggestion that the autopsy be carried out within the pressure chamber has limited application and as yet there is no published account of the procedure or its results.

There is also the possibility that bubble formation results from, or is exaggerated by, the therapeutic compression of a subject already dead. Bubbles have been found in the left side of the heart and aorta of experimental animals[23] and, clearly, their presence could be confused with the findings in death from arterial gas or air embolism. Since artefactual bubbles can be induced during any autopsy, it has been recommended that the dissection be carried out with the body, or part of it, submerged in water; the procedure is unlikely to find general favour even if it has merit.

The greatest interpretative difficulty would be encountered if a surface-orientated diver who died at pressure were recompressed after death. There would be far less difficulty in evaluating the changes in a dead scuba diver who was not at risk from decompression and who was not therapeutically compressed either before or after death. Maximum information can be obtained only by adopting a special autopsy technique and we have found the following procedure to be of value.

Radiological examination

A radiograph of the chest must be taken before the autopsy to ascertain if a pneumothorax is present; a lung lesion may be seen at the same time. The volume of a pneumothorax or bulla will be increased by post-mortem decompression when the diver has died at depth but the presence of the lesion is significant even if its size is not. Gas will regularly be seen outlining the heart chambers and major vessels whenever death has occurred at pressure but this finding is usually of no significance. The shoulder, hip and knee joints should be routinely X-rayed and if any lesion is suspected the affected bone should be removed for histological examination.

External appearances

Crepitant subcutaneous emphysema of the head, neck and chest is a common finding in cases of pulmonary barotrauma. Post-mortem evolution of gas in the tissues gives rise to a similar appearance but, in this case, crepitation will also be found over the trunk and limbs. Deep lividity of the facies is usually present on which coarse petechiae may be superimposed. Blotchy lividity presumably results from the prevention of gravitational drainage by intravascular bubbles. The state of the eardrums and middle ears must be noted.

Dissection technique

The dissection should commence with removal of the calvaria. The presence of bubbles in the pial veins can be ignored as a common artefact. The frontal lobes of the brain are then reflected; two haemostats are placed on each internal carotid artery and the vessels sectioned between them. A clamp is then placed on the basilar artery and on both the vertebral arteries before cutting the basilar artery at its origin. The brain and distal clamps can then be removed in the usual manner and placed underwater. The clamps are then removed in turn and bubbles, if present, will be seen rising from the sectioned arteries.

To gain access to the thoracic cavity, the ribs should be cut only as far as the second costal cartilages before the sternum is elevated. The pericardial sac can now be opened and the right atrium and coronary veins inspected for the presence of bubbles. A large clamp should now be placed on the superior vena cava at its junction with the heart before completing the removal of the sternum. The next step is to divide the inferior vena cava above the diaphragm between clamps and to clamp the trachea to prevent subsequent leakage of air from the lungs. Finally, a clamp is placed on the ascending aorta before removing the chest and neck organs intact in the usual way. It is an advantage to clamp also the descending aorta at the diaphragm, so that integrity of the abdominal circulation will be maintained. The neck and chest organs can then be placed underwater and the caval clamps removed, allowing any bubbles present to escape from the right atrium. The water will now be cloudy so that it is essential to place the organs in clean water before incising the aorta at its origin. Bubbles of air may appear at this stage or only after the coronary ostia have been identified and gentle pressure exerted along the course of the arteries.

In the presence of a pneumothorax, the integrity of the visceral pleura can now be tested underwater, but the lungs must not be compressed in an attempt to expel air. Rather they should be fixed by perfusion with 10 per cent formol saline at a pressure of approximately 3 kPa (30 cm H_2O) after removal of the tracheal clamp. The fixed lungs may later be thinly sectioned for evidence of barotrauma or air trapping. The ventricular walls of the heart should be weighed after fixation because it has been suggested that right ventricular hypertrophy may occur as a long-term complication of diving.

The abdominal cavity may now be examined before the distal clamps on aorta and inferior vena cava are removed. If venous bubbles are present they are readily seen within the inferior vena cava, portal and omental veins. The presence of air in the aorta can be tested by incising it after the abdominal cavity has been filled with water.

The brain and spinal cord should be preserved in fixative for later examination by a neuropathologist. Haemorrhage may be seen in the middle ears or mastoid air cells and, if so, the temporal bones should be removed intact for specialist opinion.

A sample of blood must be collected routinely for carbon monoxide estimation. There are occasions when other chemical or biochemical investigations may be required (see Chapter 15) and samples of blood, urine and vitreous humour should be collected in anticipation.

Interpretation

The post-mortem findings will have to be closely correlated with the report of the diving inspector and the results of subsequent examination of the equipment and gases. Suitable diagnostic criteria for the main dysbaric lesions can be summarized as follows:

1. A diagnosis of pulmonary barotrauma can be made confidently if a pneumothorax is confirmed radiologically or if the lungs show unequivocal evidence of interstitial emphysema.

2. Unless it is certain that the diver was not at risk from decompression sickness, and had not been recompressed either therapeutically or post mortem, the presence of bubbles in the cerebral arteries does not prove death from cerebral air embolism. In the rare event of a diver surviving a sufficient length of time, the diagnosis can be made on the presence of ischaemic cerebral lesions.

3. There is difficulty in distinguishing the lesions of decompression sickness from those of post-mortem liberation of gas. However, a diagnosis of decompression sickness will be supported by the finding of finely frothed blood in the inferior vena cava and its tributaries; petechial haemorrhages in the abdominal fatty tissues and microscopic hepatic gas/fat emboli will confirm the diagnosis and even pulmonary fat embolism will be corroborative if the diver has not been injured or resuscitated by external cardiac massage.

As the systematic post-mortem dissection of diving fatalities is a relatively recent innovation, these guide-lines should be regarded as provisional until more experience has accumulated.

References

1. Bennison, W. H., Catton, M. J. and Fryer, D. I. (1965). Fatal decompression sickness in a compressed-air worker. *J. Path. Bact.* **89**, 319.
2. Bergentz, S. E. (1968). Fat embolism. *Progr. Surg. (Basel)* **6**, 85.

3. Catchpole, H. R. and Gersh, I. (1947). Pathogenetic factors and pathological consequences of decompression sickness. *Physiol. Rev.* **27**, 360.

4. Catto, M. (1976). Pathology of aseptic bone necrosis. In: *Aseptic Necrosis of Bone*, Chap. 2. Ed. J. K. Davidson. Amsterdam: Excerpta Medica.

5. Chappell, G. L. (1963), quoted by Smith, F. R. (1967). Air embolism as a cause of death in scuba diving in the Pacific Northwest. *Dis. Chest* **52**, 15.

6. Childs, C. M. and Davidson, D. (1977). Diagnostic x-rays in hyperbaric environments. *Focus*, Ilford Ltd.

7. Clay, J. F. (1963). Histopathology of experimental decompression sickness. *Aerospace Med.* **34**, 1107.

8. Cockett, A. T. K., Nakamura, R. M. and Franks, J. J. (1965). Recent findings in the pathogenesis of decompression sickness (dysbarism). *Surgery* **58**, 384.

9. Davidson, J. K. (1964). Pulmonary changes in decompression sickness. *Clin. Radiol.* **15**, 106.

10. Davidson, J. K. (1976). Dysbaric osteonecrosis. In: *Aseptic Necrosis of Bone*, Chap. 4. Ed. J. K. Davidson. Amsterdam: Excerpta Medica.

11. Decompression Sickness Panel Report (Medical Research Council) (1966). Bone lesions in compressed air workers. *J. Bone Jt Surg.* **48B**, 207.

12. Edmonds, C. (1976). Investigation of diving accidents. In: *Diving Medicine*, Chap. 23. Ed. R. H. Strauss. New York: Grune and Stratton.

13. Elliott, D. H. and Hallenbeck, M. J. (1975). The pathophysiology of decompression sickness. In: *The Physiology and Medicine of Diving and Compressed Air Work*, 2nd edn, Chap. 23. Eds. P. B. Bennett and D. H. Elliott. London: Balliere Tindall.

14. Elliott, D. H. and Harrison, J. A. B. (1970). Bone necrosis—an occupational hazard of diving. *J. roy. nav. med. Serv.* **56**, 140.

15. Fryer, D. I. (1969). *Subatmospheric Decompression Sickness in Man.* Agardograph no. 125. Slough: Technivision Services.

16. Gonzales, T. A., Vance, M., Helpern, M. and Umberger, C. J. (1954). *Legal Medicine, Pathology and Toxicology*, 2nd edn., p. 491. New York: Appleton–Century–Crofts.

17. Halleraker, B. (1970). Fat embolism and intravascular coagulation. *Acta path. microbiol. scand., A.* **78**, 432.

18. Hanson, R. de G. and Young, J. M. (1975). Diving accidents. In: *The Physiology and Medicine of Diving and Compressed Air Work*, 2nd edn., Chap. 29. Eds. P. B. Bennett and D. H. Elliott. London: Balliere Tindall.

19. Harveyson, K. B. and Hirschfeld, B. E. E. (1956). Fatal air embolism resulting from the use of a compressed air diving unit. *Med. J. Aust.* **1**, 685.

20. Haymaker, W. (1957). Decompression sickness. In: *Handbuch der*

Speziellen Pathologischen Anatomie und Histologie, Vol. 13, pt. 1, pp. 1600–1672. Eds. O. Lubarsch, F. Henke and R. Rossie. Berlin: Springer-Verlag.

21. Haymaker, W. and Johnston, A. D. (1955). Pathology of decompression sickness. A comparison of the lesions in airmen with those in caisson workers and divers. *Milit. Med.* **117**, 285.

22. Haymaker, W., Johnston, A. D. and Downey, V. M. (1956). Fatal decompression sickness during jet aircraft flight. *J. Aviat. Med.* **27**, 2.

23. Hempleman, H. V. (1968). Bubble formation and decompression sickness. *Rev. Physiol. subaquat. Med. hyperbare.* **1**, 181.

24. Hoff, E. C. (1948). *A Bibliographic Sourcebook of Compressed Air, Diving and Submarine Medicine*, Vol. 1, p. 142. Washington DC: Department of the Navy.

25. Keatinge, W. R. (1969). *Survival in Cold Water*. Oxford: Blackwell Scientific.

26. Kidd, D. J. and Elliott, D. H. (1975). Decompression disorders in divers. In: *The Physiology and Medicine of Diving and Compressed Air Work*, 2nd edn., Chap. 25. Eds. P. B. Bennett and D. H. Elliott. London: Balliere Tindall.

27. Kinsey, J. L. (1954). Air embolism as a result of submarine escape training. *U.S. armed Forces med. J.* **5**, 243.

28. Lee, W. H., Krumhaar, D., Fonkalsrud, E. W., Schjeide, C. A. and Maloney, J. V. (1961). Denaturation of plasma proteins as a cause of morbidity and death after intracardiac operations. *Surgery* **50**, 29.

29. Liebow, A. A., Stark, J. E., Vogel, J. and Schaefer, K. E. (1959). Intrapulmonary air trapping in submarine escape training casualties. *U.S. armed Forces med. J.* **10**, 265.

30. Mason, J. K. (1962). *Aviation Accident Pathology*, p. 165. London: Butterworths.

31. Mason, J. K. (1973). Death resulting from exposure to high altitude. In: *Aerospace Pathology*, Chap. 16. Eds. J. K. Mason and W. J. Reals. Chicago: College of American Pathologists Foundation.

32. *The Medical Complications of Oil Related Industry* (1975). Scottish Council Report. Edinburgh: British Medical Association.

33. Miles, S. (1969). *Underwater Medicine*, 3rd edn., London: Staples Press.

34. Möttönen, M. and Karkola, K. (1971). The first fatal case of decompression sickness in Finland. *Med. Sci. Law* **11**, 39.

35. Muir, R. (1941). *Textbook of Pathology*, 5th edn., p. 42. London: Edward Arnold (10th edn., 1976, Ed. J. R. Anderson).

36. Okalyi, Z. (1969). Occupational mortality and morbidity among divers in the Torres Straits. *Med. J. Aust.* **1**, 1239.

37. Philp, R. B., Inwood, M. J. and Warren, B. A. (1972). Interactions between gas bubbles and components of the blood: implications in decompression sickness. *Aerospace Med.* **43**, 946.

38. Polak, B. and Adams, H. (1932). Traumatic air embolism in submarine escape training. *U.S. nav. med. Bull.* **30**, 165.
39. Schaefer, K. E., McNulty, W. P., Jr., Carey, C. and Liebow, A. A. (1958). Mechanisms in development of interstitial emphysema and air embolism on decompression from depth. *J. appl. Physiol.* **13**, 15.
40. Shim, S. S., Mokkhavesa, S., Patterson, F. P. and Trapp, W. G. (1969). Experimental fat embolism following compression-decompression in a hyperbaric chamber. *Surg. Gynec. Obstet.* **128**, 103.
41. Sillery, R. J. (1958). Decompression sickness—a review of the literature and previously unreported histological observations. *Arch. Path.* **66**, 241.
42. Snyder, R. G. and Snow, C. C. (1967). Fatal injuries resulting from extreme water impact. *Aerospace Med.* **38**, 779.
43. Strauss, M. B. and Wright, P. W. (1971). Thoracic squeeze diving casualty. *Aerospace Med.* **42**, 673.
44. Waller, S. O. (1970). Autopsy features in scuba diving fatalities. *Med. J. Aust.* **1**, 1106.

Note: A number of useful contributions have been collected under the title 'Offshore medicine'. *Proc. roy. Soc. Med.* (1976). **69**, 583—*Ed.*

18

Haemorrhage, coagulation and thrombosis

Haemorrhage and thrombosis are obvious and important pathological consequences of violence. Haemorrhage, either by its amount, induction of hypovolaemic shock or pressure effects (e.g. raised intracranial pressure, cardiac tamponade) can be rapidly lethal. Thrombosis is a later complication occurring when the more immediate effects of violence have been recognized and treated; yet it is no less lethal in its possibilities. Another more recent aspect of the story is disseminated intravascular coagulation (DIC). This causes microvascular obstruction by fibrin microthrombi as well as a haemorrhagic tendency due to consumption of coagulation factors.

Much of the subject is straightforward and well known to pathologists but certain aspects present difficulty because of the complex nature of the coagulation and fibrinolytic systems. The precise physiology of these is still uncertain and the literature on the subject has become enormous and highly technical. Understanding of the basic concepts is, however, a prerequisite for solution of the problems that arise in this field.

Normal haemostasis, coagulation and fibrinolysis

Normal haemostasis has four components—vascular contraction, platelet activity, blood coagulation and fibrinolysis. This is well seen after injury to a small artery. Transient vasoconstriction and accumulation of platelets to form a plug at the site of injury checks bleeding. These are augmented by fibrin formation. Later, fibrinolysis clears the fibrin to permit healing.

Vasoconstriction is of limited value save in the smaller vessels. Platelets are of much importance. They adhere to collagen, exposed by damage to the endothelium of the vessel wall, and a series of biochemical and structural changes follow. Platelet release of adenosine diphosphate (ADP) causes further aggregation of platelets at the site— the early stage in formation of the haemostatic plug. The platelets also release the phospholipid essential for several steps in the coagulation process proper, which is also initiated independently and concurrently by the vascular injury. Thrombin forms and fibrin formation results. Thrombin itself brings about considerable further release of platelet components and further platelet aggregation. There is thus a feedback augmentation mechanism with considerable build-up of platelets, and intervening fibrin strands, to form an efficient haemostatic plug at the site of injury. The smaller the vessel the greater will be the role of the platelets; in larger vessels the role of the coagulation process will be dominant although platelets still play a necessary part.

Normal coagulation

The simplest approach to the normal process of coagulation[1] is to consider first the appearance of the fibrin clot and the events immediately preceding it. Thereafter the more complex question of initiation of coagulation can be discussed. The internationally agreed nomenclature for clotting factors, using roman numerals, has brought some order into what was previously a confused situation. In the schematic representation of coagulation in Fig. 18.1 this nomenclature is adopted but synonyms are also given where these are still in common use.

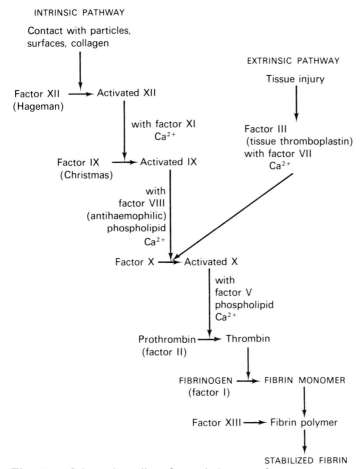

INTRINSIC PATHWAY

Contact with particles, surfaces, collagen

Factor XII (Hageman) ⟶ Activated XII

EXTRINSIC PATHWAY

Tissue injury

with factor XI
Ca^{2+}

Factor III (tissue thromboplastin) with factor VII
Ca^{2+}

Factor IX (Christmas) ⟶ Activated IX

with factor VIII (antihaemophilic) phospholipid Ca^{2+}

Factor X ⟶ Activated X

with factor V phospholipid Ca^{2+}

Prothrombin (factor II) ⟶ Thrombin

FIBRINOGEN (factor I) ⟶ FIBRIN MONOMER

Factor XIII ⟶ Fibrin polymer

STABILIZED FIBRIN

Fig. 18.1 Schematic outline of coagulation cascade.

Fibrinogen (factor I) is a large, elongated protein molecule comprising three pairs of polypeptide chains. Its molecular configuration is imperfectly understood but a good deal is known about its biochemistry. It is the most abundant clotting factor in plasma (normally 200–400 mg/100 ml). It is converted to fibrin by the enzymatic action of thrombin which splits off two pairs of small peptides (fibrinopeptides A and B) from the fibrinogen molecules. Thereafter the altered fibrinogen molecules unite by end-to-end and side-to-side linkage to form fibrin monomer and then fibrin polymer. This early polymerized fibrin is of low tensile strength and is easily disrupted. Fibrin stabilizing factor (factor XIII), present in normal plasma and in platelets, bonds the polymerized fibrin more strongly to produce haemostatically satisfactory fibrin.

The thrombin necessary for fibrinogen–fibrin conversion does not normally circulate. Indeed, there are several natural mechanisms to ensure its inactivation should this happen. Thrombin is formed by the activation of its inert precursor prothrombin (factor II), which is a normal a_2-globulin component of plasma and requires vitamin K for its synthesis; this probably occurs in the liver.

The events leading up to the conversion of prothrombin to thrombin are complex. Their biochemical nature has not yet been fully established. They involve a whole range of clotting factors normally present in plasma in an inert form but capable of activation in sequential fashion. This series of proenzyme to enzyme conversions has been termed the 'coagulation cascade'.

There are two main pathways—the extrinsic and intrinsic clotting mechanisms. They overlap and may operate together; indeed, after injury they almost certainly do.

In the extrinsic system tissue particles or tissue juice, termed 'tissue thromboplastin' (factor III), acts rapidly in the presence of ionic calcium and phospholipid together with factors VII, X and V to promote the conversion of prothrombin to thrombin. This is the system which is triggered in major tissue injury when tissue fragments or extracts enter the circulation. Brain, lung and placenta are especially rich in tissue thromboplastin.

The intrinsic system operates more slowly. When blood comes in contact with a foreign surface or negatively charged agents or surfaces, such as circulating particles or damaged endothelium with exposure of collagen, Hageman factor (factor XII) is activated. Its active form triggers a cascade through factors XI, IX (Christmas factor) and VIII (antihaemophilic factor) which, again with calcium ions and platelet phospholipid, leads into the same final common pathway of factors X and V to initiate thrombin formation. This is the system which is not dependent on major tissue injury but more on local alterations in vessel walls and circulation of particles such as micro-organisms in viraemia, bacteraemia and septicaemia, fat globules, air bubbles and immune complexes. It is altogether more subtle than the extrinsic system.

This simplified outline is far from complete and details will be modified and expanded as more becomes known of the structure of the individual factors. It does, however, illustrate the major principles underlying the two coagulation pathways. The role of the platelet must be emphasized. It serves not only to form the haemostatic plug but also, by release of its contents, to aid further aggregation of platelets (through ADP) and to promote stages of the coagulation process by phospholipid (platelet factor 3). It also seems likely that the plasma zone around the platelet and the platelet surface itself is a region in which the various clotting factors can be concentrated and/or activated to produce what might be termed a procoagulant milieu. Finally, factor XII (Hageman factor) is probably also responsible for triggering the fibrinolytic, kinin and complement systems. This demonstrates the linkage between coagulation, fibrinolysis, inflammation and immunity which is currently arousing so much interest.

Fibrinolysis
The fibrinolytic enzyme system[5] functions concurrently with the coagulation system and causes lysis of fibrin. The main components of the system are plasminogen, activators of plasminogen, the operative proteolytic enzyme plasmin and a variety of inhibitors (Fig. 18.2). It is no less complicated than the coagulation system and its biochemical nature is incompletely understood.

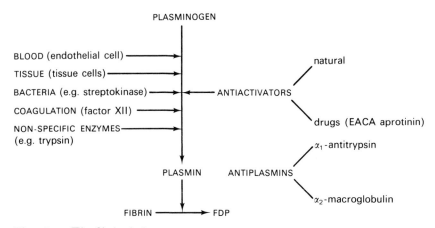

Fig. 18.2 The fibrinolytic system.

Plasminogen is a β-globulin of normal plasma. It is converted into the active fibrinolytic agent plasmin by the enzymatic action of activators which probably split a number of peptide bonds to uncover active sites.

The activators are important. They exist normally in blood and tissue. Blood activator exists in trace amounts in normal plasma. It is highly labile (half-life about 15 minutes) and is probably produced by vascular endothelium, especially in the veins. The stimulus is not known; it may be the close proximity of deposited fibrin. Most tissues other than liver and placenta produce tissue activator. Tissues especially rich in it are prostate, endometrium and lung. While some of this tissue activator may originate from the walls of blood vessels in the tissue, production by the tissue cells proper occurs; certain secretions such as milk, tears, seminal fluid and saliva also contain activator. Urinary activator, urokinase, is probably synthesized in the kidney in the vasa recta. The glomerular capillary walls are also active in producing activator. The high concentration of activator in the kidney is of great importance in determining the outcome of renal disease in which fibrin deposition occurs in the glomeruli.

In addition to these naturally occurring activators, many bacterial species produce agents which have activator characteristics. The most important is streptokinase produced by streptococci; this is widely used in fibrinolytic therapy but carries the disadvantage that it is antigenic whereas urokinase, a natural human product, is non-antigenic. Non-specific activation of plasminogen by other proteolytic enzymes such as trypsin may occur; plasmin itself can also, by autocatalysis, be an activator and thus an amplifier. It has already been mentioned that Hageman coagulation factor (XII) can initiate fibrinolysis; the mechanism is still uncertain, as is the mode of action of some steroid hormones and vasoactive agents which have the same effect.

There is thus an ample potential for the activation of plasminogen to plasmin and the fibrinolytic activity of plasma varies greatly in and between individuals. Plasmin itself is a proteolytic enzyme which can digest fibrinogen as well as fibrin though it has a relative specificity for the latter, which it digests, if it is present, in preference to fibrinogen. It also digests unstabilized fibrin more readily than stabilized fibrin.

The digestion of fibrin by plasmin results in the formation of a series of fibrin degradation products (FDP) which are fairly well characterized and can be assayed. The fibrin molecule is progressively split into smaller FDP which can be identified. These FDP have the anticoagulant side effects of impairing fibrin polymerization, inhibiting platelet aggregation and acting as antithrombin.

Inhibitors of coagulation and fibrinolysis
In systems so active and potentially so effective and universal as the coagulation and fibrinolytic systems it is evident that natural inhibitors exist. These serve to check what might otherwise be a catastrophic chain of events. In the coagulation system a range of antithrombins is known which includes certain α_2-globulins, fibrin itself (by adsorption of thrombin) and FDP. Inhibitors of the earlier stages of coagulation also exist, such as inhibitors of activated Hageman factor. Acquired anticoagulants may occasionally develop in a variety of other disorders; these are mostly directed against the antihaemophilic factor (VIII).

Controlling the fibrinolytic system are two categories of inhibitor. Antiactivators exist in plasma and check initial plasminogen conversion. Natural antiplasmins, notably α_1-antitrypsin and α_2-

macroglobulin directly inhibit plasmin. The natural inhibitors of fibrinolysis as a rule normally exceed the potential for plasmin production. The fibrinolytic system seems to possess a greater inherent lability than the coagulation system. It is well established that increased amounts of activator, denoting increased fibrinolytic potential, appear in the plasma after exercise, emotional stress, surgical operations, trauma and electric shock. What is still not clear is whether an increase in true fibrinolysis demands production of an overwhelming amount of plasmin to overcome inhibitors or preferential adsorption of plasmin without its accompanying inhibitors on to such fibrin clot as requires to be lysed.

The balance between coagulation and fibrinolysis: post-mortem *fibrinolysis*
Fibrinolysis has been known for over a century but it is only in relatively recent years that the view has been taken that it is in a loose equilibrium with coagulation. It is unlikely that the balance is a simple one. Facts that point to its existence are the occurrence of trace amounts of plasminogen activator in normal plasma and of small amounts of FDP in normal serum, the association of thrombotic disease with depression of fibrinolysis, the occurrence of thrombosis as a complication of drug antifibrinolytic therapy and the stimulus to fibrinolysis afforded by an episode of intravascular coagulation. Another aspect is the possibility that an endo-endothelial layer of fibrin constantly lines the vascular walls to permit, as a lubricant, readier microvascular perfusion at reasonable pressure. This layer has never been identified but it is claimed that it is of ultrastructural dimensions and constantly being deposited and lysed; it could well explain the normal minute levels of blood activator and serum FDP.

This equilibrium can be regarded as existing in a loose manner to maintain vascular integrity and patency. Its relevance to the thrombogenic theories of atheroma production will also be obvious. Upset in the balance in one direction will lead to possible hypercoagulability, while a swing in the other direction will evoke a fibrinolytic state.

Recognition of the importance of post-mortem fibrinolysis began with publication of the classic paper by Mole in 1948.[6] Although pathologists are aware of its occurrence they do not always fully appreciate its significance. After death blood clots; the mechanism is presumed to be spontaneous activation of the coagulation enzymes. Fibrinolytic enzyme activation also occurs and the post-mortem clot quite rapidly starts to lyse. This is especially evident if fibrinolysis has been normal or increased before death and if the subject has previously been healthy. The fact that exercise and emotional stress enhance fibrinolysis must be remembered. For practical purposes one generally finds in hospital post-mortem practice an abundance of post-mortem clot which indicates the procoagulant or fibrinolytically depressed state of the patient, who may well have suffered a more or less protracted terminal illness. Quite the opposite picture is seen in the healthy person dying rapidly as a result of injury. Here the blood is usually wholly fluid.

Measurement of post-mortem lysis is not yet possible and the variables are, in any event, too great to allow any quantification of the degree or speed of its occurrence. What can, however, be assessed, by Todd's fibrin autograph technique,[16] is the fibrinolytic potential of vascular walls. This measures in a semi-quantitative way the production of plasminogen activator by endothelium. The method works well in both biopsy and necropsy work and may give some indication of the fibrinolytic status of the subject.

The significance of post-mortem fibrinolysis is also too often ignored, especially in histological examination. Microthrombi may be difficult to find because of lytic changes. Scanty histological findings may, on occasion, assume greater meaning if this is realized.

The response of the coagulation and fibrinolytic systems to injury

After injury, and directly related to its severity, the coagulation and fibrinolytic systems show changes of much relevance to post-traumatic thrombosis.[3]

Almost immediately after injury there is a transient hypercoagulable state. Probably both the intrinsic and extrinsic pathways are stimulated and active intermediary clotting factors circulate. These are rapidly inactivated or are cleared by the reticuloendothelial system, especially in the liver; their effect is thus short-lived, but in areas of vascular stasis thrombosis could occur. However, stimulation of fibrinolysis, with increase in circulating plasminogen activator, also occurs and will, to some degree, balance this initial hypercoagulability.

Within a few hours, or less if the injury is more severe, a phase of hypocoagulability develops. This may in part be due to loss of clotting factors from continued bleeding or to compensatory haemodilution occurring naturally or as the result of transfusion. The main cause, however, is the continuing consumption of clotting factors which are still being activated by persistence of the trigger to coagulation; fibrin formation is continuing in the circulation, both locally at the injury site and also, if the injury is severe enough, systemically. There is a reduction not only in clotting factors but also in platelets and a fall in circulating plasminogen activator. This apparent fibrinolytic depression is also to be regarded as a consumption of factors. A haemorrhagic tendency may develop. The picture is essentially that of a form of DIC (see below).

This hypocoagulable phase is followed by a more prolonged period during which increased synthesis of clotting factors and replenishment of platelets occur to replace the loss. There is usually an overswing with production of an excess. Plasma fibrinogen is especially affected; it rapidly rises and may persist at high levels for several weeks. Other clotting factors will also be found to be increased for 2–3 weeks. Blood platelets rise rather more slowly so that thrombocytopenia persists for 2–3 days after injury before thrombocytosis finally develops. It is during this prolonged hypercoagulable phase that the risk of thrombosis is at its greatest and much will obviously depend upon the extent to which fibrinolytic activity increases as it is fibrinolysis that compensates for fibrin deposition by clearing it.

The changes just described have been presented in a somewhat artificial three-stage sequence. They may in practice be less clear-cut; in minor injury they may be minimal. In severe trauma, however, they are of great importance.

While there is as yet no method by which susceptibility to thrombosis can be confidently predicted and measured, it is nevertheless important to recognize at this point that certain conditions are clearly associated with an alteration in the coagulation–fibrinolysis balance in the direction of hypercoagulability. The risk of post-traumatic thrombosis is intensified in these circumstances, which include diabetes mellitus, disseminated malignancy and leukaemia, certain hyperlipoproteinaemias, pregnancy and the use of high-oestrogen oral contraceptives.

The concept of disseminated intravascular coagulation (DIC)

Disseminated intravascular coagulation (DIC) is increasingly recognized as of pathophysiological significance in a wide range of primary conditions.[4, 12] Many of these originate in, or derive from, trauma. It is defined as an acceleration of the coagulation process in the dynamic circulation with consumption of coagulation factors and platelets, microvascular obstruction by fibrin deposition and secondary activation of fibrinolysis. It has many synonyms including 'defibrination', 'hypofibrinogenaemia', 'consumption coagulopathy' and 'intravascular coagulation–fibrinolysis (ICF) syndrome'.

It is due to activation of coagulation in the circulation by the intrinsic or extrinsic mechanisms—or even by direct conversion of prothrombin to thrombin by proteolytic enzymes such as trypsin or certain snake venoms. Some of the more common causes related to injury are given in Fig. 18.3. It will be seen that they can, for simplicity, be arranged in the manner of Virchow's triad of conditions predisposing to thrombosis in major vessels—changes in the blood, in the vessel wall or in blood flow. For example, abnormalities in the blood include triggering of coagulation by thromboplastin from damaged red cells (trauma, burns, incompatible transfusion, extracorporeal circulation) or from lacerated tissues (especially in cerebral or placental injury); circulation of particulate matter activates factor XII (bacteraemia, septicaemia, air and fat embolism). The vessel wall endothelium may be injured not only by direct trauma but also by the effects of circulating endotoxin; abnormality of flow, essentially stasis with red cell injury, is considerable in shock. It is likely that combination of these factors is frequent; there is thus abundant opportunity for intravascular activation of coagulation at some stage in many cases of severe violence.

However it has been caused, once intravascular coagulation is established, it brings about the fairly characteristic chain of events which results in microvascular obstruction and a bleeding diathesis as shown in Fig. 18.3. There is free thrombin in the circulation with a fall in fibrinogen and clotting factors; platelets aggregate and may adhere to the deposited fibrin. A secondary fibrinolytic response occurs with

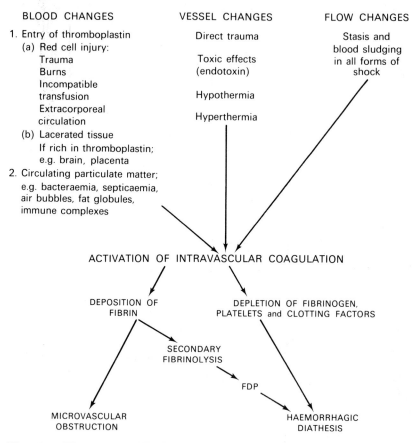

Fig. 18.3   The concept of DIC in injury.

release of plasminogen activator from endothelium. The plasmin can cause fibrinogenolysis as well as fibrinolysis and so worsen the hypofibrinogenaemia. The level of FDP rises; these FDP may worsen the bleeding tendency by complexing with fibrin monomer, thus interfering with its clotting, or by inhibiting fibrin polymerization.

The amount of fibrin that is deposited varies greatly and depends on the portal of entry of the trigger to coagulation, the state of the microcirculation at the time and the extent of the fibrinolytic response.

Detection of small amounts of fibrin in the microvasculature can be difficult because of its continuing removal by fibrinolysis. This is worsened by post-mortem fibrinolysis if there is delay between death and necropsy. Another reason for failure to detect fibrin is technical. The methods available for demonstration of fibrin histologically are at present imperfect because knowledge of the fine structure and chemistry of fibrinogen is limited. The characteristic electron microscopic appearance of fibrin, 240Å periodicity of the fibril, is seen when fibrin is formed experimentally *in vitro* but rarely when it has formed *in vivo*. Tinctorial methods give irregular results and seem to depend to a large extent on the presence of other proteins, such as albumin, associated with the fibrin. Immunofluorescent techniques are more specific but do not distinguish between fibrinogen, the various forms of fibrin and even FDP because of immunological overlap.

For these reasons considerable care is needed in interpreting the histological appearances in suspected cases of DIC. Even small amounts of fibrin in the microvasculature are of significance and must be sought carefully. The organs most commonly involved, and to which particular attention must be directed, are the lungs, kidneys, liver and adrenals.

The effects of fibrin deposition vary from minor hypoperfusion to true infarction. Another possibility is damage to red blood cells which are passing through a network of fibrin strands. This results in red cell fragmentation and abnormal red cell forms may be seen in the peripheral blood film. This red cell injury could enhance DIC, and initiate a vicious circle.

DIC is potentiated by inhibition of fibrinolysis—either natural or drug-induced—by depression of reticuloendothelial activity which reduces fibrin clearance and by a variety of conditions such as hepatic dysfunction, hyperlipaemia and pregnancy.

The real importance of DIC in cases of violence is that it may, to a greater or lesser degree according to circumstances, worsen the patient's condition as a result of continued bleeding or microvascular obstruction.

Haemorrhage

This section deals only with general aspects of haemorrhage. At post-mortem examination in cases of violence the cause of haemorrhage is generally obvious on either external or internal examination. An assessment of the amount of blood lost and the rate of loss must always be attempted although it is not always easy.[2, 8] In the case of external haemorrhage the pathologist may perhaps not have the opportunity to see and estimate for himself the volume of this blood loss. He should, however, if it is reasonable, try to do this as it is likely that the estimates of other observers at the locus will be exaggerated. In internal haemorrhage it is an easy matter to measure blood loss into the body cavities fairly accurately. A note of warning must, however, be sounded. It has been shown that from 100 to 1000 ml of blood can accumulate in a body cavity after post-mortem injury to vessels, e.g. in the chest cavity after intercostal or internal mammary vessel transection.[10]

Blood loss in closed skeletal injury and retroperitoneal haemorrhage is likely to be underestimated. The loss around a fracture of femur may amount to 1 litre or more; multiple fractures may easily mean a loss of up to half the blood volume, or even more than this; retroperitoneal haemorrhage may also be massive. Every opportunity should be taken by the pathologist of assessing the amount of tissue swelling and relating it to estimated, or better still proved, blood loss.

The victim of severe haemorrhage can live long enough to show a surprising degree of activity and movement before death occurs. This is well documented and especially true after stab wounds involving the heart and major chest vessels.[13]

Before discussing the pathological appearances in fatal haemorrhage mention must be made of the 'shock' state. This is best defined as loss of microcirculatory control with hypoperfusion.[11,15] The picture is essentially the same whether the shock is due to haemorrhage, other fluid loss, endotoxaemia or myocardial damage; haemorrhagic shock is, however, probably the best illustration of the homeostatic mechanisms concerned. Following acute blood loss and hypotension there is a rapid vasoconstrictor response with arteriolar contraction, reduced capillary bed and increase in venous return due to venospasm. There are regional variations in the degree of this adaptation, with preferential preservation of core perfusion. The arteriolar spasm fails before the venospasm and capillary engorgement results. Microcirculatory flow is sluggish. Fluid loss occurs into the tissues from these stagnant vessels in which microthrombi may form. The venocapillary blood is highly viscous as a result of red cell aggregation, or 'sludging' as it is often termed.[14] By now the hypoperfusion picture is nearing irreversibility. Core organs remain the better perfused but finally the circulation in these, too, fails and myocardial or cerebral hypoxia causes death. This brief account is, of course, applicable to the untreated case. Timely and adequate fluid replacement will reverse all but the most profound cases of circulatory failure although hypoperfusion may persist in one or several of the systems, e.g. renal, pulmonary, myocardial, endocrine or cerebral, and dominate the clinical picture. It is thought that the microvascular obstruction of DIC contributes to this persisting regional hypoperfusion.

The pathology of fatal haemorrhage depends on the time that has been available for these homeostatic responses. Rapidly fatal haemorrhage killing within minutes, and representing therefore an abrupt loss of 2–3 litres, results in the picture of exsanguination in which the bloodlessness of the tissues and organs is striking. Streaky areas of subendocardial haemorrhage may be found in the left ventricle of the heart—the so-called shock lesions. If, on the other hand, time has allowed the full range of homeostatic mechanisms to operate, i.e. haemorrhage is severe but more gradual, lesions can be found at post-mortem examination which point to irreversible shock with microcirculatory blood sludging and DIC. The subendocardial haemorrhages occur but, in addition, the tissue and organs are oedematous and show petechial haemorrhages. On microscopic examination of the myocardium tiny foci of necrosis may be found. These are best regarded as microinfarcts due to microvascular obstruction. Similar microinfarction may also be seen in the liver, especially near its surface where the possibility of collateral supply is restricted. Irregular congestion of the liver is also a feature, due to venocapillary stasis, and it contrasts with the pallor of the liver in the acutely exsanguinated patient. Another feature quite commonly observed on histological examination in shock cases is evidence of DIC as described above. Between these two examples of the pathology of fatal haemorrhage there lies a wide range of possibilities.

Major side effects of severe hypotension in acute blood loss must also be remembered in patients with pre-existing arterial disease, particularly of the coronary vessels. A degree of haemorrhage unlikely to be, of itself, lethal may then cause such intensification of myocardial hypoperfusion that true large-scale infarction follows. The same is true for the cerebral circulation.

The existence of an underlying bleeding tendency should always be considered in haemorrhage, especially if tissue injury seems disproportionally small. Haemorrhage from major vessels is unlikely to be greatly altered as it is, in any event, profound. It is haemorrhage from medium or small vessels that can be worsened. Most of the factor deficiencies are rare, apart from haemophilia (factor VIII deficiency) which occurs in about 1 in 10 000 males in Britain. Von Willebrand's disease, which is slightly more common and occurs in both sexes, is characterized by factor VIII deficiency and a concomitant capillary-type bleeding defect. These coagulation defects are generally undramatic and show prolonged oozing from small vessels. They could theoretically worsen haemorrhage from such vessels, and excessive or prolonged loss of blood from a vascular injury of this sort should alert the pathologist. There will usually be a history of previous haemorrhagic episodes and evidence of previous bleeding, notably in the joints. Bruising is not, unless truly major, a reliable pointer to a haemorrhagic disorder. Examination of post-mortem blood to assay clotting factors is pointless as the factors are so labile. Thrombocytopenic purpura, whether idiopathic or drug-induced, can produce similar accentuation of small-vessel bleeding.

Of greater significance than these is the effect of anticoagulant therapy. Whether the anticoagulant is heparin, a vitamin K antagonist such as dicoumarol or warfarin, or the more recent defibrinating agent ancrod (Arvin), a severe haemostatic defect may occur. Similarly in hypoprothrombinaemia, notably in liver disease, haemorrhage may be exaggerated. Alcohol is important not only because it causes liver disease but also because unexpectedly severe haemorrhage may occur from relatively superficial wounds in the state of vasodilatation due to alcoholic intoxication. Finally, in DIC there is, as already described, hypofibrinogenaemia and an acute bleeding state. This is, however, most likely to be seen in the forensic situation as the consequence of injury rather than as a pre-existing condition.

Thrombosis

In DIC, coagulation is widely triggered within the dynamic microcirculation while in thrombosis local circumstances, usually at one site or a restricted number of sites, determine platelet adhesion and aggregation with consequent coagulation in vessels of larger calibre.

The appearance of ante-mortem thrombi are well known. Pale firm thrombus is slowly formed in rapidly flowing blood and consists of fused platelets with some admixed fibrin. Red friable thrombus is rapidly formed in stagnant blood and shows a loose mesh of fibrin entangling the blood cellular elements. Mixed thrombus, which is the most common, forms in slowly flowing blood, mainly in the venous tree, and shows zones of fused platelets bordered by compact fibrin surrounded by areas of fibrin network containing trapped blood cells; it clearly represents episodes of slow and rapid thrombus formation.

Dating of thrombi is difficult. Almost from the onset a thrombus elicits a minor inflammatory response in the wall of the vessel containing it, especially where it adheres. This leads to eventual organization by ingrowing capillary buds and fibroblasts, and possible recanalization. It is, however, impossible to time these events precisely because of the great variation which exists both in the stimulus to organization and in the capacity of the individual to respond to it. All that can be expected is an approximation, most often expressed as 'days', 'weeks' or 'months'.

Post-mortem and agonal thrombi are unlikely sources of confusion for the experienced pathologist. Post-mortem thrombus is dark, soft, glistening-wet and non-adherent. It is common in the heart chambers and larger veins and forms a cast of the vessel in which it forms. If sedimentation of the red cells occurs quickly the uppermost part of the thrombus may appear yellow and gelatinous. Agonal thrombus occurs in the heart chambers when the circulation is failing just before death. It is composed largely of fibrin which has separated out and is yellow, wet and stringy and may be loosely attached to the heart wall. If any doubt exists about the nature of post-mortem and agonal thrombi, which will not be often, histological examination will generally settle the matter by providing evidence of foci of platelet fusion or compact fibrin.

The sites of post-traumatic thrombosis can be considered in order, bearing in mind Virchow's triad of factors predisposing to thrombosis which can be stated more precisely as:

1. changes in the coagulation–fibrinolysis balance, and in the platelets, favouring coagulation;

2. alterations in the vascular endothelium, especially exposure of collagen, causing adhesion and aggregation of platelets; and

3. stasis determining a local accumulation of procoagulant factors.

While each factor on its own might initiate thrombosis, a combination of factors is both more potent and more usual.

Cardiac and larger arterial thrombi can be considered together. A complete traumatic breach of the vessel wall will theoretically initiate formation of the haemostatic plug; this response will, in practical terms, be of no significance in view of the massive haemorrhage that rapidly kills. In smaller arteries the haemostatic plug will, of course, be found. Direct blunt trauma to the vessel, without breaching of its wall, can produce sufficient endothelial injury to initiate thrombosis; this will seldom be totally occlusive unless there is coexistent hypotension. Much more likely to be encountered is localization of thrombosis at a site of previous vascular damage, e.g. atheroma, in the hypercoagulable and hypotensive state following severe trauma.

Venous thrombi are extremely common and for all practical purposes post-traumatic thrombosis is the story of these thrombi and their consequences. While direct damage to the vein wall may occasionally play a part in their genesis, it is the combination of procoagulant activity and stasis that is important. The stasis is not only local but also, in shock, systemic. The lower limbs and the pelvic area are the common sites. Sevitt[7] found that 65 per cent of a series of 125 injured patients had deep vein thrombi in the lower limbs at necropsy dissection. The figure was even higher in the elderly (80 per cent). Many other studies show similar figures and relate the occurrence of deep venous thrombosis to bed rest, immobility and age.

Venous thrombosis commences in areas of stasis or turbulent flow, with eddy formation, such as valve pockets, junctions or angulations. Six main sites have been described by Sevitt, namely: the calf veins, especially the soleal, the posterior tibial veins, the popliteal vein below the adductor ring, the deep femoral vein, the common femoral vein where its tributaries enter and the external iliac vein. These sites may show thrombosis independently but commonly it occurs in several at the same time; it is generally bilateral.

In the first day after trauma, venous thrombi are infrequently found at necropsy but their incidence rises progressively during the next 7–10 days. This accords with the hypercoagulability which follows injury. The stages in development of venous thrombi are well known. Initially, pale platelet thrombus forms in the static areas and is covered by red fibrin-rich thrombus; successive alternating layers of pale and red thrombus are laid down as the thrombus grows. When the vessel of origin is occluded, rapid coagulation takes place up to the next junction where the episodic process recommences. Retrograde coagulation may also occur. The end result is the typical irregularly laminated mixed thrombus; its primary attachment to the vessel wall is trivial, if it occurs at all. The progressive growth of these thrombi is clearly dependent on the continued operation of the causal factors, and as stasis and hypercoagulability subside propagation will cease. It may also be checked by prophylactic anticoagulant therapy. Fibrinolytic activity will eventually lyse some of the clot but this will generally become organized and firmly adherent.

Local venous obstruction results but by far the most important consequence of deep venous thrombosis is pulmonary embolism from the iliofemoral segment. Sevitt and Gallagher[9] found major pulmonary emboli in 20 per cent of 468 patients at necropsy after a wide range of injuries. Again the incidence was greatest in the elderly; but young subjects are also commonly at risk, as studies of battle casualties have shown. When pulmonary embolism is found at necropsy its significance must be assessed. A large saddle embolus, separate emboli blocking both pulmonary arteries and large emboli in lobar arteries will cause death. Multiple small emboli in peripheral arteries will contribute to death. A few small emboli in central or peripheral small arteries will be non-fatal and may even be subclinical. Grading is, therefore, a matter of experience, bearing in mind also the general state of the patient. As a general rule, blockage of about half of the pulmonary arterial bed is regarded as lethal.

Capillary thrombi (microthrombi) are frequently found after trauma. They may be local or systemic. Local microthrombi represent the haemostatic mechanism at the injury site or are the direct result of injury of the vessel, notably in burning. Systemic microthrombi are the result of DIC, as already described, or of the irreversible shock state in which hypoperfusion, rheological changes and DIC combine as causal agents. The lung and kidney are the most common sites in which these microthrombi can be found, usually a few days after injury. They consist of platelets and fibrin. The difficulties which arise in demonstration of small quantities of fibrin histologically have already been described. The precise significance of systemic microthrombosis is debatable. It does, however, indicate that intravascular coagulation has been triggered and that the cause for this has to be sought. This cause will itself usually be of major importance, e.g. circulating thromboplastin, existence of septicaemia, or severe shock. The possibility of direct microvascular obstruction causing a variety of clinical syndromes (e.g. shock lung, renal failure, adrenal or pituitary necrosis and haemorrhage) must also be borne in mind.

References

1. Bennett, B. and Douglas, A. S. (1973). Blood coagulation mechanism. In: *Clinics in Haematology*, Vol. 2, No. 1, Chap. 1. Ed. A. S. Douglas. Eastbourne: W. B. Saunders.

2. Clarke, R, Topley, E. and Flear, C. T. G. (1955). Assessment of blood loss in civilian trauma. *Lancet* **i**, 629.
3. Flute, P. T. (1970). Coagulation and fibrinolysis after injury. *J. clin. Path.* **23**, Suppl. (Roy. Coll. Path.), **4**, 102.
4. McKay, D. G. (1965). *Disseminated Intravascular Coagulation. An intermediary mechanism of disease.* New York: Hoeber.
5. McNicol, G. P. and Davies, J. A. (1973). Fibrinolytic enzyme system. In: *Clinics in Haematology*, Vol. 2, No. 1, Chap. 2. Ed. A. S. Douglas. Eastbourne: W. B. Saunders.
6. Mole, R. H. (1948). Fibrinolysin and the fluidity of the blood *post mortem. J. Path. Bact.* **60**, 413.
7. Sevitt, S. (1970). Thrombosis and embolism after injury. *J. clin. Path.* **23**, Suppl. (Roy. Coll. Path.), **4**, 86.
8. Sevitt, S. (1974). Haemorrhage, plasma loss, oligaemia and anaemia. In: *Reactions to Injury and Burns*, Chap. 3. London: Heinemann Medical.
9. Sevitt, S. and Gallagher, N. (1961). Venous thrombosis and pulmonary embolism. A clinico-pathological study in injured and burned patients. *Brit. J. Surg.* **48**, 475.
10. Shapiro, H. A. and Robertson, I. (1962). The significance of blood in the pleural cavity observed after death. *J. forensic Sci.* **9**, 5.
11. Shepro, D. and Fulton, G. P. (Eds.) (1968). *Microcirculation as Related to Shock.* New York and London: Academic Press.
12. Simpson, J. G. and Stalker, A. L. (1973). The concept of disseminated intravascular coagulation. In: *Clinics in Haematology*, Vol. 2, No. 1, Chap. 12. Ed. A. S. Douglas. Eastbourne: W. B. Saunders.
13. Spitz, W. U., Petty, C. S. and Fisher, R. S. (1961). Physical activity until collapse following fatal injury by firearms and sharp pointed weapons. *J. forensic Sci.* **6**, 290.
14. Stalker, A. L. (1967). Histological changes produced by experimental erythrocyte aggregation. *J. Path. Bact.* **93**, 203.
15. Stalker, A. L. (1970). The microcirculation in shock. *J. clin. Path.* **23**, Suppl. (Roy. Coll. Path.), **4**, 10.
16. Todd, A. S. (1959). The histological localisation of fibrinolysin activator. *J. Path. Bact.* **78**, 281.

19

Renal failure following injury and burning

Introduction

The first reference to the occurrence of renal damage following injury appears to be that made in Edinburgh in 1823 by Cumin[5] after dissecting the bodies of burn-victims. In 1909, Colmer[4] reported the association between muscle necrosis due to compression and renal failure in patients injured during the Messina earthquake of December 1908. The German literature of World War I included reports by Frankenthal[8,9] and by Küttner[16] concerning enlargement of the kidneys following crushing of the muscles; after the war, Minami[19] published a detailed report in which he suggested that myohaemoglobin was involved in the production of renal damage. These reports went unnoticed and the syndrome was thought never to have been described before when it was rediscovered in World War II.

In a classic series of papers, in particular that published in the *British Medical Journal* in 1941, Bywaters[2] established the condition of acute renal failure in the awareness of the medical profession. As a consequence, it has gradually become apparent that acute renal failure can result from shock arising from any cause, as a complication of many illnesses and following exposure to a wide range of organic and inorganic chemicals and drugs, notably antibiotics. There is now such a vast list of causes of acute renal failure that, in a major review, Kerr[15] concluded that it would be a bold man who dogmatized as to the pathogenesis. In one study, it was found that 43 per cent of those seriously injured in World War II developed renal failure and 91 per cent of these died.

The incidence of acute renal failure in the Korean War was drastically reduced to 0·5 per cent of those seriously injured, and the mortality among these was reduced to 66 per cent by use of the artificial kidney.[21] The occurrence of the condition was lower in the Vietnam conflict than in Korea but the mortality rate could not be reduced below 66 per cent.[24] These trends are discernible in the pattern of post-traumatic acute renal failure in civilian populations.

Acute renal failure will be a rare problem to the accident service. Violent injury or burning accounts for only a small proportion of the nephrologist's patients in acute renal failure. Such cases do, however, provide some of the best examples of the condition in which the influence of age, pre-existing renal disease, other illnesses or drug ingestion can be discounted. Given a large series of such patients, it is possible to study both the uncomplicated natural history of the disease and the influence of treatment. The first part of this chapter is based on such a study. Although many of the cases described did occur during a military conflict, they do not represent the mass casualty situation seen in major wars and the patients described may be considered typical of the sporadic cases of post-traumatic renal failure which occur in a civilian population. For this reason, the American experience in Vietnam can be reviewed to provide a comparison. A discussion of the current views on pathogenesis is also given, although this has been made brief because of the several excellent reviews which have been published.[14, 15, 20]

The Halton experience

One hundred and thirty-three patients with acute renal failure following either injury or burns were treated by the Renal Unit, Princess Mary's RAF Hospital, Halton, between 1956 and 1975 (Table 19.1). Patients were admitted from a wide area and included many civilians as well as members of the armed forces. Twenty-six patients (20 injured, 6

Table 19.1   Acute renal failure in 133 patients following injury or burns, 1956–75

	Injured	*Burns*
Admitted to Renal Unit, Princess Mary's RAF Hospital, Halton	92	15
Treated by mobile haemodialysis team	20	6
Totals	112	21

burned) were not actually admitted to the renal unit but were treated at their hospital of admission by a mobile team equipped with an artificial kidney; to a large extent, these constituted the most seriously injured patients.

Sex and age distribution
Only 6 patients were female, their average age being 39 years (range 16 to 69 years). The 127 male patients were of average age 29 years (range 9 to 72 years). There was no significant difference in the average age of the patients who died and of those who survived nor between the cases treated during the periods 1956–1964 and 1965–1975.

Causes of injuries and burns
These are set out in Table 19.2. More than two-thirds of the injuries

Table 19.2 Causes of injuries and burns

Cause of injury	Number
Passenger or driver of enclosed vehicle	47
Driver of motor-cycle	19
Pedestrian hit by vehicle	11
Crush injury	5
Agricultural accident	5
Fall from a height	8
Exercise-induced muscle damage	6
Blast injury	5
Aircraft accident	2
Horse-riding accident	2
Gunshot wound	2
	112

Cause of burns	Number
Fire	10
Petrol	5
Electrical	5
Scald	1
	21

were related in some way to road traffic accidents. The remaining patients suffered injury in a variety of ways, many of them bizarre.

The patients who were burned covered a broad spectrum, including drunkards falling into the fire, children whose clothing caught alight, suicidal ritual burnings, electrical accidents at work and one patient who was buried to the waist in steam super-heated sand.

Cause of renal failure in traumatic cases

Shock

The acute renal failure was attributed to severe shock at the time of injury in 81 of the 112 patients. A bewildering variety of clinical possibilities was suggested in the remaining 31 cases. Jaundice was the commonest association in 12 out of 31 patients who were not shocked and, in these, the onset of oliguria was sometimes delayed.

Other patients sustained a defined episode of shock after the initial injury; this was caused by a variety of measures such as anaesthesia, therapeutic hypothermia and reactions to tetanus antitoxin. In 20 patients, renal failure occurred without any clear-cut episode of hypotension and some days after the initial injury in settings which included repeated anaesthetics and operations, jaundice, sepsis, hypoxia, the use of nephrotoxic drugs and the presence of indwelling catheters. Paradoxically, 10 of these patients developed oliguria at a time when they were considered to be improving.

Disseminated intravascular coagulation
Disseminated intravascular coagulation (DIC) (see Chapter 18) was not a prominent feature. It was not looked for in the early years. In later times, it was found that the levels of serum fibrin degradation products were usually raised. The values were very high (> 40µg/ml) in association with septic shock and/or pancreatitis but otherwise lay mostly between 10 and 40 µg/ml. Heparinization was never used therapeutically. Renal function regularly returned provided the patients survived their injuries, thus suggesting that, if the observed DIC was causing damage, this was naturally reversible.

Renal injury
In 2 patients both kidneys were destroyed by a crushing injury to the back. Eleven other patients suffered a loss of one kidney due to laceration, rupture or thrombosis of the renal artery; all 11 patients sustained acute renal failure in the contralateral kidney and 5 recovered. Postmortem dissection of those who died revealed 'acute tubular necrosis' in all the 'undamaged' kidneys; presumably, renal function might have eventually recovered had the patients survived. The pattern of acute renal failure in the 5 survivors did not differ clinically from that of survivors with two remaining kidneys.

Heat stroke and exercise-induced muscle damage
There were 6 patients in this group, the diagnosis being based on the typical clinical history and subsequent course. Five were soldiers undergoing unaccustomed strenuous exercise. No myoglobin was found in the urine of any patient but none was admitted to the Renal Unit within 48 hours of the exercise. One patient died in the diuretic phase but the remainder recovered. In the single post-mortem examination, necrosis of the paravertebral muscles was found and the kidney tubules contained pigmented casts.

Renal cortical necrosis
No case of renal cortical necrosis following injury was observed.

Onset of renal failure following injury

Of the 112 patients, 73 were found to be oliguric with a raised blood urea immediately following resuscitation. Out of 92 admitted to the Renal Unit, the onset of oliguria was immediate in 67 patients but occurred on the second or third days in 7 and only arose later in 4 patients.

By contrast, there was an increased incidence of late onset oliguria in the 20 more severely injured patients who were treated by mobile dialysis. Out of 19 instances, the onset of oliguria was immediate in 6, arose on the second or third day in 6 and was later in 7. This trend towards late onset oliguria following adequate initial resuscitation in a complicated clinical setting was also found in Vietnam.[17] The possible causes of acute renal failure were multiple and not necessarily mediated by the same mechanism as that occurring in shock. Nevertheless, there were instances of complete recovery of renal function, suggesting that the same tendency to natural remission exists.

Non-oliguric renal failure
It is generally thought that head injuries and burns show an increased incidence of non-oliguric (as opposed to oliguric) renal failure as compared with other forms of trauma. In this series there were 18 cases of non-oliguric renal failure, 14 following injury and 4 following burns. The incidence of head injury was 24 in 98 oliguric patients and 4 in 14 who were non-oliguric. Of the 21 burns patients, 4 were non-oliguric. These figures do not indicate a significant association between either head injury or burns and non-oliguric renal failure but it may well have been that non-oliguria led to a lower referral rate to the renal unit than did oliguria.

Deaths in the diuretic phase
There were 6 deaths in the diuretic phase. Two of these were due to abdominal sepsis; the remainder were associated with *Pseudomonas aeruginosa* septicaemia, the administration of tetracycline, fat embolism and amyloidosis of the kidneys in a patient with chronic peritoneal sepsis following peritoneal dialysis at another hospital.

Type of injury related to outcome
The majority of patients were severely injured (Table 19.3). In the period 1956–1964 dialysis was performed only according to uraemic signs or because of gross biochemical disturbances such as hyperkalaemia or a blood urea of over 58 mmol/l (350 mg/100 ml); the mortality rate was 66 per cent among admitted patients. In the period 1965–1975 haemodialysis was performed almost daily and was used to maintain biochemical normality, to minimize uraemia and to provide high calorie feeding; the mortality rate fell to 34 per cent. This improvement is largely attributable to the more frequent haemodialysis.

The results shown in Table 19.3 do not show a significant correlation

Table 19.3   Total injuries among each group

Site of injury	Admitted trauma, 1956–64 (42 patients)		Not admitted trauma, 1956–64 (4 patients)		Admitted trauma, 1965–75 (67 patients)		Not admitted trauma, 1965–75 (16 patients)	
	Lived (14)	Died (28)	Lived (Nil)	Died (4)	Lived (50)	Died (17)	Lived (3)	Died (13)
Head	nil	10	—	1	9	5	nil	3
Chest	6	4	—	3	8	7	3	7
Limbs	11	16	—	4	21	10	nil	6
Abdomen	4	6	—	2	7	9	2	6
Kidney	5	5	—	nil	4	4	nil	nil
Urinary tract	2	2	—	1	nil	nil	2	4
Pelvis	10	10	—	1	12	6	nil	7

Most patients received multiple injuries. The exact type and extent of injury are not recorded here, but all were severe.

between any particular injury, or combinations of injuries, and a fatal outcome. Detailed examination of the individual case notes provides the explanation. In the early series, several patients with apparently survivable injuries died from uraemic complications because of under-dialysis; some of these were in the diuretic phase. Some injuries, such as gross brain damage, were not survivable in either period. In the period 1965–1975, two conditions seem predominantly associated with a fatal outcome—progressive respiratory failure ('shock' lung) and gastrointestinal injury with abscess formation and septicaemia.

Burns related to outcome

Of the 21 burned patients, 20 died. Our only survivor had sustained severe burns of one arm and of the adjacent chest wall. The arm was amputated and most of the burn was excised. He recovered full renal function following a clear-cut episode of renal failure but died later from alcoholic myocarditis. There appear to be only 6 recorded survivors in the world literature. The burned area was amputated, as in our case, in 3 of these.[11, 18, 22]

The cause of this high mortality is uncertain but it suggests the presence of a toxin which inhibits recovery of renal function and is, itself, lethal. Hypercatabolism and susceptibility to infection are common. Dialysis seems to prolong life and the administration of 16·7–20·9 kJ (4000–5000 calories) per day in conjunction with haemodialysis (occasionally with peritoneal dialysis as well) has controlled the hypercatabolic state in some patients. Most patients developed pulmonary congestion together with myocardial failure expressed as hypotension, bradycardia and arrhythmias. At post-mortem, the only findings in the kidneys were 'tubular necrosis' and the presence of pigmented casts.

Recovery of renal function

It is our practice to perform an intravenous urogram (IVU), to estimate the creatinine clearance and to examine a mid-stream specimen of urine on all patients who recover. Table 19.4 sets out the results in 13 consecutive patients who recovered from severe post-traumatic renal failure. Two patients had lost a kidney from trauma but the remaining organ was normal on IVU. All the other IVUs were normal. The urines were invariably clear of protein or cellular deposits and were sterile. One patient (who had lost a kidney) had a creatinine clearance of 36 ml/min, 4 had clearances between 50 and 100 ml/min, and 8 had clearances over 100 ml/min. The occurrence of normal creatinine clearances, after 31 days of oliguria in 1 case, shows that full functional recovery is possible. While more sophisticated measurements of the glomerular filtration are desirable, it is unlikely that they would alter the conclusion that excellent recovery of renal function often occurs.

The American experience in Vietnam

The Vietnam conflict provided much information on some new problems in the management of acute renal failure.[24] The very excellence of

Table 19.4 Recovery of renal function

Patient	Age (years)	Blood urea on admission (mmol/l)[mg/100 ml]	Duration Oliguria (days)	Interval between illness and review	IVU	MSU	Creatinine clearance (ml/min)
1	66	41·7 [250]	24	3 years	N	Clear Sterile	65
2	17	69·3 [416]	21	3 years	N	Clear Sterile	117
3	63	77·5 [465]	28	2 yr 8 mth	N	Clear Sterile	54
4	18	111·7 [670]	nil	2 years	N	Clear Sterile	102
5	32	42·5 [255]	18	4 months	N	Clear Sterile	120
6	17	53·3 [320]	6	3 months	N	Clear Sterile	126
7	30	48·3 [290]	24	3 years	Normal R kidney Absent L kidney	Clear Sterile	104
8	26	95 [570]	26	2 months	N	Clear Sterile	120
9	34	25 [150]	31	5 months	N	Clear Sterile	126
10	17	40·8 [245]	18	1 yr 3 mth	Normal L kidney Absent R kidney	Clear Sterile	36
11	21	57·3 [344]	21	7 months	N	Clear Sterile	104
12	32	37·7 [226]	31	11 months	N	Clear Sterile	80
13	57	53·3 [320]	15	6 months	N	Clear Sterile	60
Averages	31	54 [324]	20	1 yr 6 mth			93

N = Normal.

evacuation procedures and of rapid volume replacement created an unusual medical situation. The patients were severely injured by high-velocity gunshot wounds, shell fragments, booby traps and napalm. Almost incredibly, the average time from injury to evacuation to a medical centre capable of definitive treatment was only 30–40 minutes. Compared to the Korean War, in which 1 in 3 seriously wounded soldiers died, only 1 in 6 died in Vietnam. The incidence of acute renal failure also fell from 1 in 200 to 1 in 600 seriously injured. However, the mortality rate of patients with post-traumatic renal failure was 66 per cent and this was not appreciably different from that which obtained in Korea. The clinicians involved concluded that there was no obvious difference in the treatment of the renal failure given to the survivors and the fatalities, and that the outcome was dictated by the primary injury and its complications. Nevertheless, they presented several remarkable case histories of survivors from which it seems evident that dialysis was invaluable.

The commonest cause of death was gram-negative septicaemia, and gastrointestinal trauma with peritonitis was the most ominous prognostic sign. Non-oliguric renal failure and late onset oliguria were frequent.

The main conclusion to be drawn from the Vietnam experience is that the incidence of acute renal failure can be drastically reduced by the prompt and vigorous treatment of initial shock caused by blood loss. This is, of course, a well known fact; it deserves emphasis here because it lends credence to the idea that acute renal failure is mediated through circulatory responses to shock.

The pathogenesis of acute renal failure (Fig. 19.1)

There is little difficulty in understanding why a kidney should fail when it is destroyed by occlusion of the arterial blood supply, or by ureteric obstruction, or by the crushing of all the glomeruli by epithelial crescents. It is much more difficult to explain the type of acute

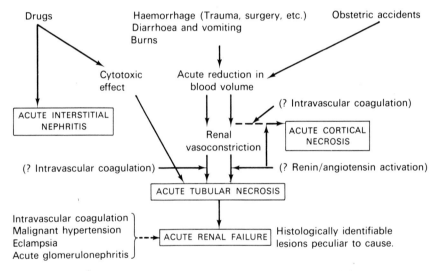

Fig. 19.1 Schematic representation of possible pathogenic mechanisms in acute renal failure.

renal failure seen in most of the patients described in this chapter. It has no agreed name, the histological findings are trivial and the pathophysiological mechanism is unproven. To avoid implying that it has a single cause or even a common pathology, it may be called the syndrome of acute renal failure and defined as:

An abrupt cessation of renal function, not reversible by fluid repletion or diuretics, which persists on average for 7–10 days (but may last several weeks) and which spontaneously, often rapidly, remits, with no evidence of renal damage other than a clinically insignificant, and non-progressive, impairment of the glomerular filtration rate.

The definition is necessarily clumsy because it concerns an observed phenomenon, the cause, persistence and reversal of which are not fully understood and which is both mimicked by, and is often associated with, other renal diseases. The main theories of causation are:

1. acute tubular necrosis with blockage by casts, with back diffusion of filtrate;
2. disseminated intravascular coagulation; and
3. activation of the renin–angiotensin system.

Acute tubular necrosis
This is both a histological description and also the most popular name by which the syndrome is known. It is closely mimicked by post-mortem autolysis. It is often associated with pigment (myohaemoglobin) casts in the crush syndrome[2] and in burns but these are by no means invariable (Figs. 19.2 and 19.3).

The study of renal biopsies taken during life quickly showed that the most striking feature was the actual paucity of changes. This *in vivo* work was begun in Denmark by Brun[13] who has recently set out the main histological findings seen by light microscopy (Table 19.5).

Experimental evidence against the importance of tubular necrosis came from studies made on salt-loaded rats poisoned with low doses of mercuric chloride.[6] These animals developed extensive tubular necrosis but maintained a glomerular filtration rate of 80 per cent of normal. The findings suggest that tubular necrosis is not necessarily accompanied by renal failure and also that passive back diffusion does not occur to any great extent in the condition—otherwise, the glomerular filtration rate (GFR), which includes urine flow rate in its measurement, would fall further.

Table 19.5 Histological appearances on light microscopy in 'acute tubular necrosis'

Bowman's capsule	Normal
Glomeruli	Normal
Proximal tubules	Often normal, but hydropic change due to mannitol may be present
Distal tubules	Focally dilated and lined with flattened epithelium. Pigmented casts are prominent and tubular necrosis, if present, is usually where a cast is located
Vessels	Normal
Interstitium	Slight focal oedema and focal infiltration of lymphocytes, plasma cells and granulocytes

Adapted from Brun.[25]

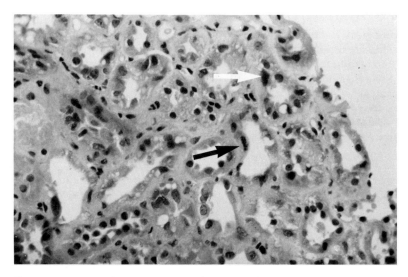

Fig. 19.2   Acute tubular necrosis without casts. Evidence of regeneration is shown by mitotic activity (black arrow) and hyperchromatic nuclei (white arrow). There is interstitial oedema. (H & E, × 300)

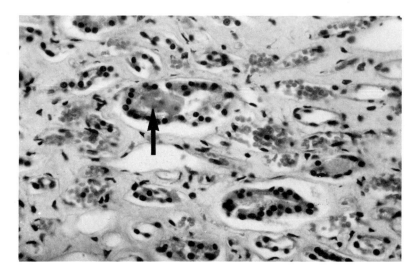

Fig. 19.3   Acute tubular necrosis with cast formation. A cast is arrowed. There is general 'flattening' on the epithelium of the distal tubules. (H & E, × 300)

Tubular blockage by casts and debris looks a more convincing aetiological factor, particularly as it probably is important in myelomatosis accompanied by Bence Jones proteinuria. Again, experimental evidence is against the concept. In anuria induced by mercury in the rat, single nephron GFR has been shown to cease before any significant tubular injury can be demonstrated while the proximal tubules are collapsed and empty;[7] casts would seem to be a consequence of filtration failure rather than the cause.[12] Filtration failure has been demonstrated in acute renal failure in man.[12]

Disseminated intravascular coagulation
Disseminated intravascular coagulation is a common finding in many of the conditions with which acute renal failure is associated. These include shock, sepsis, liver disease, pre-eclampsia, drug reactions and pancreatitis. Serum and urine levels of fibrin degradation products are raised in most cases of acute renal failure and, although the glomeruli are apparently normal when viewed by light microscopy, fibrin-like material may be seen in the glomeruli by electron microscopy.[3] There is no doubt, therefore, as to the occurrence of DIC—only as to its significance.

In those diseases in which DIC is florid and causes prominent clinical signs as a result of both thrombosis and haemorrhage, the kidneys often fail partially or completely to recover. Such conditions include haemolytic uraemic syndromes, thrombotic thrombocytopenic purpura and pre-eclampsia. But when DIC is manifested only by the presence of symptomless raised levels of fibrin degradation products (FDP), the kidney seems able to recover naturally. However, this does not preclude the possibility of initial renal thrombosis acting as a stimulus causing renal failure; the pathological state would be subsequently cleared by the kidneys' active fibrinolytic system.

The renin–angiotensin system
It is a remarkable fact that, whereas most pathologists over-emphasized the importance of tubular necrosis in the crush syndrome, they also missed a major histological change which was noted by Goormaghtigh in 1945.[10] This process was that of hypertrophy and granularity of the juxtaglomerular apparatus, appearances which are more pronounced in this condition than in any other renal lesion. Goormaghtigh postulated that a vasopressive substance is liberated in excess and causes a persistent spasm of the vascular pole of the glomerular tuft. His work was overlooked until the possibility was appreciated that renin, which is formed in the juxtaglomerular apparatus, might be involved in the causation of acute renal failure. The main experimental evidence in favour of such involvement of the renin–angiotensin system is that rats depleted of renal renin by long-term salt loading are thereby protected from the acute renal failure caused by dichromate poisoning or glycerol-induced myohaemoglobinuria.[6, 23]

Although circulating levels of renin and angiotensin are raised in renal failure it is unlikely that the action is a systemic one for the following reasons:[1]

1. Higher levels of angiotensin produced by injection do not cause acute renal failure.
2. Higher levels are found in some patients with hypertension who do not have renal failure.
3. Antagonists of circulating angiotensin do not protect against acute renal failure.

It has to be postulated, therefore, that renin is produced in the juxtaglomerular apparatus in excess, acts on available substrate and produces locally active angiotensin II.

It must be strongly emphasized that this is not a proven theory. At the present time, the most attractive hypothesis is along the following lines. There is a constriction of the preglomerular vasculature, which produces a fall in the transglomerular pressure. This constriction is presumably produced by local factors as it is not reflected by appropriately raised levels of vasoconstrictors in the systemic circulation. The fall in transglomerular pressure reduces the glomerular filtration rate to a low level, thus preventing effective clearance of solutes. Urine volume may vary from a few millilitres each day to 'normal' amounts, depending on the actual glomerular filtration rate achieved. Regardless of its volume, the osmolarity of the urine is not greater than that of the plasma. Because the stimulus is a local one, it may persist until the reflexes which work through a co-ordinated neuro–endocrine–circulatory balance can exert themselves and cause the kidney to function once more as an ultra-filter of large volumes of blood. Once the kidney is, as it were, jerked back to its correct function, it rapidly improves. Complications of the failure of filtration, such as tubular necrosis and cellular swelling, may delay recovery. Other complications such as deposition of fibrin, potassium deficiency and infection may prolong the disability or leave residual damage but, essentially, most nephrons return to normal. This theory fits most of the known facts; all that remains is to find the local vasoconstrictor. Angiotensin is the main contender.

Conclusion

Two main patterns of acute renal failure are seen following injury. The first is associated with severe shock and is usually characterized by a period of oliguria followed by almost complete recovery. As the patients are mainly young and healthy such cases provide a useful clinical model for study. The second pattern is the development of acute renal failure in a complicated clinical setting in which a large number of factors may be operating. Oliguria may be absent or late in onset. Such cases currently show a high mortality; nevertheless, full recovery of renal function may still occur. They represent the group needing the most careful study.

References

1. Brown, J. J., Gavras, H., Kremer, D., Lever, A. F., MacGregor, J., Powell-Jackson, J. D. and Robertson, I. S. (1974). *Proceedings, Acute Renal Failure Conference*, p. 143. Ed. E. A. Friedman and H. E. Eliahou. Washington DC: DHEW Publication No. (NIH) 74–608.
2. Bywaters, E. G. L. and Beall, D. (1941). Crush injuries with impairment of renal function. *Brit. med. J.* **1**, 427.
3. Clarkson, A. R., MacDonald, M. K., Fuster, V., Cash, J. D. and Robson, J. S. (1970). Glomerular coagulation in acute ischaemic renal failure. *Quart. J. Med.* **39**, 585.
4. Colmers, D. R. (1909). Ueber die durch das Erdbeben in Messina am 28 December 1908 verursachten Verletzungen. *Arch. klin. Chir.* **90**, 701.
5. Cumin, W. (1823). Cases of severe burns with dissection and remarks. *Edinb. M. & S. J.* **19**, 337.
6. Flamenbaum, W., McDonald, F. D., Dibona, G. F. and Oken, D. E. (1971). Micropuncture study of renal tubular factors in low dose mercury poisoning. *Nephron* **8**, 221.
7. Flanigan, W. J. and Oken, D. E. (1965). Renal micropuncture study of the development of anuria in the rat with mercury-induced acute renal failure. *J. clin. Invest.* **44**, 449.
8. Frankenthal, L. (1916). Über Verschüttungen. *Virchows Arch. path. Anat.* **222**, 332.
9. Frankenthal, L. (1918). Die Folgen der Verletzungen durch Verschüttung. *Bruns' Beitr. klin. Chir.* **109**, 572.
10. Goormaghtigh, N. (1945). Vascular and circulatory changes in the anuria crush syndrome. *Proc. Soc. exp. Biol. Med.* **59**, 303.
11. Hartford, C. E. and Ziffren, S. E. (1971). Electrical injury. *J. Trauma* **11**, 331.
12. Hollenberg, N. K., Epstein, M., Rosen, S. M., Basch, R. I., Oken, D. E. and Merrill, J. P. (1968). Acute oliguric renal failure in man: evidence for preferential renal cortical ischaemia. *Medicine (Baltimore)* **47**, 455.
13. Iverson, P. and Brun, C. (1951). Aspiration biopsy of kidney. *Amer. J. Med.* **11**, 324.
14. Kerr, D. N. S. (1972). *Renal Disease*, 3rd edn., pp. 417–461. Ed. Sir Douglas Black. Oxford: Blackwell Scientific.
15. Kerr, D. N. S. (1973). In: *Acute Renal Failure*, pp. 9–36. Ed. C. T. Flynn. Lancaster: MTP Co. Ltd.
16. Küttner, H. (1918). Beiträge zur Kriegschirurgie der grossen blutigen Fasstomme. II. Die Verschüttungsnekrose ganzer Extremitäten. *Bruns' Beitr. klin. Chir.* **112**, 581.
17. Lordon, R. E. and Burton, J. R. (1972). Post traumatic renal failure in military personnel in S.E. Asia. *Amer. J. Med.* **53**, 137.

18. Marshal, V. C. (1971). Acute renal failure in surgical patients. *Brit. J. Surg.* **58**, 17.
19. Minami, S. (1923). Über Nierenveränderungen nach Verschüttung. *Virchows Arch. path. Anat.* **245**, 247.
20. Muehrcke, R. C. (1969). *Acute Renal Failure: Diagnosis and Management*, pp. 167–261. Ed. R. C. Muehrcke. St Louis: C. V. Mosby.
21. Smith, L. H., Jr., Post, R. S., Teschan, P. E., Abernathy, R. S., Davis, J. H., Gray, D. M., Howard, J. M., Johnson, K. E., Klopp, E., Mundy, R. L., O'Meara, M. P. and Rush, B. F. (1955). Post-traumatic renal insufficiency in military casualties. II. Management, use of an artificial kidney, prognosis. *Amer. J. Med.* **18**, 187.
22. Stephens, F. O. and Stewart, J. H. (1965). Burns complicated by anuria. Recovery after radical surgery and haemodialysis. *Lancet* **ii**, 15.
23. Thiel, G., McDonald, F. D. and Oken, D. E. (1970). Micropuncture studies of the basis for protection of renin depleted rats from glycerol induced renal failure. *Nephron* **7**, 67.
24. Whelton, A. and Donadio, J. V., Jr. (1969). Post-traumatic acute renal failure in Vietnam. A comparison with the Korean experience. *Johns Hopk. med. J.* **124**, 95.
25. Brun, C. (1973). In *Acute Renal Failure*, pp. 46–52. Ed. C. T. Flynn. Lancaster: MTP Co. Ltd.

20

The forensic significance of fat and bone marrow embolism

The subject of fat embolism (FE) has fascinated traumatologists since it was first described in 1862 by Zenker.[39] A recent bibliography[5] lists no less than 965 references since 1927 and some of the early dilemmas are still far from clarification.

General considerations

Many of the arguments generated in the literature stem from a failure to distinguish between the two very different aspects of fat embolism—the pathological finding and the clinical syndrome. Peters,[23] for example, spoke in 1942 of fat embolism being responsible for 22 per cent of 'immediate' accidental deaths; this would now be regarded as a clear contradiction in terms. Apart from a possible association with medical negligence, the clinical syndrome, which generally develops only following a latent period after injury of some 24 hours, has no major medicolegal importance. It will not be discussed in this chapter; the interested reader is referred particularly to the definitive work by Sevitt.[32]

It is intended rather to consider the interpretation of the pathological findings from the forensic aspect. In this context, bone marrow embolism (BME)—i.e. the presence of recognizable particulate bone marrow in the vessels—is inseparable from fat embolism. Some of the principles discussed could be applied to other tissues—e.g. liver—but while such conditions do occur, they are so rare as to have only minimal forensic interest.

Fat emboli can be discovered in the lungs—pulmonary FE—or in the tissues supplied by the major circulation—systemic FE—of which the brain and the renal glomeruli are the most constantly affected. It is imperative that this anatomical distinction, which is fundamental to the forensic applications, be made clear in any discussion. Systemic bone marrow embolism has been reported (see below) but must be extremely rare; for all practical purposes, BME is a pulmonary phenomenon.

Some attempt at quantification of pulmonary fat embolism is also essential to its understanding. An acceptable, and at the same time simple, system is not easy to achieve. The author has used a grading based on the ease of discovery of emboli in frozen sections stained with Oil Red O;[17] the classification adopted is shown in Table 20.1. The

Table 20.1 A simple classification of pulmonary fat embolism⋆

Grade 0	No emboli found
Grade 1	Emboli found after some searching
Grade 2	Emboli easily found
Grade 3	Emboli present in large numbers
Grade 4	Emboli present in potentially fatal numbers

⋆ Based on the microscopic appearances in Oil Red O stained sections.

subjectivity of the method is obvious and it fails to allow for variations in technique; it is, however, useful in practice, particularly in making the important distinction between grade 1 and grade 2 appearances. No similar grading of systemic fat embolism has been used; emboli are generally either widespread in the brain and/or kidney or they are found only after much searching. Table 20.2 shows the attempt at quantification of pulmonary bone marrow embolism made during the same study. This is of far less significance. All authors agree that the incidence of pulmonary embolism by fragments of body tissue depends greatly upon the avidity with which it is sought—'we see what we look for'.[8] The failure to discover bone marrow emboli may be no more than an artefact of block selection—a particularly disappointing conclusion in so far as the medicolegal significance of a single embolus is similar to that which can be attributed to the presence of many. It will be seen later that marked positivity for BME tends to correlate with grade 3 FE but the relationship is uncertain and is largely of restricted academic interest.

Interpretation of the pathological appearances is essentially a problem of fat embolism; much confusion in this respect has arisen from the failure of observers to quantify their findings. Fat emboli discovered in

Table 20.2 A method of indexing the severity of pulmonary bone marrow embolism⋆

Each slide examined gets a 'score' (s) allocated as follows:

Equivocal but acceptable	1 point
Positive 1–2 emboli	2 points
Positive 3–5 emboli	4 points
Positive 6 + emboli	6 points

$$\text{Index of embolism severity} = \frac{(s_1 + s_2 \ldots + s_n) \times 5}{n}$$

Where n = number of slides examined.
A score of 1–4 = mildly positive;
5 and above = markedly positive.

⋆ The figure 5 is chosen because that was the number of slides examined in normal circumstances during the study.

the lungs may be incidental only or they may be the result of disease affecting the body fat depots; in either case, they are likely to be few in number. Alternatively, they may be considered as markers of ante-mortem trauma when the quantitative relationship might be expected to be variable. Finally, the emboli could be present in such numbers as to be fundamentally related to the cause of death. These distinctions must be taken into account when attributing medicolegal significance to the findings.

Origins of fat emboli

Pulmonary fat embolism has been associated aetiologically with injury from the time it was first described. There is, however, evidence that it may occur in other circumstances.

Some pulmonary fat embolism can be found in a proportion of routine autopsies in which death was apparently not connected with violence. The reported incidence varies according to the source of the material; in the author's unselected series, it was 20 per cent.[17] All observers agree, however, that the emboli are few in number; greater degrees discovered in 'hospital' post-mortem material are almost always associated with surgery involving damage to adipose tissue—the only grade 3 case in the series quoted followed radical mastectomy.

Specific diseases have been incriminated as producing fat emboli. Other than those which are likely to disrupt fat depots—for example, osteomyelitis and gas gangrene—these are mostly associated with abnormalities of lipid storage or metabolism; diabetes, pancreatitis and chronic alcoholism are the most obvious. There is certainly a possibility that a few emboli may be shed from a grossly fatty liver but the concept that this can be of significant degree has received little support; some recent experimental work has suggested an indirect association between the liver and the production of emboli through the medium of unstable hepatic lipoproteins.[21]

Burning is also said to be associated with the presence of emboli. The present author has been unable to confirm this in persons dying rapidly in conflagrations. Sevitt,[32] whose experience in this field must be unique, found emboli in 37 per cent of fatal cases; moderate numbers were found only once out of 43 instances. It could be that persons dying in hospital after treatment present a different picture from those dying immediately.

It is possible that day-to-day trauma to the soft tissues is responsible for minor degrees of pulmonary fat embolism but, again, it is unlikely that *significant* embolism can be produced from simple damage to adipose tissue.[37]

Systemic fat embolism in the absence of trauma must be excessively rare. It has been reported as occurring in chronic alcoholics and has even been suggested as a possible cause of alcoholic psychosis.[16] The only non-injurious condition in which it occurs with relative constancy is the rare syndrome of post-decompression[17] or, better, post-descent[9] shock; the nature of this condition has considerable bearing on the pathogenesis of systemic fat embolism due to trauma and it is discussed later.

It cannot be over-emphasized that the pulmonary findings discussed thus far relate to trivial degrees of embolism (grade 1 in Table 20.1). When the more gross forms are considered (grade 2 or greater), only injury to bone—and particularly fracture—has an authentic correlation with pulmonary fat embolism; it is logical to suppose that the embolic fat comes from the local source of traumatized marrow.

It is well known that this simple concept was opposed with surprising success by Lehman and Moore in 1927.[15] These authors believed that the emboli were derived from the normal plasma fat and represented the products of chylomicron aggregation. Despite the widespread attention given to this theory, the protagonists were unable to produce experimental proof save through the addition of ether to plasma *in vitro*. Moreover, the theoretical objections raised to a local origin of embolic fat, which were based largely on quantification of the fat available in the bone and present in the lungs, were later challenged.[22] Variations on this theme, including attempts to relate post-traumatic lipaemia to the production of emboli, have been proposed from time to time but, while their relevance is less certainly defined as regards systemic embolism, they cannot explain the primary pulmonary condition. There seems no doubt that the early workers did not distinguish between true embolic particles and a sudanophil plasma.

There is very adequate clinicopathological and experimental evidence[14, 32, 33, 37] that significant pulmonary fat embolism is due almost exclusively to bony injury and that the emboli come from the injured part. No other mechanism would explain the vast preponderance of pulmonary over systemic embolism in fatal violent deaths with negligible survival time—indeed, no other theory would account for the presence of *any* embolic fat in these circumstances; the same applies to the rapid appearance of emboli during orthopaedic operations of a relatively localized nature or those involving rib traction. Perhaps the local origin of fat is most strongly indicated by the very frequent concurrence of pulmonary bone marrow emboli, the origin of which cannot be in doubt. Bone marrow emboli were found in 81 per cent of cases showing grade 2 or more fat embolism in the author's series of cases.[19] These results have been confirmed more recently in other centres.[3, 11]

There is, therefore, every reason to suppose that pulmonary fat and bone marrow emboli can be used as markers of bony injury in life and that this may be their main forensic application. The precise conditions which affect their significance must be considered.

Pulmonary embolism as a marker of ante-mortem violence

The relatively obvious theory as to the medicolegal value of the finding is shown in Fig. 20.1. The present concern is to distinguish post-mortem

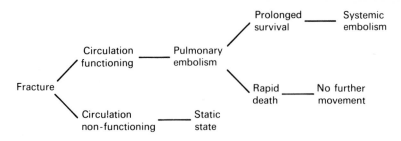

Fig. 20.1   Theoretical evaluation of tissue metabolism as a marker of ante-mortem violence.

injury from that inflicted only a short time before death. The occurrence of emboli in those who have survived to be treated in hospital is not relevant; the most appropriate study involves those dying at, or nearly at, the scene of the accident.

The author has previously published such a survey of aircraft accidents;[19] the results of this are summarized in the succeeding paragraphs.

Incidence of emboli
Taking aviation fatalities as a whole, significant—that is, easily discernible—pulmonary fat embolism is present in 37 per cent of those showing fractures, and bone marrow embolism in 33 per cent. This last figure, which, with the exception of a more recent paper,[12] is higher than has been reported elsewhere in accidental death, results from the usual examination of five slides from each case. Although there is no essential forensic significance in the degree of bone marrow embolism —one embolus is theoretically as indicative of ante-mortem injury as are several—there is a correlation between the degree of FE and that of BME. Ten per cent of cases showing grade 1 fat embolism were positive for bone marrow and in none of these was the latter of major proportion; at the other extreme, 93 per cent of grade 3 fat embolism cases showed bone marrow embolism and 62 per cent of these were described as major (Table 20.3). The occurence of emboli was modified by several factors.

Number of fractures
Surprisingly, it was found that the incidence of embolism fell with the degree of bony injury; this was very evident when long bone fractures and rib fractures were considered (Table 20.4). Sevitt[32] had previously found a close positive correlation between the severity of bony injury and the severity of pulmonary embolism and had used the finding as evidence of the local origin of the embolic fat. This represented the only major discrepancy between Mason[17] and Sevitt who, publishing

Table 20.3 Correlation of pulmonary fat and bone marrow embolism in 400 cases of death involving fracture of bone

Grade of FE	Total cases	No. +ve for BME			Maj./Min.	% +ve for BME
		Total	Minor	Major		
0	148	0	0	0	—	0
1	103	10	10	0	0	10
2	92	68	41	27	0·66	74
3–4	57	53	20	33	1·65	93
Totals	400	131	71	60		33

their findings simultaneously, had otherwise achieved remarkable agreement. The explanation lies in the nature of the fatalities—Sevitt's cases survived for comparatively long periods in hospital whereas Mason's died very rapidly; in the latter series, therefore, the extent of the injury would probably do no more than reflect an inverse relationship with the length of the agonal period.

Length of the agonal period
The precise time to die is difficult to establish in accidental deaths, particularly when these occur far from assistance as was usually the case in the aviation accidents. Nevertheless, a good correlation with the degree of embolism was observed when the agonal period was divided into immediate death, survival for minutes and survival for hours on the basis of the circumstantial evidence. Of the immediate deaths, 24 per cent showed significant pulmonary fat embolism and 21 per cent bone marrow embolism; all those surviving for hours showed widespread FE, and 87 per cent showed BME. Clearly, the longer the interval between injury and death, the greater was the chance of a positive finding; nevertheless, emboli were produced with sufficient speed to identify between one-quarter and one-fifth of those persons who were alive at the moment of sustaining severe, rapidly fatal injury, including injury to bone.

Table 20.4 Pulmonary embolism in the presence of long bone and rib fractures

	Long bone fractures		Rib fractures	
	1 or none	6, 7 or 8	6 or less	7 or more
Total cases	97	119	143	238
Percentage FE grades 2–4	62	9	71	16
Percentage +ve for BME	57	3	67	11

An interesting anomaly became apparent in the series—the longer the survival period beyond 5 hours, the less was bone marrow embolism evident despite the continuing presence of severe fat embolism (Table 20.5). This finding was not new and served only to confirm results from earlier and smaller series analysed by Sevitt.[2,8] The evidence strongly suggests that there is a rapid resorption of bone marrow em-

Table 20.5 Pulmonary embolism and the interval between injury and death

	Significant fat (%)	Bone marrow (%)
'Immediate' death	24	21
Minutes	78	77
Hours	100	87
More than 24 hours	100	50

boli from the lungs; indeed, the finding of severe FE in the absence of BME indicates positively a prolonged agonal period. No modern observers seem to have been able to confirm the contention by, for example, Rappaport et al.[28] that marked bone marrow embolism can be found in the absence of fat embolism following trauma uncomplicated by disease. The author has noted such a tendency only in those cases of pulmonary marrow and fat embolism which result from effective postmortem external cardiac massage accompanied by stress forces on the ribs.

Cardiovascular competence
If the theoretical basis of this medicolegal sign is correct, there should be a positive association between pulmonary embolism and competence of the cardiovascular system.

Table 20.6 Pulmonary embolism and competence of the cardiovascular system (CVS)

	Fat embolism			Bone marrow embolism		
	Grades 0–1 (No.)	Grades 2–4 (No.)	(%)	Absent (No.)	Present (No.)	% +ve
Laceration of atria, ventricles and/or aorta (total no. = 219)	190	29	13	199	20	9
Major CVS intact (total no. = 181)	61	120	66	70	111	61

In some 14 per cent of those showing CVS rupture, only the atria were involved. There was a strong possibility of several moments of injury in many of the fatal accidents, e.g. those involving inflight escape attempts.

This proved to be the clear trend (Table 20.6). Of the aircraft accident fatalities examined, 13 per cent showed significant pulmonary fat embolism when the cardiovascular system was damaged, as compared with 66 per cent in those whose circulation was intact.

The evidence therefore indicates that pulmonary fat and bone marrow embolism are associated with fracture—or, at least, trauma to bone —and that the appearance of particles in the lungs is dependent upon a combination of a competent circulation and the time for which that circulation continued after injury. There is a *prima facie* case for regarding pulmonary fat and bone marrow emboli as acceptable markers of ante-mortem injury.

Relative merits of fat and bone marrow embolism in forensic work

In reaching similar conclusions, Sevitt[32] made two important provisos: first, that pulmonary fat emboli must be present in significant numbers and, second, that there must be evidence from their shape that the emboli had reached the lungs under pressure—i.e. that they were 'moulded' rather than appearing as simple globules. It is also important that the very real hazards of technical artefact should be eliminated.

It is tempting to suggest that, by contrast, bone marrow emboli will provide totally objective evidence of ante-mortem violence. Against this view must be balanced the problem of sensitivity. Although no special histological techniques are required for their demonstration, bone marrow emboli are far harder to find than are those due to fat—there is no immediately obvious contrast in their staining properties in haematoxylin and eosin sections and not all particles contain Oil Red O positive material. Experience has shown that, to achieve anything approaching a guarantee of a positive finding in all 'positive' cases, a minimum of three lung sections must be examined on a square search basis; this is time consuming and false negatives cannot be excluded with certainty. It follows that specificity can be obtained only at the expense of sensitivity—approximately 12 per cent of cases of rapid accidental death showing significant fat embolism are, in practice, negative for bone marrow embolism.

The specificity of BME has also been recently denied.[12] Norwegian workers have claimed that pulmonary bone marrow emboli are present in 8·3 per cent of random autopsy material in which there has been no bone involvement in life. They considered it probable that bone marrow embolism is a natural event and concluded that emboli could no longer be considered of medicolegal consequence. It is disappointing that this study, which produced what must be regarded as unusual results, was not undertaken in parallel with an evaluation of fat embolism. There is some additional evidence from the author's own material to indicate that the specific relationship between BME and fracture is not absolute. Out of 22 aircraft accident fatalities in whom fractures were not demonstrated at post-mortem, 4 showed both fat and bone marrow emboli in the lungs. None of these cases was examined by X-ray and all had been subjected to severe crash forces; they could, therefore, be accepted as instances of ante-mortem trauma as opposed to ante-mortem fracture but, nevertheless, have to be regarded as anomalous.

Weighing up the evidence and taking all these factors into account, it is concluded that grade 2 fat embolism represents an effective way in practice of indicating ante-mortem violence to bone. The finding of bone marrow emboli is strongly corroborative of that interpretation but, when using this parameter, one must be prepared for false negative results and, with less certainty, for an occasional false positive.

Importance of the emboli discovered

If pulmonary fat and bone marrow emboli are to be regarded as true indicators of life at the time of injury, their finding will be of medicolegal importance in three main areas.

In the criminal sphere, the presence of emboli should clearly differentiate between the body which was injured in life and one which was traumatized during the process of disposal. Thus, it should be possible in bodies recovered from the water to distinguish fracture due to post-mortem buffeting from those inflicted before immersion; emboli may be found even in the presence of considerable putrefaction.[18] The distinction of post-mortem fire fractures from true injury may be equally important in the case of bodies recovered from conflagrations.

There are two interesting aspects associated with civil litigation. First, many life insurance policies are effected against accidental death and carry very high benefits in relation to premium; the pathologist therefore has an essential duty to decide upon the role of any disease state discovered at autopsy. The precise wording of the agreement may be important—in some instances, benefits may not be payable if death, although due to accidental injury, was precipitated by disease. Nevertheless, the finding of pulmonary emboli in, say, an automobile accident, is tenable evidence that, at least, the victim was not dead before the crash. This observation may be of fundamental importance to insurers and beneficiaries alike but, even so, it may still be questioned whether death was ultimately due to injury or to disease; an opinion would have to be based on the nature and extent of each.

Second, embolic phenomena may be used in the solution of *commorientes* or disposal of estates in the event of apparently simultaneous death. The importance of the pathological evidence in this situation is emphasized in Chapter 4. Two particular caveats as to interpretation must be stressed. In the first place, quantitative comparisons are seldom valid in indicating either the extent of injury or the duration of the agonal period; differences between the subjects are indicated only by presence of emboli on the one hand and absence on the other. Secondly, any attempt to interpret the agonal period through the study of emboli presupposes that there has been no attempt at external cardiac massage. Resuscitation is frequently accompanied by rib fracture and always by mechanical strain on sternum and ribs; if it is effective, a circulation is simultaneously established. The presence of emboli would then be an expected post-mortem artefact, the occurrence of which has been well documented.[30,38]

Systemic fat embolism
Systemic bone marrow embolism can, for practical purposes, be ignored; it has been very occasionally reported as occurring but the finding is so uncommon as to be without forensic significance.

Systemic fat embolism, on the other hand, is important as an actual cause of death. A 'pulmonary syndrome' undoubtedly occurs but is essentially a condition of the elderly and previously infirm. Pulmonary fat embolism *may* be fatal in such persons—witness the high incidence of severe symptoms in those undergoing total hip replacement;[13] the literature also contains reports of six unusual deaths attributed to pulmonary bone marrow embolism, which are summarized by Pyun.[27] In general, however, systemic involvement is essential to the diagnosis of the full-blown clinical syndrome and, certainly, to its autopsy diagnosis.

Systemic embolism is extremely rare in very rapid deaths—the author has seen only two cases; a traumatic interatrial communication had been established in both. Clinical symptoms associated with systemic spread are typically delayed for about 24 hours. Thus, while asymptomatic pulmonary fat embolism is almost invariable following injury to bone, clinical manifestations are uncommon; it is of obvious medicolegal significance to establish what transforms the innocuous pulmonary condition to the potentially fatal systemic state.

Attempts have been made to invoke a simple pathway for emboli through natural arteriovenous connections. Pulmonary shunts have been proposed as the route taken by such emboli[26] but, if these connections are always present, one might question why systemic embolism should be so rare. The significance of a patent foramen ovale is referred to later; for the present it need only be noted that fatal cases of fat embolism are commonly seen in persons with an intact interatrial septum—a defect may facilitate but is not essential to the process. It is far easier to conceive simply of a build-up of hydrostatic pressure in the lungs so that, eventually, the fat is squeezed through the arterioles as they become increasingly blocked. Such a theory would explain the delayed onset; it would correlate with the observation that manipulations—which would be expected to produce further showers of emboli—predispose to the clinical syndrome and persuasive experimental evidence of its validity has been produced.[10] It is also found that the occurrence of cerebral fat embolism is proportional to the pulmonary concentration.[7] The difficulty in accepting the concept lies in the fact that, far from maintaining a satisfactory cardiac output, the patient developing clinical fat embolism is almost invariably in a state of shock; this objection is supported by experimental work.[34]

Pulmonary induced hypoxia has been suggested as an important precipitant by some[29,35] but has been denied by others.[1] Nevertheless, the concept of systemic fat embolism as being a concomitant of, or even the result of, hypovolaemic shock is gaining ground;[4,36] there may be an intimate association with intravascular coagulation.[24,31] Some evidence for a resultant relationship of systemic embolism to shock is to be found in its remarkable clinical similarity to the very rare condition of post-descent shock.[9,20] Numerous papers refer to the occurrence of systemic fat embolism during surgery requiring an extracorporeal circulation and the presence of bubbles in blood for transfusion has been suggested as a predisposing cause.[6] The experimental association of gas bubbles, microthrombi and fat emboli reported, *inter alia*, by Philp and his colleagues[25] is, therefore, of very great importance.

Post-descent shock and pathogenesis of systemic fat embolism

Fatal post-descent shock always was a very rare condition and is eliminated by modern aviation technology; the syndrome is, however, similar to cerebral fat embolism. A few apparently hypersusceptible individuals suffer a premonitory attack of decompression sickness at a height of some 8800 m (29 000 ft): they then pass into coma with or without a lucid interval and the mortality is very high. Post-descent shock and cerebral fat embolism are similar in the presence of skin manifestations, pyrexia, haemoconcentration and leucocytosis. At autopsy examination of 12 aviation cases, some degree of pulmonary fat embolism was almost invariable and well marked systemic embolism was found in 4, with equivocal emboli in a further 5 cases; the intensity of study was, however, by no means uniform. A patent foramen ovale was present far more often than would be expected by chance; again, however, cases occurred in which the septum was normal and it is possible that the apparent correlation reflects only on the care with which the examination was conducted.

The controversy surrounding the pathogenesis of post-descent shock has been as intense as has that concerning fat embolism and has followed much the same line—is the embolism the primary pathological trigger or is it the result of the severe accompanying shock? For many reasons, the present author is now persuaded that the latter is probably the case; the general similarity between the two conditions would then suggest that the same may be true of systemic fat embolism. If this be so—and it is by no means certain—the development of clinical fat embolism is essentially an unusual manifestation of severe surgical shock. The uncertainty lies, of course, in the reason for its invariable association with severe pulmonary fat embolism which clearly has a different pathogenesis. It is, therefore, perhaps true to say that the major medicolegal significance of systemic fat embolism is of a negative character—since its cause is unknown and its occurrence capricious, there can be no question of a relationship with medical negligence.

The suggestion that bubbles may form niduses for embolic particles in the blood has its greatest potential significance in the field of decompression and one wonders why fat embolism has been a feature of post-descent shock and not of death due to rapid ascent from increased atmospheric pressure. It is now reported (Chapter 17) that fat embolism is to be found in diving fatalities when it is sought. This observation may do much to clarify the understanding of these unusual deaths in aviators and divers. Meantime, it has obvious forensic importance as being an indication of the mode of death in diving fatalities which are becoming of increasing industrial concern.

References

1. Allardyce, D. B., Meek, R. N., Woodruff, B., Cassim, M. M. and Ellis, D. (1974). Increasing our knowledge of the pathogenesis of fat embolism: a prospective study of 43 patients with fractured femoral shafts. *J. Trauma* **14**, 955.
2. Armin, J. and Grant, R. T. (1951). Observations on gross pulmonary fat embolism in man and the rabbit. *Clin. Sci.* **10**, 441.
3. Bhaskaran, C. S., Reddy, A. S. and Rao, A. A. (1971). Pulmonary fat embolism in accident fatalities. *Indian J. Path. Bact.* **14**, 75.
4. Durst, J., Knodel, W., Heller, W., *et al.* (1973). Zur Lipasetheorie Kronkes und ihrer Bedeutung für die Pathogenese der posttraumatischen Fettembolie. *Mschr. Unfallheilk.* **76**, 193.
5. Eckert, W. G. (Ed.) (1974). *Literature Compilation on Fat Embolism*. Wichita: Inform.
6. Fadali, A. and Walstad, P. M. (1972). In-vacuo blood collection: a possible cause of fat emboli. *Surgery* **71**, 738.
7. Fischer, H. (1972). Pathologisch-anatomische Untersuchungen über Häufigkeit und Schwere der Fettembolie. *Actuel. Traumatol.* **2**, 197.
8. Fisher, J. H. (1951). Bone marrow embolism. *Arch. Path.* **52**, 315.
9. Fryer, D. I. (1969). *Subatmospheric Decompression Sickness in Man*. Agardograph no. 125. Slough; Technivision Services.
10. Gee, D. J. (1967). Cerebral fat embolism: its experimental production. *J. forensic Med.* **14**, 60.
11. Giusti, G. V. and Panari, G. (1971). Embolie polmonari di tessuto middolare. *Minerva med.-leg.* **91**, 52.
12. Havig, O. and Gruner, O. P. N. (1973). Pulmonary bone marrow embolism. *Acta path. microbiol. scand.* **81**, 276.
13. Jones, R. H. (1975). Physiologic emboli changes observed during total hip replacement arthroplasty. *Clin. Orthop.* **112**, 192.
14. Kerstell, J., Hallgren, B., Rudenstam, C. M. and Svanborg, A. (1969). The chemical composition of the fat emboli in the post-absorptive dog. *Acta med. scand.*, Suppl. **499**, 1.
15. Lehman, E. P. and Moore, R. M. (1927). Fat embolism including experimental production without trauma. *Arch. Surg.* **14**, 621.
16. Lynch, M. J. G., Raphael, S. S. and Dixon, T. P. (1959). Fat embolism in chronic alcoholism. *Arch. Path.* **67**, 68.

17. Mason, J. K. (1962). *Aviation Accident Pathology*, pp. 134, 146, 242. London: Butterworths.
18. Mason, J. K. (1965). The importance of the histological examination in death from accidental trauma. *Med. Serv. J. Can.* **21**, 316.
19. Mason, J. K. (1968). Pulmonary fat and bone marrow embolism as indicators of ante-mortem violence. *Med. Sci. Law* **8**, 200.
20. Mason, J. K. (1973). Death resulting from exposure to high altitude. In: *Aerospace Pathology*, Chap. 16. Eds J. K. Mason and W. J. Reals. Chicago: College of American Pathologists Foundation.
21. Pauley, S. M. and Cockett, A. T. K. (1970). Role of lipids in decompression sickness. *Aerospace Med.* **41**, 56.
22. Peltier, L. F. (1956). Fat embolism—1. The amount of fat in human long bones. *Surgery* **40**, 657.
23. Peters, G. (1942). Die Gehirnveränderungen bei stumpfer Gewalteinwirkung von vorn (auf die Stirn). *Luftfahrtmedizin* **7**, 344.
24. Philp, R. B., Gowdey, C. W. and Prasad, M. (1967). Changes in blood lipid concentration and cell counts following decompression sickness in rats and the influence of dietary lipid. *Canad. J. Physiol. Pharmacol.* **45**, 1047.
25. Philp, R. B., Inwood, M. J. and Warren, B. A. (1972). Interactions between gas bubbles and components of the blood: implications in decompression sickness. *Aerospace Med.* **43**, 946.
26. Prinzmetal, M., Ornitz, E. M., Simkin, B. and Bergman, H. C. (1948). Arteriovenous anastamoses in liver, spleen and lungs. *Amer. J. Physiol.* **152**, 48.
27. Pyun, K. S. and Katzenstein, R. E. (1972). Widespread bone marrow embolism with myocardial involvement. *Arch. Path.* **89**, 378.
28. Rappaport, H., Raum, M. and Horrell, J. B. (1951). Bone marrow embolism. *Amer. J. Path.* **27**, 407.
29. Ross, A. P. J. (1970). The fat embolism syndrome: with special reference to the importance of hypoxia in the syndrome. *Ann. roy. Coll. Surg.* **46**, 159.
30. Sack, K. and Wegener, F. (1968). Artifizielle postmortale Fettembolie. *Zbl. allg. Path. Anat.* **111**, 24.
31. Serck-Hanssen, A. (1965). Post-traumatic fat embolism. Red cell aggregation, hylaine microthrombi and platelet aggregates in 5 fatal cases. *Acta path. microbiol. scand.* **65**, 31.
32. Sevitt, S. (1962). *Fat Embolism*. London: Butterworths.
33. Sherr, S. and Gertner, S. B. (1974). Production and recovery of pulmonary fat emboli in dogs. *Exp. molec. Path.* **21**, 63.
34. Soloway, H. B., Hufnagel, H. V. and Huyser, K. L. (1969). Experimental fat embolism. *Arch. Path.* **88**, 171.
35. Szabo, G. (1970). The syndrome of fat embolism and its origin. *J. clin. Path.* **23**, Suppl. (Roy. Coll. Path.), **4**, 123.
36. Tedeschi, C. D., Walter, C. E. and Tedeschi, L. G. (1968). Shock and fat embolism: an appraisal. *Surg. Clin. N. Amer.* **48**, 431.

37. Watson, A. J. (1970). Genesis of fat emboli. *J. clin. Path.* **23**, Suppl. (Roy. Coll. Path.), **4**, 132.
38. Yanoff, M. (1963). Incidence of bone marrow embolism due to closed chest cardiac massage. *New Engl. J. Med.* **269**, 837.
39. Zenker, F. A. (1862). *Beiträge zur normalen und pathologischen Anatomie der Lunge*, p. 31. Dresden: Braunsdorf.

21

The psychopathological effects of violence

This chapter will deal with two psychological aspects of violence—first, psychological factors leading to violence, and then the psychological effects of violence and the interaction between aggressor and victim. It is important to make clear, however, that, of itself, violence is not a pathological phenomenon. Very occasionally, and only occasionally, it can be generated by a pathological process and it can produce pathology in the assaulted individual.

It may seem odd to suggest that an aspect of biology which produces so much pathology is not in itself pathological. The important consideration is, of course, pathological to whom? For the winner, a violent encounter may be one aspect of his success in dealing with his environment. It is only in very recent times that the use of violence has been questioned. Somebody else's violence to us has always been undesirable, even 'wrong', but warfare, violent punishments and the like have usually been regarded as necessary, often laudable, ways of maintaining social order.

It is often claimed that man is a particularly violent creature. This is probably not true in the sense that he fights particularly frequently. It is only true in the sense that he uses his special facility of high intelligence as much in violence as in all activities and he thereby increases his destructiveness. This very increase of destructiveness, which comes with technology, is probably the basis of our modern questioning of violence. With the aid of nuclear weapons, we are now capable of destroying all living things on Earth. The outcome of a fight when firearms are available is horrific and frequently goes far beyond the original intent.

The word 'violence' is usually used loosely, as if we all clearly understood its meaning. In fact, violence is a very diverse concept embracing boys fighting, warfare, corporal punishment, homicide, forceful sexual assault, baby battering, road accidents, football hooliganism, boxing and so on. Many of these forms of violence are situationally and individually specific. A baby batterer, for example, may be no good as a soldier and it is unlikely that boxers are especially prone to commit murder. Not all of these situations can be considered below and it should be remembered that generalizations cannot easily be made from specific illustrations.

It is absurd to look for *the* cause of violence, even if the type of violence is very clearly specified. Complex behaviour has complex origins. If we were to examine why a particular road accident took place at a particular time at a particular spot, we could be superficial and say that one of the cars had faulty brakes. Faulty brakes would indeed be an important factor but closer examination would reveal many others, such as poor visibility around a bend, a slippery road surface, loose steering in the other car, one fatigued driver, another partially intoxicated, and so on. This is not the place to delve into all the complexities behind violent behaviour—it has been done elsewhere;[16] attention is drawn, however, to some of the factors which are frequently involved in human violence—frustration, hatred, anger, paranoia, prejudice, animalization, training, other forms of learning, obedience, anomie, intoxication, disease, etc. Rarely, if ever, is one of these factors sufficient to produce a violent attack; it usually requires the coincidence of several, maybe many, before there is an outburst. If none of the factors predominates, or if the predominant one is misunderstood, then the so-called 'motiveless' attack occurs.

Role of the victim

One factor obviously missing from the above list is the victim. The choice of victim is rarely a chance matter although, sometimes, the reason can be far from obvious until the precipitating factors are understood. The usual victim of violence is a friend, a relative or some other person closely involved with the assailant. In Wolfgang's study of murder in Philadelphia,[41] only 12 per cent of murders were committed by strangers; in an analysis made in England and Wales[14] it was also found that most persons murdered, especially women and children, were the victims of spouses, lovers, relatives and friends. Similar patterns are also found in other violent crimes such as assault and rape.[27, 32]

It takes at least two to make a fight and an exact analysis of a violent event would need a review of the psychological and social factors affecting all the parties concerned. An example will illustrate the point. Mr A has a bad day at the office. For reasons he cannot control, his firm is losing money. This had made his boss irritable and Mr A is blamed, sometimes justly sometimes unjustly, for a series of mistakes. Mr A has never liked his boss but dare not respond too directly because he might lose his job. He had hoped to leave work on time but he is given a late task which delays him. He realizes that he is tense and he knows this may cause difficulties in the home, so he stops at the pub for a pint, or two . . . . When he finally arrives home, he finds his wife in considerable agitation. She has had a bad day herself, one of the children is ill and she needs to talk about it but, in trying to get things off her chest, she has had a row on the telephone with her mother and now feels very guilty. Mr A's late homecoming has alarmed her. Has he had an accident, has he finally run off as he has been threatening lately? When he arrives he has clearly been drinking, enjoying himself and ignoring her. As dinner is put on the table, he asks her whether she has remembered to phone the gas company. She has not; an argument ensues which quickly breaks into a shouting match. Eventually in fury she throws an empty tea-cup at him and he does something he used to see his father do a great deal—he loses self-control, knocking his wife across the room so that she receives a black eye and a cut arm.

At the hospital she is regarded as a potential battered wife and he as an aggressive man. Both are correct assessments but the incident needs more understanding. Several factors have been involved—frustration, fear, hatred (of the boss—perhaps temporarily displaced to the wife), alcohol, learning. More importantly, the choice of victim, whilst not directly related to some of the causative factors, is not random; she played her part in this commonplace drama.

Even in rape, where an assailant might be expected to choose a partner as randomly as possible, it seems that this is not often the case. In an American study, Amir[1] found that white men usually chose white women and black men black women, and that over one-third of all rapes were between acquaintances; one-fifth of the victims had police records themselves. Even in the apparently totally casual rape the victim may remind the assailant of some despised woman such as his mother.[28] The interaction between assailant and victim is again of importance. A rapist on the author's files, seeking distorted revenge for being jilted, carried out three attacks on strangers. Each time he attacked it was with a knife on a dark common. The first woman screamed, fought him, ran faster than he could and escaped with a severe fright and a cut hand. The second woman struck a terrorized bargain with him in which she offered to masturbate him; he agreed. The third woman agreed to intercourse, sat talking with him about his distress afterwards and persuaded him to go to the police. Clearly, the response of the women to the situation was critical in determining the outcome.

This observation should not surprise us. When animals of other species fight, the victim or loser can stop the contest by submitting or giving in and there is usually a well defined signal system concerning this between the contestants.[38] A goose, for example, stretches out its neck in a vulnerable way so that the victor could strike and kill; it does not, but the loser retreats. One of man's unique difficulties may be related to this phenomenon. We are very weak fighters without our technology surrounding us; it is difficult for a naked man to kill another in the same state. Perhaps we have not evolved a very effective submission signalling system because it has not been a biological necessity. Suddenly, in terms of evolution, we have developed highly lethal weapons. Maybe we are prepared to use these on one another to the detriment of our species because we have no deep-rooted and effective surrender mechanism. We can also kill at a distance (e.g. by dropping bombs) so that another person's surrender signals could not even reach us.

Morris and Blom-Cooper[33] summed up the victim's contribution to murder quite bluntly and vividly in their *Calendar of Murder*. Heterosexual relationships can sometimes be fraught with potential violence. 'Desdemona, had she been unloved by Othello, might have lived,' they tell us. A cornered burglar may panic, especially if the householder defends his property vigorously, and he may inflict severe injuries. The murder 'out of the blue', in which a victim is struck down without reacting in any way, is a rarity; almost invariably there are words or actions which precipitate the killer into greater force than was intended. Morris and Blom-Cooper believed that disastrous consequences could more often be avoided if calmness always prevailed when assault was threatened; they accepted this as a pious counsel of perfection because victims, like attackers, are human beings and, as such, are only partly able to control their behaviour.

Effects on the victim

When we consider the amount of supposed concern about the problem of violence, it is really quite staggering how little we really know of its psychological and social consequences. Perhaps this is because violence has only become a subject of real scientific interest in recent years, certainly within this century. Whatever the reason, the fact must be accepted that long-term follow-up studies of the victims of violence are not available. Systematic studies of the short-term psychological effects of violence are also missing. We are in an extraordinary state of civilized development. When violence occurs we preoccupy ourselves, reasonably enough, with preventing further incidents; but we then go on to discuss what harmful things, including further violence, can be done to the perpetrators without offering any substantial psychological or social assistance to the victim. In recent years, the British Parliament has debated the issue of capital punishment at length; it does not devote the same degree of attention to the subject of help for victims. Our collective ignorance of this problem unfortunately makes me fall back on analogies, anecdotes and clinical experience for the discussion of the psychological effects of violence on the victim.

The first important effects of violence are physical and it is with these that this book is largely concerned. Here it is intended to emphasize that physical damage can include brain damage. Many battered babies, for example, end up with permanent brain damage. In a recent survey of epileptic prisoners,[17] one or two men were found who claimed that their brain dysfunction, and hence their fits, related to assaults from their parents when they were children. Kempe *et al.*[22] reported in their classic paper on 302 battered children. Of these, 33 had died and 85 had suffered permanent brain injury; they noted that 'subdural haematoma with or without fracture of the skull is ... an extremely frequent finding'. Clearly any victim of violence is a potential victim of brain damage. The effects of brain damage are complex and are dealt with in more detail in Chapter 12. For present purposes, it is stressed that psychological damage can follow brain injury and that this damage can manifest itself in many ways. The epileptic group of prisoners referred to above did not have a particularly high quota of violent offences when compared with other prisoners but some of them had been violent and, in one or two cases, the disinhibiting effects of the brain damage—especially to the frontal lobes—seemed to be an important factor in that violence. An important collection of Second World War brain injury cases at Oxford has proved a fruitful source for the study of the later effects of brain damage. Jarvie[21] described six cases of penetrating brain wound in which 'disinhibition' occurred after involvement of the frontal lobes. One man was changed from 'shy' and 'not interested in sex' to 'garrulous', 'immodest', and 'constantly talking about sex'. A quiet but ambitious man lost control of his sexual behaviour after his injury and was convicted for indecent exposure. Lishman[24] studied the same material and has shown that brain damage plays a part in the genesis of a wide range of psychiatric problems. He demonstrated that both the depth and the quantity of brain damage each make an independent contribution to psychiatric disability. He also found a clear relationship between severity of psychiatric disability (a composite of intellectual, behavioural and emotional disturbances) and temporal lobe damage. However, affective disorders, behavioural disorders and somatic complaints were all more frequent after frontal lobe damage in the 21 per cent of the cases who showed severe post-traumatic disturbances.

While it is true that almost no follow-ups have been carried out on victims of criminal violence, there have been one or two surveys of the psychological effects of natural disasters and of warfare. Such disasters are important in their own right; they may even give clues to the psychological effects of all forms of violence but extrapolations have to be drawn with caution because interpersonal violence is preceded by emotional conflict which may significantly affect the aftermath of violence.

Two major surveys of the psychiatric health of the civilian population were carried out during the Second World War.[3,23] Both these studies suggested that, if the war produced a rise in psychiatric ill-health, then that rise was a minimal one. However, it was shown that Londoners suffered a considerable increase in peptic ulceration during the bombing.[31] It is physical disorder which seems to be the long-term result of this kind of stress—as, indeed, it is after bereavement.[35] Bennet[2] conducted an investigation into the health of people in Bristol who had suffered flooding two years previously. The floods caused no deaths but 3000 properties were flooded, many to a depth of 1·8–2·1 m (6–7 ft). It was found that, when compared with a matched non-flooded group, there was a 50 per cent increase in the number of deaths among those whose homes had been flooded, with a conspicuous rise in deaths from cancer. Surgery attendances rose by 53 per cent; referrals to hospital and hospital admissions were more than doubled. A study of Belfast by Lyons[26] has suggested that the violent troubles there have actually reduced the level of psychiatric illness. He came to this conclusion after noting that psychiatric referrals from the badly affected areas have fallen, but, of course, other factors—such as anxious people moving away or being too afraid to make excursions to the psychiatric outpatients' clinic—may account for this fall. Fraser[11] had previously shown that there was no increase in the psychiatric referral rate when areas of Belfast were affected by riots but there was a considerable increase in the number of prescriptions for tranquillizers. Lyons himself[25] had also previously noted that when patients were affected by the riots they usually developed acute anxiety states.

Perhaps, then, we should look at some of the anecdotal and clinical material which is available in relation to disasters. 'Acute anxiety state' is not very descriptive of what an individual feels although it may indicate to the doctor that large doses of tender loving care, plus small doses of sedatives, will suffice while the natural healing processes take place. Following the Summerland disaster on the Isle of Man, two patients had to be admitted to hospital because of their emotional distress and many others showed symptoms such as persistent vomiting, urinary incontinence and mental withdrawal.[18] Tucker and Lettin[39] described the effects of a bomb explosion on 37 casualties; 4 of these had symptoms such as anxiety, agoraphobia and hysterical deafness. All improved with reassurance and tranquillizers. Wolfenstein[40] has attempted to describe the effects of disaster in detailed psychoanalytic terms. She draws attention to the 'disaster syndrome' in which individuals are described by themselves and by others as 'shocked', 'stunned' or 'dazed'. People showed little outward emotion at earthquakes or following the A-bomb attacks on Japan or after the Worcester tornado. A witness at Hiroshima described 'the silence in the grove by the river, where hundreds of gruesomely wounded suffered together ... The hurt ones were quiet; no one wept, much less screamed in pain; no one complained; none of the many who died did so noisily; not even the children cried; very few people even spoke'. Wolfenstein suggests that the disaster victim has been forced to take in more than he can assimilate and there is a compensatory resistance to taking in any more stimuli; hence the insensitivity of the disaster victim to what is going on around him. The unawareness of wounds is another denial, as is fainting which may occur in the impact of the disaster or sometimes days later as the overwhelming nature of the disaster threatens to emerge into consciousness. Wolfenstein goes on to suggest that panic is a reaction to disaster which is frequently anticipated but rarely encountered. It seems to occur when the way to safety seems so close at hand but the escape route is found to be partially or totally blocked. Being trapped, she suggests, rouses intense terror and this, in turn, may impair judgement; for example, seamen on a burning ship have sometimes jumped into water covered with flaming oil and burned to death.

Wolfenstein's next point is that an experience of extreme danger is not over once the danger is past, even for those who survive it intact. 'Following a catastrophic event people are apt to find themselves forced to relive it over and over again in memory.' An alternative mental process is suppression or amnesia (partial or complete) for the event. Usually, people recover psychologically from disasters. But this does not always happen, and agitated depression, excessive preoccupation and unjustified guilt feelings may all persist. Indeed, according to Wolfenstein, a feeling that it may all happen again is a fairly common reaction, while anxiety at separation from loved ones is intensified.

Rape victims seem to comprise one of the few categories of sufferers from individual violence who have been subjected to any sort of psychological study. Fox and Scherl[10] described three phases following a rape attack: the acute reaction lasting several days in which there is shock, dismay, disbelief and fear; the outward adjustment phase when denial, suppression, and rationalization take place; and, finally, integration when there may be depression, guilty feelings, a desire to talk or feelings of being damaged or unclean. These workers suggested that the professional can help the rape victim by understanding these phases and going through a routine of (1) medical attention, (2) legal and police contacts, (3) notification of family and friends, (4) dealing with current practical matters, (5) clarifying the factual details, (6) daily guidance if possible, steering between simple passive listening and too active an intervention, and (7) psychiatric consultation—usually a routine requiring only occasional active assessment or treatment. Greer[15] believes that nightmares, depression, pathological shyness, or inability to leave the house, a terror of darkness and attempted suicide are all possible consequences of rape. Clearly these possibilities must be borne in mind as the consequences of any assault. Cohn[7] has drawn attention to a special problem—the sexual act may be perpetrated by terror and the victim left with little or no sign of struggle or resistance; this should not persuade observers that no rape was committed or that the psychological concomitants will not follow. Burgess and Holmstrom[5,6] have set up a counselling service for rape victims and have studied 92 victims. They have described a 'rape trauma syndrome' which they classify into an acute or disorganization phase characterized by emotional reactions of various kinds, tension symptoms together with feelings of guilt and humiliation and a long-term or reorganization phase during which the victim readjusts her life as far as possible; she sometimes moves house* and may complain of nightmares and various phobias during this phase.

As already emphasized, the commonest forms of violence in peacetime are sexual and domestic. A good account of the worst effects of domestic violence has been given by Pizzey[36] in her account of the refuge for battered wives she has set up in Chiswick. She describes the terror many of the women live through and the disturbances, particularly aggressive behaviour, which are manifest in their children. 'Anyone who has been badly knocked about loses all sense of reality and ability to cope. Battered women are almost permanently in a shocked state. The constant fear of another beating leaves them very

---

* She may, indeed, be forced to do so by the reaction of friends of a convicted assailant—*Ed.*

tense and nervous. Some can't eat, others sleep little. Even the toughest find it hard to fight off the depression which has overwhelmed (them).' Gayford[13] has interviewed 100 of these severely battered women at Chiswick. He found that, apart from trauma, 18 were suffering from chronic physical illness. The majority attended their general practitioner frequently and 71 were taking antidepressants or tranquillizers. A psychiatric opinion was sought for 46 wives; 21 were told that they were depressed and were treated with either drugs or ECT. Thirty-four attempted suicide by poisoning, 7 mutilated themselves and 9 harmed themselves in other ways. All workers draw attention to the shame, rather like that noticed in the rape victim, which these women experience. They feel in some way responsible for the assaults and they try to hide the facts, even from their doctor, saying that they fell over or had a trivial accident. Fonseka,[9] examining 88 women attending a casualty department for injuries following domestic violence, found them to be in acute distress but they changed their stories about the injuries as the initial shock wore off and they rationalized the event more and more as it receded; 25 per cent of this sample had had previous injuries and 25 per cent were being treated for 'depression'.

A Parliamentary Select Committee[19] has recently begun an investigation into the problem of violence in marriage. Among other recommendations they suggest that each large urban area should have a well publicized family crisis centre continuously open (see also Gunn[16]) and that medical schools and nursing colleges should give special attention to the social dynamics of family life and to the medical—both physical and psychiatric—correlates of marital disharmony.

The increasing interest in domestic violence shown by the medical profession began with the so-called 'battered baby syndrome'. One of the most remarkable features of the battered baby story is that it was overlooked as a problem until 1946 although injured children must have been attending doctors for hundreds of years. Most of the literature has concentrated on the physical and social aspects of baby battering but, in 1966, Galdston[12] reported his psychiatric observations on children who had been physically abused ranging in age from 3 months to $3\frac{1}{2}$ years. He noticed that some of the children showed extreme fright upon all and any contact, others were apathetic to the point of apparent stupor as they lay or sat about motionless, devoid of facial expression and unresponsive to all attempts at evoking recognition. Pizzey noticed that children subjected to violence, either directly or vicariously, were seriously disturbed—boys were especially aggressive and destructive, breaking walls, stoning puppies, fighting and sometimes needing exclusion from school. Observations such as these lead to a consideration of what might be the long-term psychological effects of baby battering on the individual. There have been no really long-term follow-up studies published yet but Martin,[30] in a 3-year follow-up study, has reported that one-third of all the babies failed to thrive and that many showed significant delays in language development. MacKeith[29] has reviewed this subject recently and speculates that 'non-accidental injury' may account for 6 per cent of new cerebral palsy cases each year. He quotes Elmer and Gregg[8] as indicating that only a few out of 20 abused children gave promise of becoming self-sufficient adults. MacKeith drew attention to the general belief that many battering parents were themselves maltreated as little children and this is certainly supported by other workers.[37] 'Hence,' he argues, 'one late sequel of NAI (Non Accidental Injury) is that the child who has had NAI is at high risk for injuring his or her own child. This risk is largely the consequence of the deprivation or maltreatment, but any person with brain injury is probably more vulnerable to untoward environmental stresses.' Martin also reviewed the literature on this point and came to the same conclusion; in his own work he has sometimes been able to trace a pattern of violence through three or four generations.

Effects on the family

Plainly, the individual victim is the main point of concern after a violent episode but the effects of the episode on the family should not be disregarded. Burgess and Holmstrom[4, 5, 6] described the difficulties some women have in resuming normal sexual relationships after a rape attack and, indeed, the difficulties some men have in accepting their sexual partners back again after they have been raped. The most obvious problem for the family is the horror and shock they sustain when one of their number has been attacked. This is particularly pronounced when the victim dies. First, there are all the usual effects of bereavement such as intense anguish, somatic symptoms, feelings of disbelief and unreality and identification with the victim—sometimes amounting to suicidal ideas.[34, 35] In addition, there are the special problems peculiar to the homicide situation in which another human being is clearly culpable and is the focus of anger and aggression. Burgess[4] has also studied this kind of victim reaction. She again divided the phenomena following the homicide into an acute phase and a reorganization phase, and she stressed the intense fear which is sometimes engendered in the families of victims so that they may develop phobias (e.g. about not letting people walk behind them); they may buy guns and burglar alarms, and they may require sedatives. She noted that a homicide family may be deliberately or unwittingly shunned by others, and the value systems of members of the family may be completely altered—for example, from conservative to radical.

Role of medical services

The scanty evidence which is available about the effects of violence on individuals and families, added to a little simple observation, makes it clear that victims sometimes need psychological and social support over and above the services provided for their physical trauma. The experiments tried in the USA, where emergency consultation and advice is used in the casualty department and is followed by the offer of more extended contact over the next few weeks, seem eminently sensible. Nowhere is it suggested that the services need be specially sophisticated, although sensitive support may minimize anguish. Burgess and Holmstrom used a system of nurse counsellors with arrangements for referral to gynaecologists, psychiatrists and the like when necessary. Very few would argue against the type of system they advocate; it cannot be very expensive in resources and yet it is so often overlooked simply because it is not part of the routine.

General effects of violence

This subject cannot be left without a few words on the general effects of violence. Once again, most of what is said has to be speculative but that, in itself, is worth noting. There is great concern in the press that violence is on the increase and that, in some way, this heralds the destruction of our society. This is not the place for a detailed debate of the subject but one or two simple issues need to be clarified. First, whether 'violence' is increasing or decreasing depends very much on definitions. Do we include or exclude acts of war or terrorism—e.g. the casualties due to the conflict in Northern Ireland? Do we include or exclude road casualties? A road 'accident' may not be a true accident at all and, even if it is, it may be related to antisocial behaviour such as selfish driving or excessive drinking. More people are killed on the roads of Northern Ireland than are killed by firearms and bombs. Should one include or exclude institutionalized or state violence? Even if an agreed definition of violence is reached, it must be faced that the total amount of violence in a society can never be accurately measured because the vast majority is domestic in nature and occurs behind closed doors. Secondly, the time-scale employed makes an enormous difference to the conclusions. It may be true, for example, that violence has increased or decreased over the past decade but does that mean very much in terms of the social history of a nation?—the trend over the past 100 years may have been in the opposite direction.

It is worth noting that the press concept of violence is gleaned from rare, noteworthy events on the one hand and from official figures, such as the criminal statistics, on the other. The major sources for official figures are the police returns on offences reported to them. It is clear that only a small proportion of the large number of violent incidents which technically breach the law ever reach police notice. It is possible that an upswing in the number of cases reported to the police is actually reflecting a lowering of public tolerance towards this kind of behaviour. There is at present a great increase in the number of battered babies and battered wives being brought to the attention of the authorities. This does not necessarily mean an increase in this type of crime— although it might. Nobody now believes that parents never attacked their children before the Second World War, yet a crude analysis of the statistics would reveal just that. History books can be at least as valuable as statistics in gaining insight into social trends. London is a relatively safe place to walk about in provided you do not cross too many roads. This was not true at the beginning of the nineteenth century when people did not willingly walk in the streets after dark; if they had to, they carried truncheons called 'protectors'. The statistical chances of being killed on the roadways between towns are not insignificant but, in contemporary terms, this is because of 'accidents'. In the eighteenth century, highway robbery was a serious risk; it hardly occurs at all now.

Nevertheless, all observers are agreed that the forms of violence are changing. As mentioned earlier, technology has always determined the pattern of violence in an age. We are now in an era where powerful technology is relatively easily available. One or two people can hijack an aeroplane. A small group of fanatics can kill many people with a bomb based on fertilizers and an alarm clock. Accurate firearms are freely available to every United States citizen. Given a successful raid on a plutonium store, one or two people could, without much difficulty, construct a nuclear bomb. I believe that it is the power of the new technology which is causing the new concern with violence. It may be, therefore, that the change in the pattern of violence has made us take it seriously and forced us, perhaps for the first time, to regard it as a threat to the species rather than as a tool to be used for particular purposes.

Suppose, however, that in addition to a change in the form of violence there is an increase in the absolute amount committed. Suppose that more people are being robbed, raped and murdered; more are fighting in the streets, beating their wives, battering their children. What general effects will this produce? Will society be unaffected, strengthened or endangered? The answer to this question is at present unknown. It is difficult to think of a scientific or experimental way in which it can be solved. Violence is sometimes met by counter-violence; at other times it is met by submission and conflict resolution. Violence can increase frustration in a society, leading to more violence, but it can also reduce tension. Some people will learn violent behaviour from seeing it all around them. Others will be revolted and made pacific by an increase. However, the fact that what is happening cannot be measured exactly will not be of great consequence because government policies and public pressures will not be determined by scientific data— they will reflect contemporary mores.

In the speculative, and sometimes heated, debate on the general effects of violence, television often gets a special mention. Presumably this is because it is still a new invention and because it seems to intrude, so successfully, into the heart of almost every family in the land. The fear is that it may be able to influence millions of people in a particular way simultaneously. This fear, which totally neglects the diversity and resilience of human personality, is surprising; it ignores the balance that occurs even in the most TV-addicted household between family influences and other influences of which TV is only one. Certainly TV must affect our behaviour to some extent or else advertisers would not buy time on it; but they would be amazingly successful if they could really make us change our basic habits and attitudes. Suppose that, just by advertising, a French producer could turn us from beef eaters to snail gourmands? Fortunately, people are not so easily influenced and habit patterns can only be slightly modified by TV advertising—as, for example, in inducing a switch from one breakfast cereal to another.

The research which has been conducted on the effects of TV violence tend to bear this out. A recent review of this research[20] concluded that 'the Mass Media do not have any significant effect on the level of violence in society'. The authors reviewed the relevant literature on a variety of mechanisms which have sometimes been incriminated as ways in which television violence can increase the general level of violence; e.g. imitation, identification, triggering, desensitization or attitude change. There is no substantial evidence for the effectiveness of any of these mechanisms. It is also pointed out that there are no reliable correlational studies showing an association between television exposure and such things as aggressiveness or delinquency. There is evidence for a relationship between cinema attendance and delinquency—although not necessarily aggressive delinquency—but this is, of course, open to many interpretations.

References

1. Amir, M. (1971). *Patterns in Forcible Rape*. Chicago: University Press.
2. Bennet, G. (1970). Bristol floods 1968. Controlled survey of effects on health of local community disaster. *Brit. med. J.* **3**, 454.
3. Blacker, C. P. (1948). Neurosis and the Mental Health Services. Oxford: Oxford University Press.
4. Burgess, A. W. (1975). Family reaction to homicide. *Amer. J. Orthopsychiat.* **45**, 391.
5. Burgess, A. W. and Holmstrom, L. L. (1973). The rape victim in the emergency ward. *Amer. J. Nurs.* **73**, 1741.
6. Burgess, A. W. and Holmstrom, L. L. (1974). Rape trauma syndrome. *Amer. J. Psychiat.* **131**, 981.
7. Cohn, B. N. (1975). Succumbing to rape. In: *Rape Victimology*. Ed. L. G. Schultz. Springfield: Thomas.
8. Elmer, E. and Gregg, G. S. (1967). Developmental characteristics of abused children. *Pediatrics* **40**, 596.
9. Fonseka, S. (1974). A study of wife-beating in the Camberwell area. *Brit. J. clin. Pract.* **28**, 400.
10. Fox, S. S. and Scherl, D. J. (1972). Crisis intervention with victims of rape. *Soc. Work* **17**, 37.
11. Fraser, R. M. (1971). The cost of commotion: an analysis of the psychiatric sequelae of the 1969 Belfast riots. *Brit. J. Psychiat.* **118**, 257.

12. Galdston, R. (1966). Observations on children who have been physically abused, and their parents. *Amer. J. Psychiat.* **122**, 440.
13. Gayford, J. (1975). Wife battering: a preliminary survey of 100 cases. *Brit. med. J.* **1**, 194.
14. Gibson, E. and Klein, S. (1969). *Murder.* London: HMSO.
15. Greer, G. (1975). Seduction is a four-letter word. In: *Rape Victimology.* Ed. L. G. Schultz. Springfield: Thomas.
16. Gunn, J. (1971). Forensic psychiatry and psychopathic patients. *Brit. J. Hosp. Med.* **6**, 260.
17. Gunn, J. (1978). *Epileptic Prisoners.* New York and London: Academic Press.
18. Hart, R. J., Lee, J. O., Boyles, D. J. and Batey, N. R. (1975). The Summerland disaster. *Brit. med. J.* **1**, 256.
19. House of Commons (1975). *Report from the Select Committee on Violence in Marriage.* London: HMSO.
20. Howitt, D. and Cumberbatch, G. (1975). *Mass Media, Violence, and Society.* London: Elek Science.
21. Jarvie, H. F. (1954). Frontal lobe wounds causing disinhibition. *J. Neurol. Neurosurg. Psychiat.* **17**, 14.
22. Kempe, C. H., Silverman, F. N., Steele, B. S., Droegemueller, W. and Silver, A. K. (1962). The battered-child syndrome. *J. Amer. Med. Ass.* **181**, 17.
23. Lewis, A. (1942). Incidence of neurosis in England under war conditions. *Lancet* **ii**, 175.
24. Lishman, W. A. (1968). Brain damage in relation to psychiatric disability after head injury. *Brit. J. Psychiat.* **114**, 373.
25. Lyons, H. A. (1971). Psychiatric sequelae of the Belfast riots. *Brit. J. Psychiat.* **118**, 265.
26. Lyons, H. A. (1972). Depressive illness and aggression in Belfast. *Brit. med. J.* **1**, 342.
27. McClintock, F. H. (1963). *Crimes of Violence.* London: Heinemann.
28. MacDonald, J. M. (1971). *Rape, Offenders and their Victims.* Springfield: Thomas.
29. MacKeith, R. (1975). Speculations on some possible long term effects. In: *Concerning Child Abuse.* Ed. A. W. Franklin. Edinburgh and London: Churchill Livingstone.
30. Martin, H. (1972). The child and his development. In *Helping the Battered Child and his Family.* Eds C. H. Kempe and R. H. Helfer. Philadelphia: Lippincott.
31. Morris, J. N. and Titmus, R. M. (1944). Epidemiology of peptic ulcer. *Lancet* **ii**, 841.
32. Morris, N. and Hawkins, G. (1969). *The Honest Politician's Guide to Crime Control.* Chicago: University Press.
33. Morris, T. and Blom-Cooper, L. (1964). *A Calendar of Murder.* London: Michael Joseph.
34. Parkes, C. M. (1964). Effects of bereavement on physical and men-

tal health—a study of the medical records of widows. *Brit. med. J.* **2**, 274.

35. Parkes, C. M. (1975). *Bereavement.* Harmondsworth, Middx: Penguin.

36. Pizzey, E. (1974). *Scream Quietly or the Neighbours will Hear.* Harmondsworth, Middx: Penguin.

37. Steele, B. F. and Pollock, C. B. (1968). A psychiatric study of parents who abuse infants and small children. In: *The Battered Child.* Eds R. E. Helfer and C. H. Kempe, Chicago: University Press.

38. Tinbergen, N. (1964). *Social Behaviour in Animals,* 2nd edn. London: Chapman & Hall.

39. Tucker, K. and Lettin, A. (1975). The Tower of London bomb explosion. *Brit. med. J.* **3**, 287.

40. Wolfenstein, M. (1957). *Disaster.* London: Routledge & Kegan Paul.

41. Wolfgang, M. E. (1958). *Patterns in Criminal Homicide.* New York: Wiley.

THE BRITISH SCHOOL OF OSTEOPATHY
14 SUFFOLK STREET, LONDON SW1Y 4HG
TEL: 01-930 9254-8

THE
8-8
TEL. 01-930

Index

The British School of Osteopathy

* 2 2 9 1 *

**This book is to be returned on or before
the last date stamped below.**

F1 OCT 1984

-7 DEC 1984

15 MAY 1985

2 7 MAY 2010

MASON